# Interpersonal Psychotherapy for Adolescents

Interpersonal psychotherapy for adolescents (IPT-A) is a comprehensive guide for clinicians. It will enable readers to add IPT-A to their clinical repertoire or to deepen their existing practice of IPT-A, using a time-limited, evidence-based intervention that is engaging for young people.

The guide outlines the structure, skills, and techniques of IPT-A, utilising real-life encounters in the therapy room that reflect the diverse nature of adolescents and young adults who present for therapy. It provides the reader with a bird's-eye view of how IPT-A works. It expands the range of IPT-A clinical tools, techniques, and models to assist the reader to work effectively with a wide range of clients. The book provides a new protocol for the psychological assessment of young people, acknowledging the importance of culture and spirituality alongside the biological, psychological, and social dimensions that have previously comprised assessment. The importance of the clinician forming a transitory attachment relationship with the client is emphasised throughout.

The target audience for this book is mental health clinicians, including psychologists, psychiatrists, social workers, mental health nurses, occupational therapists, general practitioners with a mental health focus, and students from these professions.

**Robert McAlpine, PhD, MAPS, FACCLP**, is a clinical psychologist who works with adolescents and adults in regional New South Wales, Australia. He also teaches introductory and advanced courses in Interpersonal psychotherapy and supervises therapists who are using IPT and IPT-A in their clinical practices.

**Anthony Hillin, B Soc Stud (SW), M Adol MH,** has 30 years' experience as a clinician and trainer, emphasising holistic approaches to change. He specialises in the impact of loss, transition and conflict on the wellbeing of individuals and organisations. Anthony provides introductory and advanced level training and supervision in IPT, IPT-A and related topics worldwide.

# Interpersonal Psychotherapy for Adolescents
A Clinician's Guide

Robert McAlpine
and Anthony Hillin

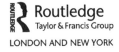

LONDON AND NEW YORK

First published 2021
by Routledge
2 Park Square, Milton Park, Abingdon, Oxon OX14 4RN

and by Routledge
52 Vanderbilt Avenue, New York, NY 10017

*Routledge is an imprint of the Taylor & Francis Group, an informa business*

© 2021 Robert McAlpine and Anthony Hillin

The right of Robert McAlpine and Anthony Hillin to be identified as authors of this work has been asserted by them in accordance with sections 77 and 78 of the Copyright, Designs and Patents Act 1988.

All rights reserved. No part of this book may be reprinted or reproduced or utilised in any form or by any electronic, mechanical, or other means, now known or hereafter invented, including photocopying and recording, or in any information storage or retrieval system, without permission in writing from the publishers.

*Trademark notice*: Product or corporate names may be trademarks or registered trademarks, and are used only for identification and explanation without intent to infringe.

*British Library Cataloguing-in-Publication Data*
A catalogue record for this book is available from the British Library

*Library of Congress Cataloging-in-Publication Data*
A catalog record has been requested for this book

ISBN: 9780367332877 (hbk)
ISBN: 9781482227178 (pbk)
ISBN: 9780429272394 (ebk)

Typeset in Goudy
by MPS Limited, Dehradun

# Contents

| | |
|---|---|
| *List of clinical tools* | vii |
| *List of figures* | viii |
| *Acknowledgements* | x |
| *Foreword* | xi |

**PART I**
**Introduction** — 1

| | | |
|---|---|---|
| 1 | Introduction and orientation to this guide | 3 |
| 2 | A model of holistic assessment | 16 |
| 3 | Attachment in young people | 49 |
| 4 | Clinical techniques | 74 |

**PART II**
**The Initial Phase of IPT-A** — 117

| | | |
|---|---|---|
| 5 | The Initial Phase of IPT-A | 119 |

**PART III**
**The Middle Phase of IPT-A** — 159

| | | |
|---|---|---|
| 6 | The Middle Phase of IPT-A | 161 |
| 7 | Complex Grief | 169 |
| 8 | Interpersonal Disputes | 205 |
| 9 | Role Transition | 241 |
| 10 | Interpersonal Gaps | 278 |

## PART IV
**Consolidation Phase of IPT-A**    313

11  Conclusion of Acute Treatment    315

12  Continuation and Maintenance Therapy    331

## PART V
**Closing thoughts**    337

13  Closing thoughts    339

*Index*    344

# List of clinical tools

| | | |
|---|---|---|
| 2.1 | Resilience grid | 24 |
| 2.2 | Suicide risk assessment protocol | 26 |
| 2.3 | Ethno-cultural identity matrix (ECIM) | 31 |
| 2.4 | Stages of change | 41 |
| 2.5 | Case formulation checklist | 42 |
| 3.1 | The Clinicians Response Scale | 64 |
| 3.2 | Working with the young person's attachment style | 67 |
| 4.1 | Feelings Diary | 88 |
| 7.1 | My tasks following loss | 196 |
| 7.2 | Helpful things I can do after loss | 196 |
| 9.1 | Role Transition | 249 |
| 10.1 | Social skills list | 286 |
| 10.2 | Practice sheet for a single skill | 297 |
| 10.3 | Practice sheet for a conversation or complex interaction | 298 |
| 10.4 | Practice sheet for a specific social skill | 299 |
| 10.5 | Questions for a young person's significant others about social competencies | 310 |

# List of figures

| | | |
|---|---|---|
| 1.1 | Stepped care for depression in adolescents | 7 |
| 1.2 | Sequential stages of an IPT-A intervention | 10 |
| 2.1 | Summary of the model of holistic assessment | 18 |
| 2.2 | Model of holistic assessment | 19 |
| 2.3 | Key and Associated Symptoms | 25 |
| 3.1 | The four-dimensional model of attachment | 54 |
| 3.2 | Clinicians Response Scale: Tracey | 65 |
| 4.1 | Monitoring communication patterns | 79 |
| 4.2 | Personal Diagram (Part 1) | 84 |
| 4.3 | Personal Diagram (Part 2) | 85 |
| 4.4a | Interpersonal Incidents grid | 92 |
| 4.4b | Interpersonal Incidents: General statements | 93 |
| 4.4c | Interpersonal Incidents: General affect | 93 |
| 4.4d | Interpersonal Incidents: Specific incident | 94 |
| 4.4e | Interpersonal Incidents: Specific affect | 95 |
| 4.4f | Interpersonal Incidents: Identifying misunderstandings | 97 |
| 4.4g | Interpersonal Incidents: Affective shift | 100 |
| 4.5 | Identification of Conflict-Solving Styles | 103 |
| 5.1 | Erin—holistic assessment summary | 123 |
| 5.2 | The Closeness Circles | 126 |
| 5.3 | Erin's Closeness Circle | 127 |
| 7.1 | The arc of therapy for Complex Grief in the Middle Phase of IPT-A | 173 |
| 7.2 | Different experiences of grief | 191 |
| 7.3 | Mei's handout: My tasks now mum has died | 197 |
| 7.4 | Jake's handout: Helpful things I can do after moving | 197 |
| 8.1 | Seven stages for working on Interpersonal Disputes | 209 |
| 8.2 | Admir—holistic assessment summary | 212 |
| 8.3 | Admir's Conflict Curve | 218 |
| 8.4 | Jan's Conflict Curve | 222 |
| 8.5 | Manu's dispute map | 232 |
| 8.6 | Gina's dispute map | 235 |
| 9.1 | Family structure Role Transition—Pippa old role | 251 |

| | | |
|---|---|---|
| 9.2 | Family structure Role Transition—Pippa | 255 |
| 9.3 | Grant—holistic assessment summary | 269 |
| 9.4 | Same-sex attraction Role Transition—Grant | 273 |
| 10.1 | Ava's anger chart | 300 |
| 10.2 | Identifying blind spots | 303 |
| 11.1 | Bill's Care Map | 328 |
| 12.1 | IPT-A as modular therapy | 335 |

# Acknowledgements

I am indebted to all the young people I have had the privilege of working with. I never cease to be amazed at the openness and generosity with which you share your lives. Thank you. I am equally amazed by the insight and determination you display, often in the face of extremely tough life stories. Your resilience constantly reminds me that the seeds of your healing lie within you. I am just the gardener who waters the plants and who, as you often tell me, provides (sometimes too much) fertiliser. Although fertiliser is not the word you use.

Many thanks also to my friend and colleague Nisha Dhani for reading the manuscripts and providing balanced editorial advice.

Finally, thanks to Wendy. With love and gratitude.

R.M.

This book is not just the product of recent years. My part in it springs from my personal and professional experience dating back to my adolescence. From my first interest in social work, through the challenges of the HIV epidemic, and into more recent decades addressing young people's mental health and wellbeing, I have been inspired by clients, colleagues and friends. They have shown me the transformative power of listening, respect, and kindness in the face of death, uncertainty and the many challenges of life. Knowing you has provided some of the richest lessons of my life and led me to IPT and its potential for young people.

I'm also indebted to the many people who have helped with this book, directly and indirectly. My thanks to the late Professor Beverley Raphael, Professor The Honourable Dame Marie Bashir AD CVO, Dr Ros Montague, Professor Louise Newman, Dannielle Byers and Dr Simone Cayes, for their support for our work and their passion for young people's well-being; to Professor Scott Stuart for encouraging us to write this book; to our publishers, Joanne Forshaw, Alec Selwyn, Daradi Patar, Naomi Wilkinson, and Charlotte Taylor, for their availability and patience with our delays; to my parents, who died during the writing of this book, for their love and support, which continues to sustain me; and to my partner, Colin, for his love, humour and editing skill.

Anthony

# Foreword

Experience strongly suggests that when participating in a psychotherapy seminar, a student makes several very rapid judgments within the first one or two minutes. The first is whether or not the teacher would be someone he or she would go to see should they need a therapist him or herself. The research credentials of the expert, his or her prestige, and his or her academic affiliations make no difference at all. What matters is whether the presenter is a real human being, who can convey empathy, who listens well, and who will take the time to understand others. In essence, whether the expert presenter is also an expert therapist.

The second judgement is whether the material presented makes intuitive sense. Does the approach fit real patients, or is it simply an esoteric "ivory tower" approach that has no real relevance? Does the therapy involve theory far too complex for therapists to grasp, much less patients, or does it involve simple life principles? And does the approach make unrealistic claims to be superior to other approaches, or is it open to recognising the value of other therapies or combinations of therapies for the variety of patients encountered in real clinical practice?

The third judgement is whether or not the patients presented are real and whether they are like the patients that the learner encounters every day. In other words, do the approach and the patients presented have relevance to clinical practice? And is the presenter speaking clinically of "cases" or relating the stories of the real people who come to see him or her for help?

All of these judgments apply equally to psychotherapy textbooks. They, too, must be authentic and touch on the real experiences of the people we work with daily. They must be flexible; unlike many of the research manuals that require rigid application, the psychotherapy texts that make a difference are guides to practice, assisting the learner to apply the approach using clinical judgement rather than dictating the structure and techniques to be used. And most importantly, the authenticity of the authors needs to shine through in the stories told, the empathy conveyed, and the emphasis on caring and relationship that is necessary to do psychotherapy. We must first come to understand and care for our patients; then we can help them.

We have desperately needed a psychotherapy guide like this for the treatment of adolescents, particularly for the work being done using interpersonal psychotherapy.

There is a great deal of research involving IPT for adolescents, and it is fine work. Evidence-based practice rests on such empirical research. But the foundation of evidence-based practice, when it is applied with real people in real clinical settings, must be the therapeutic alliance and caring for and understanding our patients. That is the essence of this guide.

There are several critical elements of the book that build upon the empirical research in IPT for adolescents. The first is that the clinical work is based on attachment theory, reflecting the importance of relationship in adolescent development. The need for attachment is reflected both in the clinical approach to IPT as well as its application to the therapeutic alliance. To listen and care, to convey to adolescents that they are heard and that they matter—that is the therapist's first task.

The second element is the emphasis on a holistic model of care and conceptualisation. Hillin and McAlpine were responsible for introducing the broader biopsychosocial/cultural/spiritual model of understanding the people we work with in IPT nearly a decade ago; their innovation has led to a far greater ability to understand the people with whom we work. And the holistic model explicitly emphasises to the therapist the need to listen to and understand the patient, particularly the way in which his or her distress is expressed culturally and spiritually. It would be nearly impossible to work with adolescents experiencing grief and loss, debilitating conflicts, difficult life changes, and gaps in their capacity to relate to others without understanding their cultural and spiritual backgrounds.

The authors' emphasis comes from personal experience as well, as much of their work over several decades has been with distressed and traumatised adolescents from minority and Aboriginal communities. Their empathy and willingness to be present with others from all different walks of life shines forth in their writing.

A third critical addition the authors have made is the emphasis on collaborating with the patient in care. In their guide, IPT (as should be the case with all other therapies) is done *with* the patient, not *to* the patient. This is reflected in the emphasis on psychoeducation so the young person understands the process of therapy. It is reflected in clinical decisions being made with the patient and even in their use of the term treatment *agreement* rather than treatment *contract*. The work is collaborative and encourages the participation of the patient. This, too, rests on the therapist's ability to understand and listen and is especially important for work with adolescents.

Finally, the authors present IPT as a treatment that provides continuity of care rather than a terminable treatment. The empirical data are clear that maintenance treatment with IPT is effective in preventing relapse; that data alone suggest that clinicians should not be terminating treatment, particularly with individuals at high risk. More important, however, is the authors' recognition that the relationship we form with our patients, particularly with adolescents, is critically important to them and that termination of treatment is a real abandonment of the patient. To terminate treatment is to effectively undermine all of the attachment work and corrective therapeutic experience that occurs in a good working relationship in therapy, whereas providing the opportunity to return to treatment as needed, and maintenance therapy as necessary, provides a secure base—a real supportive relationship—for the adolescent.

On a personal note, I have had the opportunity to work with Rob and Anthony over many years, conducting training with them, observing their work, and collaborating with them on various projects. What they convey in this book is authentic to their work as therapists and to who they are as individuals. Listening well, understanding and appreciating diversity, caring for others, and acting with consistent integrity are qualities that are conveyed in their writing as well as their relationships. And those qualities, more than research credentials or even clinical experience, make a fine therapist and a fine clinical guide. They also make fine human beings.

I have no doubt that readers will find the book extremely helpful with their work with IPT generally and with adolescents specifically. The structure and techniques of IPT are well described; the theory and conceptualisation are important additions to previous work in the field. But most importantly, the need to listen well, to be real, and to truly care for others is clear throughout the guide. That is the essence of IPT.

Scott Stuart, Director, IPT Institute

# Part I
# Introduction

# 1 Introduction and orientation to this guide

**Contents**

| | |
|---|---|
| Welcome and introduction | 3 |
| Aims for the book | 4 |
| The authors | 5 |
| The target audience and how to use this book | 5 |
| Introducing the case studies | 6 |
| Locating IPT-A within a stepped care approach | 7 |
| Personalised treatment | 8 |
| Terminology | 8 |
| Overview of IPT-A | 9 |
| *Assessment and formulation* | 9 |
| *The Initial Phase of IPT-A* | 10 |
| *The Middle Phase of IPT-A* | 12 |
| *The Consolidation Phase of IPT-A* | 13 |
| Summary | 14 |
| References | 14 |

## Welcome and introduction

Welcome to *Interpersonal Psychotherapy for Adolescents—A Clinician's Guide*. This introduction provides a brief overview of the content and layout of this book and offers some suggestions on how it can be used.

Interpersonal Psychotherapy for Adolescents (IPT-A) is an evidence-based intervention that is intrinsically engaging for young people and is generally straightforward for clinicians to learn. It teaches things about which young people are interested to learn: about themselves, relationships, emotions, and how to communicate effectively. It also teaches young people about their distress and symptoms and the connection between these and interpersonal issues. IPT-A develops interpersonal competencies that many young people are keen to acquire.

One of the key messages of IPT-A is that if clients can communicate their needs for closeness and support to others effectively, the likelihood of their attachment needs being met will increase. This is a revolutionary concept for some young people, especially those with a limited sense of their own ability to create the type of relationships they want. It will be life changing for many to discover ways that they may be able to proactively create and orchestrate the nature of their relationships and the quality of support available to them. IPT-A not only encourages this hopeful view of the possibility for successful relationships, it also teaches the required skills and provides the necessary support for young people to integrate these competencies in their important relationships.

## Aims for the book

This book builds on the work of Mufson and others (Mufson et al., 1993, 2004), who initially developed IPT-A. The intervention is still relatively new, and clinical work subsequent to the publication of the original manuals provides the *practice-based evidence* to balance and enhance the *evidence-based practice* outlined in the research. (See Pu et al., 2017, for example, for a review of this research.)

This Clinician's Guide aims to enhance the engaging nature of IPT-A to make this treatment even more accessible to a broad range of young people from early adolescence to early adulthood. There are several major new additions to IPT-A provided in this book:

1. We extend the biopsychosocial model to include the role of cultural and spiritual dimensions in assessment and treatment in IPT-A. These domains of experience can have a far-reaching effect on the interpersonal world of young people but are often overlooked in clinical practice (e.g., Proctor, 2011).
2. We demonstrate the assessment of attachment behaviours and how to adapt IPT-A to address the adolescent's attachment style. A central aim of IPT-A is to improve interpersonal functioning by enhancing communication skills in significant relationships. Another way of stating this is "to assist clients to meet their attachment needs more effectively". In addition, a sound understanding of attachment can greatly assist therapists to avoid colluding with the client's dysfunctional and habitual ways of interacting that are interrupting their relationships and thus contributing to psychological distress and symptoms.
3. We expand the use of IPT-A to include young adults. The previous IPT-A literature focussed on 12- to 18-year-olds. Some young adults are better accommodated within an adolescent assessment and treatment framework for a number of reasons. The boundary between adolescence and young adulthood is somewhat arbitrary. The timing and particular dynamics of development and maturity play out in different ways, depending on a range of individual and external factors. For an increasing number of young people, independence, economic self-sufficiency and leaving their parent's home is delayed well into the third decade of life. In many parts of

the world, it is not uncommon for people in their twenties to continue to deal with life circumstances that were once associated predominantly with the second decade of life. For some of these young people, the accompanying developmental dynamics and the impact on their relationships continue well beyond 18 years.

For these reasons, and to ensure better continuity of care, some mental health services have moved away from a model of separate adolescent and adult services, which requires the transfer of cases at 18 years, to a youth mental health service model that provides care for an age range of 12 to 25.

4   We include the key roles of Continuation and Maintenance as core components of therapy included in a revised third phase of treatment, the Consolidation Phase. An important characteristic of IPT-A is its time-limited nature. It may not be appropriate, however, to terminate treatment for some young people solely because a prescribed number of sessions has been reached.
5   We substantially expand the range of IPT-A clinical tools and techniques. The techniques are integrated throughout the book, and the clinical tools are found throughout the book.

## The authors

Rob and Anthony came to IPT-A with many years' experience using other approaches to working with young people and adults. Our work in school settings, public mental health services, and private practice has encompassed a wide range of populations who are often reluctant to seek help from mental health services and who experience elevated risk of suicide, depression, or other adverse outcomes. This has included young people who are Indigenous, culturally and linguistically diverse, LGBTQIA,[1] homeless or living in out-of-home care, and those involved in the criminal justice system.

The challenge of making therapy accessible and engaging for a diverse range of young people has been central in our work. Our conviction in the value of IPT-A for a wide range of young people has been further reinforced by our work in different corners of the globe: Australasia, Europe, and USA. This has driven our desire to disseminate this developmentally engaging intervention.

## The target audience and how to use this book

This book has been written for mental health clinicians, including psychologists, social workers, psychiatrists, mental health nurses, occupational therapists, psychotherapists, counsellors, general practitioners with a mental health focus, and students of these professions. It will also be useful for people who provide training and clinical supervision for these clinicians.

Some readers will want to work their way through each chapter. The book is also presented in a way that will enable the reader to dip into sections that may be of particular interest—for instance, when you want to prepare for a next session with a client. The contents are listed at the beginning of each chapter, together with subheadings and cross-referencing, to make it easy to locate particular information.

## Introducing the case studies

Throughout the book, a suite of major case studies is presented that incorporate a broad range of characteristics and circumstances that adolescents and young adults experience. In each chapter you will see how IPT-A can be tailored to the individual needs of particular young people. In addition to our major case studies, numerous brief case examples appear throughout the text to illustrate the diversity of client presentations and applications of IPT-A. The case studies have been developed based on themes from real cases. The information has been changed to ensure confidentiality.

Brief descriptions are included here to help orient you to the major cases.

**Erin**, aged 16, developed depression after discovering that she was colourblind. She was devastated to learn that she was no longer eligible for the career that she had her hopes set on. Erin felt that her family and friends dismissed the impact of this and other losses. She withdrew and became increasingly isolated.

**Michelle,** aged 14, identifies as Aboriginal. She developed depression following multiple losses. Spiritual and cultural factors, as well as the impact of loss on her extended family and community, added to the complex nature of her grief.

**Admir**, aged 16, experienced significant conflict with his mother Fatima, which escalated prior to the onset of his depression. Fatima also experienced mental health issues but refused a mental health referral.

**Manu**, aged 20, lived with his mother. He was keen to leave home but felt responsible for looking after her, particularly as they lived in an unsafe neighbourhood. He felt embarrassed in front of his friends by the way his mother treated him. A combination of guilt about his desire to leave and about conflict with his mother contributed to Manu's depression.

**Pippa**, aged 14, became depressed after her parents separated. Pippa missed the way things used to be and feared being supplanted in her father's affections by his new family. She did not see how she could adjust to the new expectations imposed on her by her new family structure.

**Grant**, aged 15, developed depression and anxiety, in relation to his growing awareness of his sexuality. He was gay but this was ego dystonic. He experienced bullying and feared rejection by his father and his church.

**Tanya,** aged 14, presented for therapy after a suicide attempt following disputes with her mother that left her with a sense of disconnection and hopelessness.

**Crystal**, aged 22, developed depression and anxiety after her relationship with her boyfriend ended. She was surprised by the ending of the relationship and also by difficulties in her friendships. The Initial Phase of ITP-A revealed significant gaps in Crystal's ability to maintain relationships.

**Steph**, aged 16, was referred by her family doctor after she disclosed to him that she had been self-harming. In the initial session, the therapist identified significant depressive mood, but without enough symptomatology to warrant a diagnosis of major depressive disorder.

These cases will be progressively developed in subsequent chapters, demonstrating the application of IPT-A to a wide range of young people and clinical presentations. The book explores how IPT-A helped reduce these young people's symptoms as they learned new ways to cope with these experiences.

## Locating IPT-A within a stepped care approach

The role of specific interventions, such as IPT-A, is best understood when it is located within the spectrum of interventions for mental disorders.

Providing mental health treatment when mental disorder is not present may pathologise normal adaptive processes. A stepped care approach suggests that tailoring the level of care to the degree of severity will be effective, provide a better use of scarce resources, and often be more acceptable to the young person and his or her family (Cross and Hickie, 2017). This may be especially true in cultures and contexts where mental illness is stigmatised.

Figure 1.1 represents a stepped care approach adapted from the UK's National Institute for Health and Care Excellence (NICE) guidelines for adolescent depression (2017). The left side of the figure represents prevalence as an inverse iceberg, with incidence decreasing and levels of distress and impact on functioning increasing towards the bottom of the figure.

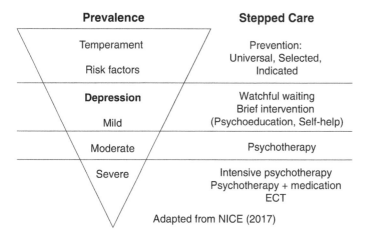

*Figure 1.1* Stepped care for depression in adolescents.

The spectrum of intervention (from low to high intensity) matched to client need may include prevention programs, watchful waiting, psychoeducation, social support, non-directive supportive therapy, guided self-help, group programs, psychotherapy, medication, electroconvulsive therapy (ECT), and inpatient care. Low intensity options may include online interventions. Attention to suicide risk is required in all presentations of depression.

Within this stepped care approach, IPT-A is an appropriate intervention for young people with moderate to severe depression and related presentations and can be delivered in ways that are acceptable to the young person and his or her parents.

Early intervention is crucial for young people's mental health and wellbeing (RANZCP, 2010). Programs that educate people who are in a position to notice early signs and symptoms of mental disorder such as parents, young people, teachers, and other service providers are a key part of early intervention—for example, Youth Mental Health First Aid (Gryglewicz et al., 2018). Collaboration between mental health services and these other stakeholders can enhance early intervention and increase the capacity of these staff to support young people with mental disorders. This in turn can free up mental health clinicians to work with more severe cases (McAlpine et al., 2008).

## Personalised treatment

One of the reasons that IPT-A is engaging for young people is that it provides numerous opportunities to tailor psychotherapy to each client's individual circumstances. This guide outlines how IPT-A is delivered in different ways according to the following:

- the nature of the young persons' interpersonal skills and the level of support currently available to them
- the Problem Area associated with the onset of their depression or other disorder
- their attachment behaviours
- their level of engagement
- the appropriateness of involving their parents or others in treatment

These factors for individualising the intervention are intrinsic to IPT-A. We also demonstrate how additional considerations can suggest specific avenues for personalising IPT-A, including those arising from holistic assessment, the young person's readiness for change, self-help strategies, and the need for continuing or maintenance treatment.

## Terminology

For convenience, we use the terms adolescent, young people, young person, or client throughout the book to refer to a broad age range comprising adolescents and young adults.

The people who are important to the young person are sometimes referred to as their significant others. This may include parents, caregivers, extended family, friends, teachers, sports coaches, or other people who play a significant role in the young person's life. For the sake of fluency, the term "parents" is sometimes used to denote "parents or caregivers".

## Overview of IPT-A

Mufson et al. (2004) described a three-phase model of IPT-A comprising an Initial Phase, a Middle Phase, and a Termination Phase. Each phase consisted of four sessions, providing a twelve-session intervention. Whilst the present book retains some core elements of Mufson's model, we have removed Assessment and Formulation from the Initial Phase and replaced the Termination Phase with a Consolidation Phase, which includes Conclusion of Acute Treatment followed by Continuation and Maintenance treatment. These changes reflect the sequence of therapy: a therapist would not choose IPT-A as an intervention until a thorough assessment has been completed. Nor would a therapist "terminate" an intervention merely because twelve sessions have elapsed. Figure 1.2 shows the sequential stages of an IPT-A intervention.

### Assessment and formulation

Chapter 2 describes assessment and formulation in detail. In most cases, assessment will include interviews with the young person and his or her parents or other significant people (if appropriate) separately and together.

Engel in 1977 proposed the biopsychosocial model of assessment that, since that time, has been adopted as the gold standard of comprehensive assessment, exploring how biological, psychological, and social factors interact to shape the individual (Engel, 1977). More recently, this model has been expanded to include Cultural and Spiritual domains (APA, 2013; Ravishankar, 2012; Hillin and McAlpine, 2005), to acknowledge the centrality of these factors in the lives of many of our clients and the role they play in mental health and wellbeing.

The exploration of these five domains proceeds so that factors that predispose, precipitate, perpetuate, or are protective of distress or disorder are canvassed in order to develop a picture of the young person that includes, but is not limited to, symptomatology. Young people are much more than a collection of symptoms. The goals of this process are to (1) arrive at a wide-ranging formulation that will help the client understand their current distress and its context, (2) begin to achieve a level of hope and belief that things can be better, and (3) determine the nature of the intervention to follow: will IPT-A be the intervention of choice? Or will a longer-term dynamic intervention—or a cognitively focussed intervention, for example—be more appropriate?

Prior to beginning the Initial Phase of IPT-A, the therapist will discuss with the young person a preliminary formulation. The remainder of the formulation,

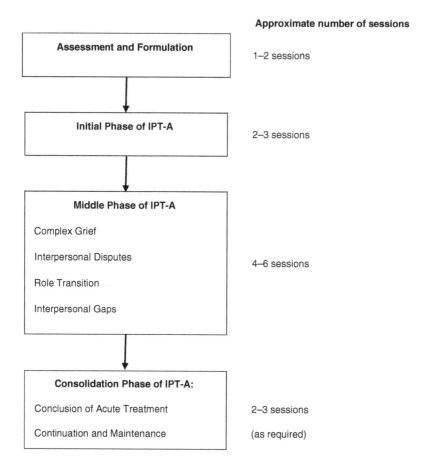

Figure 1.2 Sequential stages of an IPT-A intervention.

the Interpersonal Formulation, will be discussed following the exploration of the young person's interpersonal world, conducted in the Initial Phase of IPT-A.

During the Assessment and Formulation and the stages that follow, the therapist will strive to develop a strong therapeutic alliance with the young person. The nature of this relationship is best described as that of a transitory attachment figure. (See Chapters 2–4; 11–12.)

### The Initial Phase of IPT-A

The Initial Phase provides psychoeducation to help the young person understand more about her symptoms, how these originated, how therapy works and how therapy will help her. Once the young person *understands* how she became distressed and begins to see a plausible pathway forward, she will be more likely to *believe* that the therapeutic process will benefit her. These two consequences of psychoeducation, understanding and believing, together enhance the prospect of optimal clinical outcome.

Central to the Initial Phase is the Interpersonal Inventory, which consists of five tasks. The aim of the inventory is to place the young person's distress or symptomatology within an interpersonal context.

The first task is to explore in detail the young person's significant relationships. The therapist will facilitate discussion of specific relationships, how relationships might change, and individuals to whom the young person might turn for support and care.

The second task of the Interpersonal Inventory involves placing the young person's symptoms in a time frame. A timeline is employed to record the impact of significant events on the young person's life as well as exploring any interpersonal consequences.

The third task represents a major departure from other therapeutic interventions. It consists of the therapist and young person collaboratively identifying which of four Problem Areas is most closely associated with the client's distress:

1  **Complex Grief** is identified when the young person's distress or symptoms are most closely linked to significant loss. This Problem Area includes bereavement and a range of other forms of loss including loss of a relationship, a pet, friendship, culture, loss due to change of location, migration, etc. This often presents when the young person has not had an opportunity to grieve the loss and the unresolved grief has progressed into depression or other symptoms (Chapter 7).
2  **Interpersonal Disputes** are identified as the Problem Area when unresolved conflict dominates the clinical picture. The critical feature of Interpersonal Disputes is that the client feels "stuck", unable to move due to intransigence. The disputes are usually between the young person and people who matter, including his parent, sibling, boyfriend or girlfriend, teacher, employer, peer, or sports coach. Often, unmet expectations about others feature in this Problem Area. The dispute leads to distress and with no end in sight the distress progresses to symptomatology (Chapter 8).
3  **Role Transitions** occur when a new role in life is cast, a role that causes the young person significant distress. Examples include family breakup, arrival of a new sibling, a new job or school, becoming a parent, parent illness, leaving home, finishing school, and loss of health. When young people lack psychosocial support and have compromised attachment needs, these changes can precipitate debilitating stress that may progress into disorders such as depression or anxiety. Role Transition is usually accompanied by ambivalence about the new role, grief about the loss of the old role, loss of social support associated with the old role, anxiety due to lack of familiarity

with the new role, and the need to develop new skills and social support (Chapter 9).
4 **Interpersonal Gaps** refer to a lack of social and communication skills that impair the young person's ability to initiate and maintain relationships. Although they may crave relationships, these young people experience repeated failure in their attempts to connect with others and become depressed or anxious within the context of rejection and loneliness (Chapter 10).

In the fourth task of the Interpersonal Inventory, the therapist emphasises the link between the Problem Area and psychological distress or symptoms, explaining that as the Problem Area becomes the focus in therapy, the symptomatology will begin to resolve. Through discussion of real-life interpersonal incidents, the young person comes to better understand this link and consequently develops the understanding that as the Problem Area is addressed so his or her distress will lessen.

The fifth task of the Interpersonal Inventory, a task that actually begins the first time the therapist meets the young person, is to develop an hypothesis about the client's attachment style. An understanding of the primary attachment style of the young person is an integral part of IPT-A. Psychological problems occur and interpersonal relationships break down when a client's needs for attachment are not being adequately met. The goal of IPT-A is not to change clients' attachment style but to help them develop interpersonal skills that will assist them to meet their attachment needs more effectively. The young person's attachment style will influence how IPT-A is individualised for each client, including expectations about therapy, the rate therapy progresses, client-therapist relationship strategies, and the specific therapeutic techniques employed. Attachment is addressed in Chapter 3 and elsewhere in the book.

Following the five tasks of the Interpersonal Inventory, the therapist is in a position to discuss the Interpersonal Formulation (Chapter 5), adding to the initial formulation that followed the holistic assessment (Chapter 2).

The final task of the Initial Phase of IPT-A is to discuss the responsibilities of the young person, his or her family, and the therapist and to prepare the young person for the next stage of therapy: the Middle Phase.

### *The Middle Phase of IPT-A*

In the Middle Phase of IPT-A, the therapist and young person work together to address the Problem Area identified in the Initial Phase. The therapist uses strategies relevant to the particular Problem Area—for example, to

- help clients effectively grieve their loss and connect to their new life without the lost person or object (Complex Grief).
- promote insight to understand conflicts and develop skills to resolve them (Interpersonal Disputes).

*Introduction and orientation to this guide* 13

- assist the young person to disconnect from the old role and develop interpersonal skills relevant to managing the new role (Role Transition).
- develop social and interpersonal skills for initiating and maintaining relationships (Interpersonal Gaps).

The therapy room becomes a laboratory for the young person to explore his existing interpersonal strategies and explore potential new ones. The therapist will then assist the young person to identify "safe others" with whom he can rehearse these new relationship skills, then discuss and process these when back in the therapy room. Clinical techniques used in the Middle Phase, including role play and chair work, are described in Chapter 4.

## *The Consolidation Phase of IPT-A*

Once the work of the Middle Phase has progressed sufficiently, usually within about four to six sessions, therapy moves into the Consolidation Phase, during which the Problem Area remains the focus of treatment, but therapy takes on a different emphasis. The Consolidation Phase constitutes Conclusion of Acute Treatment and Continuation and Maintenance Treatment. In Conclusion of Acute Treatment the therapist has four primary tasks:

1 stepping back from the role of transitory attachment figure
2 facilitating independent functioning through assisting the young person to internalise and generalise the psychosocial gains made in treatment to date
3 preparing the young person and parents so that they can recognise early warning signs of relapse or recurrence, and build a plan to deal with this, should it eventuate
4 assessing the need for Continuation and Maintenance treatment

These goals are addressed in Chapter 11.

The Conclusion of Acute Treatment offers an opportunity to address dependence the young person may have developed on the therapist (or on therapy) by strategically retreating from the role of transitory attachment figure, whilst maintaining a therapeutic alliance that may be reactivated if necessary. As the therapist retreats, others fill this space. The therapist and the young person collaboratively work out how this can be achieved.

The second task of the Conclusion of Acute Treatment is to strengthen new interpersonal behaviours the young person has developed during therapy with a view toward independent functioning. This task is aimed at assisting the young person to internalise gains, i.e., to incorporate the psychosocial gains made during therapy into her interpersonal repertoire. The therapist will assist the young person to generalise these gains when confronted with psychosocial challenges that occur outside the therapy room.

Third, the therapist will assist the young person and parents (if appropriate) to be alert for changes that may indicate increased risk of relapse (or recurrence) and develop plans to deal with these possibilities. An individual Care Map (see Chapter 11) may be used to identify if signs of depression or other disorders are returning and appropriate steps that can be taken to prevent relapse or recurrence.

Fourth, during the last sessions of Conclusion of Acute Treatment, the therapist will assess the need for and plan Continuation and Maintenance therapy. Although IPT-A is a time-limited model of therapy, research suggests that, in order to reduce the likelihood of relapse or recurrence, Continuation and Maintenance are required over an extended timeframe but with reduced contact (Birmaher et al., 2007).

Continuation therapy is negotiated when the young person has not achieved significant symptom resolution. Maintenance, on the other hand, will be a part of all IPT-A interventions, even for young people who have achieved complete symptom resolution. The aim of Maintenance sessions is to provide continued support so that the gains made during the previous stages of treatment minimise the likelihood of relapse or recurrence. The Continuation and Maintenance stages of IPT-A are described in Chapter 12.

**Summary**

Interpersonal Psychotherapy for Adolescents is a time-limited, evidence-based intervention. IPT-A proceeds from an holistic assessment, through an Initial and Middle Phase to a Consolidation Phase, which includes Conclusion of Acute Treatment and Continuation and Maintenance therapy. After this, the young person is encouraged to be alert for signs of recurrence and to re-connect with therapy should this occur. The collaborative nature of the therapeutic relationship underpins the entire therapeutic process.

This clinician's guide provides step-by-step assistance for clinicians using IPT-A. It offers a timely expansion of the clinical techniques and activities that can be used to achieve the goals of IPT-A with a diverse range of young people.

**Note**

1 LGBTQIA (lesbian, gay, bisexual, transgender, queer or questioning, intersex and asexual).

**References**

American Psychological Association. (2013). *Diagnostic and statistical manual for mental disorders: Fifth edition*. Washington, DC: American Psychiatric Association.

Birmaher, B., Brent, D., et al. (2007). Practice parameter for the assessment and treatment of children and adolescents with depressive disorders. *Journal of the American Academy of Child and Adolescent Psychiatry*, 46(11), 1503–1526.

Cross, S. & Hickie, I. (2017). Transdiagnostic stepped care in mental health. *Public Health Research and Practice*. E7(2):e2721712. http://dx.doi.org/10.17061/phrp2721712.

d'Souza, R. (2002). Do patients expect psychiatrists to be interested in spiritual issues? *Australasian Psychiatry*, 10(1), 44–47.

Engel, G. (1977). The need for a new medical model: A challenge for biomedicine. *Science*, 196, 129–136.

Hillin, A. & McAlpine R. (2005) *Interpersonal psychotherapy for adolescents: Workshop handouts*, Sydney, Australia. Hillin and McAlpine.

Gryglewicz, K., Childs, K., & Soderstrom, M. (2018). An evaluation of youth mental health first aid training in school settings. *School Mental Health*, 10(1), 48–60. https://doi.org/10.1007/s12310-018-9246-7.

McAlpine, R., Hillin, A. and Montague R., 2008, The NSW school-link training program: The impact of training on mental health service provision to adolescents in New South Wales, Australia, *International Journal of Mental Health Promotion*, 10, 5–13.

Mufson, L., Moreau, D., Weissman, M. & Klerman, G. (1993). *Interpersonal psychotherapy for depressed adolescents*. New York: The Guilford Press.

Mufson, L., Dorta, K., Moreau, D. & Weissman, M. (2004). *Interpersonal psychotherapy for depressed adolescents (2nd Edition)*. New York: The Guilford Press.

Mufson, L., Gallagher, T., Dorta, K. & Young, J. (2004). A group adaptation of interpersonal psychotherapy for depressed adolescents. *American Journal of Psychotherapy*, 58(2), 220–237.

National Institute for Health and Care Excellence (NICE) (2017). *Depression in children and young people: Identification and management*. London (UK): NICE.

Procter, E. (2011). *The spiritual and religious beliefs of adolescents. Royal College of Psychiatrists*, Monograph. Available at https://www.rcpsych.ac.uk/docs/default-source/members/sigs/spirituality-spsig/elizabeth-procter-the-spiritual-and-religious-beliefs-of-adolescents-x.pdf?sfvrsn=211cd18a_2.

Pu, J., Zhou, X., Liu, L., Zhang, Y., Yang, L. et al. (2017) Efficacy and acceptability of interpersonal psychotherapy for depression in adolescents: A meta-analysis of randomized controlled trials. *Psychiatry Research*, 253, 226–232.

Ravishankar, S.S. (2012). Interview by Russell daSouza. *Asian Journal of Psychiatry*, 5(4), 358–359.

Singhal, M., Manjula, M. & Sagar, J. (2015). Adolescent depression prevention programs—A review. *Journal of Depression and Anxiety*, 4(197), 1–7. doi:10.4197/2167-1044.1000197.

The Royal Australian and New Zealand College of Psychiatrists (RANZCP). (2010). *Prevention and early intervention of mental illness in infants, children and adolescents. Planning strategies for Australia and New Zealand*. RANZCP.

Young, J., Mufson, L., & Davies, M. (2006b). Efficacy of interpersonal psychotherapy-adolescent skills training: An indicated preventive intervention for depression. *Journal Child Psychology and Psychiatry*, 47(12), 1254–1262.

# 2  A model of holistic assessment

**Contents**

| | |
|---|---|
| Introduction | 16 |
| The holistic model of assessment | 17 |
|    *The Biological Domain* | 18 |
|    *The Psychological Domain* | 21 |
|    *The Social Domain* | 28 |
|    *The Cultural Domain* | 30 |
|    *The Spiritual Domain* | 33 |
| Distress and impairment | 39 |
| Readiness to change | 40 |
| The formulation | 40 |
| References | 46 |

## Introduction

While assessment and formulation are central components of mental health intervention, even experienced mental health workers run the risk of developing shortcuts in this area that may lead them to miss key information about a client and thereby choose a less than optimal course of treatment. The general aim of this chapter is to provide therapists with a framework to assist them in their continually evolving skills of assessment and formulation.

Specifically, this chapter provides an assessment process that does not view psychological distress or psychiatric problems narrowly as a medical disease or merely a cluster of symptoms but conceptualises the young person's functioning as the integration of her biological, psychological, social, cultural, and spiritual domains. This model of assessment is congruent with the theoretical underpinnings of IPT-A and leads directly to specific techniques and interventions used in IPT-A. In addition, it focuses not only on risk factors for mental distress and disorder but also on the strengths and protective factors that may constitute a significant part of the young person's psychological and interpersonal world.

When the young person first arrives for consultation, the therapist begins an information gathering process common to many psychotherapeutic approaches to determine what intervention, if any, will best suit the client's needs.

At this initial point, the therapist will in most cases meet with the young person; one or both parents, if appropriate; and, on some occasions, other family members. The therapist will explain assessment and therapy to the client and parents. Apart from providing relevant psychoeducation about assessment and therapy, this session is also an opportunity to access the parents' perspective on the young persons' difficulties and to obtain an indication of the duration and frequency of the presenting problems as well as the parents' perspective on the degree of distress and impairment these problems are causing the young person. As it is helpful to engage parents as collaborative therapists, this first meeting also presents an initial opportunity to gauge how effectively the parents may be able to embrace this role once therapy begins.

After this initial meeting with the young person and her parents, which usually occupies a part of the first session, the therapist then begins meeting with the young person alone. The approach to the assessment of adolescent clients described below is based on the notion that in an assessment interview, two experts come together. The client is the expert on the raw material of her life: no one else has this expertise. The second expert, the therapist, brings a specific set of skills to the session: first, his or her ability to help the client understand her life more effectively and, second, to collaboratively plan a future course of action.

## The holistic[1] model of assessment

In 1977 George L. Engel proposed a model for assessment that included biological, psychological, and social domains of human functioning (Engel, 1977). Holistic assessment acknowledges the importance of these three domains but contends that whilst the exploration of these domains may lead to an accurate understanding of a client, this understanding may still not be enough. Holistic assessment extends the biopsychosocial model and proposes two additional domains that also exert significant influence on clients: the Cultural and the Spiritual domains.

Holistic assessment shifts the focus away from the presence of symptoms of mental disorder to a comprehensive exploration of the lived experience of the young person and to how biological, psychological, social, cultural, and spiritual domains interact to shape this experience. In addition to exploring the five areas of functioning, the therapist enquires about levels of distress and impairment that may be implicated in the current expression of symptoms and the young person's readiness to change. Finally, the therapist constructs with the young person a formulation that will, first, help the young person to better understand his current life experience and, second, guide the therapy toward a positive outcome. The model of holistic assessment is summarised in Figure 2.1.

18  Introduction

Movement away from but includes symptomatology

Encompasses:

- Biological
- Psychological
- Social
- Cultural
- Spiritual

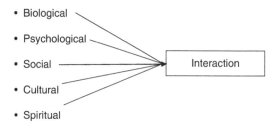

Distress and impairment

Readiness to change

Formulation

*Figure 2.1* Summary of the model of holistic assessment.

The five domains within the holistic assessment model and some suggestions for exploration are described below. Using these five as guidelines, the therapist encourages the young person to tell her story in such a way as to elicit the necessary and sufficient information for the construction of an holistic formulation. Whilst this model presents five discrete domains, in reality they are not mutually exclusive. There will be overlap between them, and some of the related suggestions for exploration may occur within more than one domain.

Within each of these five domains, factors that may predispose, precipitate, perpetuate, or protect distress or mental disorder will be considered. Figure 2.2 illustrates these and proposes examples of enquiry relevant to each.

## *The biological domain*

An exploration of the role of any biological factors that may be contributing to the distress or disorder is an essential component of an assessment interview. Parental depression, for example, is the most consistently replicated risk factor for depression in their offspring (Collishaw et al., 2016; Tharpar et al., 2012).

Another prominent risk factor for depression and related disorders is substance use (Torikka, 2017). For example, has substance use been involved in predisposing the young person to mental disorder? Have substances been involved in precipitating the current episode? Is substance use implicated in perpetuating the current episode? Additionally, is there any protective value in the current use of substances, and, if so, how might this be the case?

The case of Sarah, a 16-year-old student, illustrates how a wide range of factors, beginning with those from the Biological Domain, interact to shape her wellbeing.

A *model of holistic assessment*  19

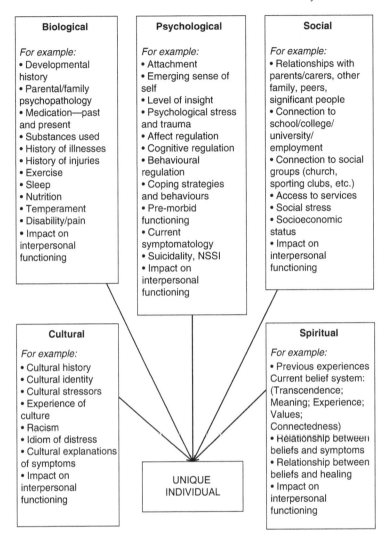

*Figure 2.2* Model of holistic assessment.

**Sarah**, in her last year of secondary school, was experiencing symptoms of depression and anxiety. Her general practitioner prescribed fluvoxamine (150 mg daily), which she had been taking for six weeks with no apparent improvement in mood. Sarah was smoking small amounts of cannabis daily and binge drinking most Friday nights. In her initial assessment, Sarah revealed that both her mother and father drank heavily and that her father had spent several months in a drug and alcohol rehabilitation facility in the previous year. Sarah's parents reported her developmental history was normal; they reported usual childhood illnesses and only minor injuries; confirmed their own substance use problems and reported no additional family psychopathology. They described Sarah as being "highly strung", a characteristic they had noted since her early childhood.

Sarah's parents' excessive alcohol use suggests the possibility that Sarah may have a vulnerability to substance misuse (Vassoler et al., 2014), which may act to predispose her to problematic use. The therapist would explore the relationship between Sarah's cannabis use, her alcohol use, and the symptomatology of both depression and anxiety to determine if this use had a role in precipitating the depression and anxiety. The therapist would additionally explore if the substance use was perpetuating the symptomatology; in addition, the therapist would enquire if Sarah was self-medicating with either substance in attempt to alleviate symptoms. In this case, her substance use may, at least in the short term, be protective of distress or symptomatology, in a similar manner to which diazepam may be protective of symptomatology.

The additional information provided by Sarah's parents, that she was "highly strung" and had been so for much of her life, may indicate that her current depression and anxiety were occurring within the context of an anxious temperament (Cloninger et al., 2006). Regarding a family history of mental disorder, although Sarah's parents did not report any family psychopathology, the therapist would exercise caution in concluding too much from this because the parents' substance use may be masking temperamental vulnerabilities, if not symptomatology, of their own or within their extended family.

As part of the exploration of the Biological domain, the therapist would ask Sarah about sleep patterns as well as about diet and exercise, to establish how these variables were acting to predispose, precipitate, perpetuate, or be protective of Sarah's current symptom profile.

Sarah had neither disability nor a history of illness, surgery, or brain injury. However, for some young people, each of these can impact on mental distress and disorder. Physical and intellectual disabilities have both been shown to be associated comorbidly with mental (especially affective) disorders and substance use (MacCulloch, 2004; Tonge et al., 2009) and as such should not be overlooked as possible biological contributors to distress. Likewise, other biological variables may not be recognised by the young person as relevant to functioning in everyday life. Examples include past viral illnesses, physiological changes such as menarche or menstrual hormonal fluctuations, and childhood accidents that may have had neurological implications. Corticosteroids, antidepressants, contraception medication, and some antibiotics may have unexpected but significant impact on functioning, while even moderate use of alcohol and even caffeine may alter the effect of some prescription medications such as antidepressant or antipsychotic medication (Stahl, 2011). These should be explored in ways that are appropriate to gender and cultural sensitivities.

Finally, how do the variables explored within the Biological domain impact the young person's interpersonal functioning? For example, how does Sarah's binge drinking affect her relationship with her mother and father? Does her drinking cause conflict with her parents but confer a level of acceptance with her peer group? Do her friends encourage or discourage her cannabis use? Is Sarah's difficulty falling asleep related to a hypervigilance around her mobile phone or social media expectations? Does Sarah's fear of missing out on social interactions within her peer group drive behaviours, such as keeping her mobile phone on and by her bed at night, which then significantly reduces the amount and quality of restful sleep she gets each night?

*The psychological domain*

In a similar manner to which the Biological domain is central to understanding the young person's current life experience, the role of psychological factors that may be contributing to symptoms or mental disorder remains an equally essential component of an assessment interview. How may the young person's attachment style, for example, predispose her to mental disorder? How have her attachment-related behaviours had a role in precipitating the current episode? Is her attachment style implicated in perpetuating the current episode, or is there any protective value in the young person's attachment behaviours? (The role of attachment is discussed in detail in Chapter 3.)

Similarly, the young person's sense of self can have significant impact on the experience of distress and disorder as well as on the direction that therapy takes. Sowislo and Orth (2012) in a meta-analysis of 95 studies, observed that decreased self-esteem significantly increased risk of depression and anxiety through both internal and external channels: young people with low self-esteem seem to ruminate and focus on negative thoughts and simultaneously tended to seek out negative feedback from others. Both pathways were shown to raise vulnerability to depression and perpetuate the depressive episode. These authors conclude by suggesting that therapeutic strategies that increase self-esteem may well have positive impact on both anxiety and depression. This illustrates how a thorough assessment may not only clarify the processes that underlie the young person's distress but also suggest therapeutic directions.

Understanding the young person's level of insight into his current distress can be useful in two ways. First, understanding the young person's insight allows the therapist to see the problem from the client's point of view, which facilitates rapport and engagement. Second, the young person's degree of insight into his current problem can be seen as one measure of their appraisal of reality. The level of insight into his or her current situation can be assessed along a continuum as

| Little or no insight | Partial insight | Mature insight |

←——————————————————————————————→

Part of the therapeutic goal of IPT-A is, through psychoeducation, to correct any distortion and help the young person achieve a more mature insight into her psychological and interpersonal world. However, the level of psychoeducation is moderated by the client's level of insight. Getting this right is not solely a task of assessment but remains a continual challenge for the therapist. Advancing too quickly with psychoeducation increases the risk of damaging engagement, whereas proceeding too slowly risks reducing potential therapeutic gain. The therapist can use the young person's movement towards a more mature insight during therapy to guide the rate and timing of psychoeducation.

Continuing the case of **Sarah**, her initial denial of the impact of her alcohol consumption on her depression and anxiety is characteristic of a young person who lies towards the left-hand end of the insight continuum. However, the fact that she was seeking help for her problems rather than denying their existence is indicative of at least some degree of insight. Because of Sarah's partial insight, the therapist decided to go gently with psychoeducation rather than compromise engagement with too much information.

The traumatising effects of experiences such as physical or sexual abuse, domestic violence, community violence, adverse drug experiences, multiple or significant losses, repeated exposure to negative experiences, and the like can affect individuals from the immediate aftermath of the event and for years afterwards. For some young people, symptoms following traumatic events may not appear for months or even years after. Unresolved trauma can predispose young people to psychological symptoms, traumatic events can precipitate symptoms, and the continued impact of traumatic memory can perpetuate symptoms. However, symptoms associated with traumatic events may appear quite differently from symptoms of, for example, depression or anxiety. Themes of guilt and self-blame, self-disgust, self-hatred, low self-esteem, powerlessness, profound mistrust of others, fear of intimacy, and fears about the safety of self and others may be associated with the clinical picture following trauma, even when other symptoms do not reach threshold for a *Diagnostic and Statistical Manual for Mental Disorders: Fifth Edition* (DSM-5) diagnosis of post-traumatic stress disorder (PTSD; APA 2013). In this respect, the experience of trauma may be underestimated or even missed completely during assessment. However, until the traumatic experiences are identified and managed, their impact may continue to subvert any attempts to deal with other symptomatology.

For many years, psychological assessments have focused on symptomatology young people are currently experiencing. Of equal importance, though, are the strengths our clients manifest, often in the face of considerable adversity. For many young people, their distress is an indication that they do not have well developed strategies for coping with life's problems (McAlpine, 1999). Frydenberg and Lewis (2012) described coping strategies as constituting a set of cognitive, affective, and behavioural actions that arise in response to a particular concern or problem. These strategies represent an attempt to restore equilibrium or to remove the turbulence, and this may be done by attempting to solve the problem (problem-focused coping) or managing the emotional responses to the

A model of holistic assessment  23

problem without necessarily arriving at a solution (emotion-focused coping). Assessing a young person's coping strategies includes an appraisal of his skills of both problem- and emotion-focused coping. As young people can actively learn productive coping strategies that can then impact on their negative affectivity, the assessment of functional and dysfunctional coping behaviours can be a key component in understanding the etiology of psychological disorder and in promoting more positive mental health and lifestyles.

Related to this, resilience, or the individual's capacity to cope with stress and adversity, has also been associated with positive and negative mental health (Anyan and Haemal, 2016; Maston, 2008; Rutter, 2008). In an early report from The International Resilience Project, Grotberg (1996) identified fifteen personal characteristics that differentiated resilient children and adolescents. These characteristics factored into three clusters:

1   External supports and resources
    I have ...

    - People around me I trust and who love me, no matter what
    - People who set limits for me, so I know when to stop before there is danger or trouble
    - People who show me how to do things right by the way they do things
    - People who want me to learn to do things on my own
    - People who help me when I am sick, in danger, or need to learn

2   Internal personal strengths
    I am ...

    - A person people can like and love
    - Glad to do nice things for others and show my concern
    - Respectful of myself and others
    - Willing to be responsible for what I do
    - Sure things will be all right

3   Social and interpersonal strengths
    I can ...

    - Talk to others about things that frighten me or bother me
    - Find ways to solve problems that I face
    - Control myself when I feel like doing something not right or dangerous
    - Figure out when it is a good time to talk to someone or to take action
    - Find someone to help me when I need it

These three clusters of resilient characteristics have been developed into a two-dimensional model based on competence and connection[2] (Clinical Tool 2.1).

The competence dimension comprises the ten characteristics from *Internal personal strengths* (I am ...) and *Social and interpersonal strengths* (I can ...), while the connection dimension comprises the five characteristics from

## Clinical Tool 2.1  Resilience grid

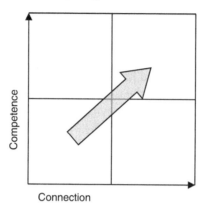

### Competence

*Internal personal strengths*  (I AM)

- A person people can like and love
- Glad to do nice things for others and show my concern
- Respectful of myself and others
- Willing to be responsible for what I do
- Sure things will be all right

*Social and interpersonal strengths*  (I CAN)

- Talk to others about things that frighten me or bother me
- Find ways to solve problems that I face
- Control myself when I feel like doing something not right or dangerous
- Figure out when it is a good time to talk to someone or to take action
- Find someone to help me when I need it

### Connection

*External supports and resources*  (I HAVE)

- People around me I trust and who love me, no matter what
- People who set limits for me so I know when to stop before there is danger or trouble
- People who show me how to do things right by the way they do things
- People who want me to learn to do things on my own
- People who help me when I am sick, in danger or need to learn

*External supports and resource (I have ...).* This tool can assist the therapist and young person to identify areas of resilience and sets a clear direction towards increased competence and increased connection (towards the top right corner of the grid).

Including resilience in assessment and in therapy brings about a significant shift within the clinical environment from the traditional focus on deficit to a focus on ability, which then facilitates the therapist and young person to explore and develop personal strengths that may have been largely invisible and unacknowledged. Discovering these strengths can then create a new set of options for dealing with life's difficulties rather than reacting to these difficulties symptomatically or resorting to substance use to block them out.

As illustrated above, within an holistic assessment, the young person is seen as much more than just an aggregation of symptoms. However, an examination of current signs and symptoms of psychological disorder still constitutes a necessary component in understanding the young person's current suffering.[3] Detecting depression and other mental disorders in adolescence can be difficult because troubled young people are often dismissed as having problems related to bad behaviour, a "phase" they may be going through, or sometimes to the normal experience of adolescent angst. Exploring the frequency, intensity, and duration of symptoms will help differentiate psychological disorder from normative adolescent experience.

Depression, like other disorders, is not an all or nothing diagnosis. The NICE guidelines (NICE, 2019) identify Key and Associated symptoms that adolescents with depression may experience:

| Key Symptoms | Associated Symptoms |
| --- | --- |
| • Depressed or irritable mood most of the day, nearly every day<br><br>AND/OR<br><br>• Marked diminishment in pleasurable activities and interests<br><br>• Fatigue or low energy, low motivation | • Poor or increased sleep<br>• Diminished ability to think and concentrate<br>• Loss of confidence and low self-esteem<br>• Poor or increased appetite<br>• Suicidal thoughts or acts<br>• Agitation or slowing of movements<br>• Guilt or self-blame |

*Figure 2.3* Key and Associated Symptoms.

These guidelines suggest mild depression is associated with up to four of these symptoms, moderate depression with five to six symptoms, and severe depression with seven to ten. But in addition to the number of symptoms experienced, young people also experience varying degrees of impairment and distress associated with their symptoms. The parameters of distress would include the frequency, duration, and intensity of the symptoms, whilst impairment would include (1) social impairment: that is, the degree that significant relationships (for example with family, friends and teachers) have been impacted by the disorder, and (2) educational impairment, for example, school attendance, grades, connectedness with school, behaviour, and extracurricular activities.

In summary, an exploration of current symptomatology constitutes a key element within the holistic assessment of young people. A systematic assessment will include an evaluation of the presence of symptoms; the frequency, duration, and intensity of these symptoms; and the degree of distress and impairment the experience of symptoms is causing the young person.

As there is significant evidence that the risk of suicide attempt and other suicidal behaviour increase with the presence of mental disorder or anxious distress, and increase further with the use of substances (Tharper et al., 2012) any assessment of young people should include a competent and comprehensive assessment of suicide risk. Clinical Tool 2.2 is a suicide risk assessment protocol that many mental health professionals find useful. This protocol is intended to act as an adjunct to the clinical interview, certainly not to replace it. The primary value of this tool is to help the therapist ensure primary risk factors are covered in the enquiry. The therapist can then make a clinical judgement of the current level of suicide risk on the basis of comprehensive assessment and develop an action plan.

---

### Clinical Tool 2.2   Suicide risk assessment protocol

**Assessing Suicide Risk**

Name:                                                                                              Date:
                                                                                                   Comments

Current ideation (including ambivalence)
Current plan—details, means, time, lethality, chance of intervention
Previous attempts
Family history/climate
Recent history in peer group
Recent stressors
Sense of burdensomeness
Disconnection from support
Psychosocial resources
Mental health status (including comorbidity, substance use,
   impulsivity, and aggression)
Other issues (including sexual orientation, rural or remote setting,
   homelessness)
Medical status
Access to means (especially firearms)

When **Sarah's** therapist asked about suicidality, she spoke openly about having thought about taking her life several times in the past year. It emerged that talk about suicide was fairly common within her peer group and two of her friends had taken overdoses of paracetamol in the past six months. Although Sarah had no current plan and had not thought about suicide in the past few months, recent episodes of self-harm alerted the therapist that Sarah was experiencing levels of intolerable affect that she was regulating by cutting her arms. Previous suicidal ideation seemed to be linked to psychosocial stressors, especially perceived rejection by significant members of her peer group. It appeared these same stressors were triggering the self-harm. While the therapist determined Sarah's current suicide risk was low to medium, she was concerned about the easy availability of paracetamol and agreed with Sarah to discuss current suicidal ideation at the beginning of each session. In addition, the therapist and Sarah discussed strategies Sarah could employ if she did feel suicidal and gave Sarah her own phone number and a 24-hour help line for emergency use.

Suicidal behaviour needs to be differentiated from other types of self-harm that do not have suicidal intent. Non-suicidal self-injury (NSSI) has been defined by Nock and Favazza (2009) as "the deliberate committing of direct physical harm to one's own body in the absence of suicidal intent and for purposes not socially sanctioned" (p. 9). NSSI occurs relatively frequently in adolescents. One year prevalence rates of approximately 7000 per 100000 per year and lifetime prevalence rates of approximately 13% have been widely reported (Hawton, Rodham, & Evans, 2006; Lawrence et al., 2015). Young women aged between 16 and 17 are at highest risk of NSSI, with lifetime prevalence for this group reported to be 22.8% (Lawrence et al., 2015).

For many young people who do self-harm, NSSI is an effective albeit dysfunctional way of relieving intense distress. For some young people, their self-harm is episodic, that is, occurs irregularly, whilst for others this behaviour is more predictable and repetitive. For some young people, especially those for whom self-harm is episodic and who have not developed an identity as a "cutter", their self-harm is ego-dystonic. However, for others, especially for those who do identify as a cutter, their self-harm may be ego-syntonic and often more resistant to change. NSSI may, for some young people, contribute to precipitating and perpetuating depression or other disorder.

**Leon** found cutting his calves was the only way he could manage his intense feelings of anger, frustration, loneliness, and helplessness. But for Leon this behaviour was ego-dystonic: he saw his NSSI as necessary but contemptible. Managing these powerful feelings by cutting contributed to his sense of helplessness and hopelessness, which intensified his depression and provided further evidence for his emerging belief that he had no control over his life.

Some young people, though, claim that their NSSI is protective.

**Jane** managed explosive feelings of anger towards herself and others by cutting her arms and thighs. During these episodes of overwhelming affect, Jane had the pervasive belief that the intensity of her escalating state would lead to her own destruction or the annihilation of others. She found that the only way she could reduce the intensity of her affect to manageable levels was by cutting. She believed her cutting had, on many occasions, saved her life. Jane likened her cutting to the pressure relief valve on a pressure cooker.

When assessing NSSI as a component of a mental disorder or as an effective but dysfunctional coping strategy in a young person without disorder, understanding the meaning of the self-harm behaviour for the young person is key. An assessment characterised by respectful curiosity may help the young person discuss this aspect of her life which, for many, is accompanied by an expectation and fear of being judged by others.

An exploration of how the young person's psychological domain impacts his interpersonal functioning will complete this domain.

*Therapist:* *Del, one of the things we've been talking about today is how you deal with sad and angry feelings, and you've told me that when these feelings are around you prefer to be alone. I'm just wondering, when you are sad or angry, does this change things between you and your Mum?*
*Del:* *Just that we don't talk much.*
*Therapist:* *And you're used to talking a lot with your Mum. Are there other people you talk to when you feel like this?*

### The social domain

The movement from early adolescence through middle to late adolescence and finally adulthood is a period normatively characterised in many cultures by a movement towards independence and a firmer identity. During this time, the family plays less of a role as the primary source of nurture and belonging, and the peer group begins to take up much of this role. The family, the peer group, and the school—and for some, social, sporting, religious or other groups—provide an interactive social context as the young person is progressing through adolescence.

Whilst some families offer connection and support for young people with mental health problems and may be keen for involvement in the assessment and management of their family member, other families are less accommodating or available. Some family structures confer on their members genetic loadings for psychological and substance-related difficulties and also model ineffective coping strategies often associated with mental ill-health and problematic levels of substance use.

Young people raised within a family structure characterised by mental disorder and/or high levels of substance use are also more likely to develop insecure attachment styles. Bowlby (1988) suggests that a close link exists between the young person's social support structure and their attachment style. Adolescents with anxious attachments styles are in effect doubly disadvantaged. First, they are likely to have experienced inconsistent or absent care during their early years, which may impact on their capacity to trust others to help meet their attachment needs. Second, because young people with anxious attachment are more likely to have reduced capacity to care for others or to form fulfilling intimate relationships, their social support networks are often undeveloped.

Although **Sarah's** mother and father had problems with alcohol, they were both concerned about Sarah's drinking and cannabis use. Sarah described them as overprotective to the point of wanting to know her every movement. She felt they genuinely cared about her but over recent months, because of their excessive involvement with her life, Sarah was taking less notice of their wishes and they seemed powerless to control her. However, Sarah believed if things went wrong, her parents would always be there for her.

Sarah was ambivalent about her relationship with her peer group. She reported that they were the most important thing in her life, yet she could find very little positive to say about them. She often hated being with them but felt miserable when she was away from them. Most of her peer group drank heavily when they were out, and all smoked cannabis. Sarah saw no future for herself in this group if she gave up cannabis.

Whilst peer groups may provide positive opportunities to negotiate normative tasks of adolescence, they also provide opportunities for dissatisfaction and distress. Ego-dystonic peer pressure, face-to-face and online bullying within the peer group, and the inability of some young people to initiate and maintain relationships may be central in precipitating or perpetuating mental health problems.

Both mental disorder and substance use individually impact on education and employment. The co-occurrence of the two adds another layer of complexity to this relationship. Consistent attendance in an educational setting or workplace has been shown to be protective against development of both mental and substance use disorders (Zubrick, 2014). Conversely, non-attendance has been shown to be a risk factor. However, the relationship between education/work and comorbid disorder is complex. Mental disorder and problematic substance use make it difficult to attend to the demands of study or employment. These issues make it difficult to access the protection education or employment offer (Lawrence et al., 2015).

Due to the significance of the social domain during adolescence, changes in the social world can have considerable impact on the young person's life experience, distress, and symptomatology and on the young person's interpersonal relationships.

*Therapist:* Hayley you told me that Tegan, your best friend, has now left school because of her sickness and I know you spent a lot of time with her when she was at school. Has Tegan leaving changed things much between you and the other kids at school?

*Hayley:* Well over the last year or so I spent nearly all my time with Tegan and now it's like I have to start all over again. And they've all got their own friends now. In class I sit with other kids but at recess and lunch I mostly go to the library.

*Therapist:* So Tegan leaving has meant that now you're spending a lot of time by yourself?

*Hayley:* Yeah, most of the time really.

*Therapist:* Do you miss hanging out with other kids?

*Hayley:* Yeah but what can you do? You can't just go up to someone and say, "Can I be your friend?"

### The cultural domain

Culture is defined by Matsumoto (1996) as "the set of attitudes, values, beliefs and behaviour shared by a group of people, but different for each individual, communicated from one generation to the next" (p. 16). The experience of culture for young people can have significant impact on their mental health, whether it be Big C culture (that is, cultural differences defined by ethnicity and race) or small c culture: differences in attitudes, values, beliefs, and behaviours encountered when negotiating the various groupings and points of connection during the adolescent years.

The impact of Big C culture on the young person may be influenced by many factors such as cultural norms, expectations, language/s spoken, and racism. If migration is part of the young person's experience or his family's experience, then additional influences can include country of birth, recency of arrival, age at arrival, circumstances of migration, parental attitudes, impact of migration on the young person's cultural identity, and the extent of affiliation the young person and his family have with their new community and with the culture of origin.

When the young person's family culture is a minority in their society, it can be helpful to assess the relative connectedness the young person has with his family culture and the majority culture. This exploration can be facilitated by Clinical Tool 2.3, rather clumsily named the Ethno-Cultural Identity Matrix, (ECIM) modified from a model developed by Kitano (1989) cited by Marsella (2001). In the clinical Tool 2.3, the horizontal axis represents connection to the traditional, or family culture, (or culture of origin), and the vertical axis represents connection to the host or majority culture. Often, when used transparently with young people, clients come up with quadrant descriptions that are meaningful for them. For example, an Australian/Chinese young man who found this tool helped him understand the context of his distress a lot better, labelled the top left quadrant "Bit of both," the top right "Aussie", the bottom left "Chinese", and the bottom right "Out of both".

## Clinical Tool 2.3 Ethno-cultural identity matrix (ECIM) (adapted from Kitano, 1989)

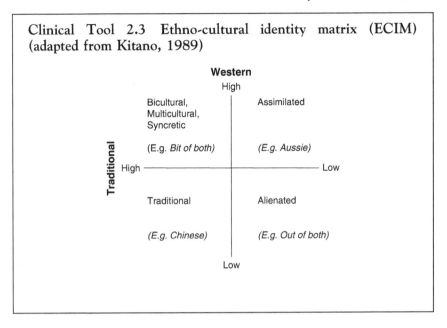

This matrix represents the young person's connectedness to the traditional and to the mainstream culture and illustrates the extent to which young people negotiate their cultural identity. While there are risk and protection factors associated with each quadrant, research suggests the Bicultural quadrant is associated with adaptive psychosocial adjustment and the Alienated quadrant is associated with higher levels of isolation, stress, and maladjustment (Bashir, 2000; Klimidas and Minas, 1995). This model is dynamic rather than static: young people may move between quadrants dependent on circumstances. For some young people, this balancing act is maintained seamlessly, whilst for others the inherent stressors may increase vulnerability to mental health difficulties and/or substance use problems.

This model can apply to Indigenous young people attempting to negotiate their traditional norms and those of the dominant culture, it can shed light on the struggle of some same-sex attracted young people negotiating the differences between the culture around same-sex attraction and that of the dominant heterosexual paradigm, and it may also assist in the assessment of a young person who is attempting to navigate the expectations and behaviours of her family compared to those of her peer group.

Culture can affect the development and communication of symptoms of mental health problems. Depression, for example, is expressed and manifested in a variety of ways in individuals from differing cultures and ethnic backgrounds. Depression as a syndrome is a commonly occurring disorder in all cultures and the core symptoms of depression vary little from country to country (Kessler and Bromet, 2013). However, some cultural variations do exist in two primary areas: (1) recognition of the disorder as a problem and (2) the subjective experience. In most Western cultures, depression is described in terms of mental suffering, sadness, despair, or pessimism. Depressive disorders occur along a broad continuum from mild mood disturbances to major depressive disorders with psychotic symptoms. However, in non-Western cultures, depression is often expressed through various somatic symptoms (Marsella, 2001; Salzman, 2018). Feelings of being unwell and wanting to die, common in depression, are often expressed through a range of ailments such as headaches, stomach upsets, or back pain (Minas and Lewis, 2017; Marsella, 2001). Culture may influence how the behaviours and feelings associated with disorder are explained and displayed. The different ways emotions are displayed in non-Western cultures may lead to an incorrect diagnosis if viewed from a Western perspective. For example, Manson (1995) illustrates cultural mores around expressions of sadness: "Some middle-eastern cultures encourage the display of extreme sadness and sorrow; some Native American cultures discourage the display of extreme sadness and sorrow; in some Indochinese cultures the expression of emotion is seen as private and limited so as to not harm the family/society as a whole" (p. 127).

The word depression is absent from some languages, and there are considerable variations in the language of affect across cultures. Manson (1995) identifies that some cultures prefer to express affect using personal "I" statements, whereas other cultures prefer more collective expressions, using "we" statements. Some cultures prefer nonverbal expressions, believing that silence, meditation, and acceptance are the keys to mental health. Vocabulary used in expression of emotions and feeling states varies greatly across cultures. Some cultures have a large and rich vocabulary containing words to represent even the subtlest differences. Others have few words to express and describe emotional feelings and states.

Culturally competent assessment will include attending to the young person's cultural frame of reference, taking care not to judge as psychopathology those normal variations in behaviour, belief, or experience that are particular to the individual's culture, while at the same time attending to symptom patterns that are contributing to the young person's impairment and distress.

Cultural expectations can impact on relationships with significant others:

**John** was a 12-year-old school student originally from Greece and now living with his family in Australia who developed symptoms of social anxiety when he began secondary school. Although John was fluent in English, his parents only spoke Greek and had strong expectations that John would speak Greek when he was at home, instructing him that to speak English whilst at home was disrespectful to them and to John's grandparents, who lived with them. When John brought some soccer friends from his new school home after a game one weekend, he noticed they were laughing whilst he was talking to his parents. This event triggered a sensitivity in which John began to constantly interpret others' behaviour as assessing him. As a counter, John began to deliberately develop anti-Greek behaviours at home, which clearly distressed his parents and grandparents, and at school, according to his teachers, alienated himself from his peers by trying too hard to be accepted. The expected rejections supported John's hypothesis that he was, in his terms, "a loser" and he retreated into his bedroom.

John's school counsellor conceptualised these behaviours using the Ethnocultural Identity Matrix (ECIM). John initially was able to negotiate his bicultural heritage by keeping the quadrants separate. Whilst at home, he spoke Greek and conformed to his parents' (and grandparents') expectations. That is, he was comfortable in the Traditional quadrant of the ECIM. While he was at school, John left his Greek-ness at home and was at ease in his role as an Australian adolescent—the Assimilated quadrant. However, when friends from his Assimilated world entered his Traditional world, John was unable to negotiate a smooth amalgamation (which would have been the Bicultural quadrant), preferring instead, after an abortive attempt to force acceptance, to retreat to the safety of isolation in his bedroom—the Alienated quadrant of the ECIM.

John's cultural struggles impacted his relationship with significant others in his life and in so doing left him without the support he was accustomed to—that of his parents and his friends—and strengthened a fear of negative evaluation by others, which was reinforced by reactions to his self-defeating attempts to put things right.

## The spiritual domain

> "Many of the things you can count don't count; many of the things you can't count really count".– Albert Einstein

The term spirituality is derived from the Latin *spiritus*, which equates to breath or breathing. By extension, spirituality contains elements of that which gives life and, by further extension, that which gives meaning and purpose.

Whilst it is difficult to clearly define spirituality, an overview of the literature suggests that the term embraces concepts such as transcendence, meaning, experience, values, and connectedness. Spirituality includes but is not limited to religion or religious experience, as demonstrated by a working definition of spirituality proposed by Goldstein (2010): "spirituality is defined as meaning-making, feelings of connectedness to others, self, and/or a higher power and the openness to and search for self-transcendence" (p. 3).

In 2002 Australian psychiatrist Russell d'Souza found in a survey of adult mental health patients that 79% of these patients rated spirituality as very important and 82% thought their therapists should be aware of their spiritual needs and beliefs. Some 67% of these patients believed their spirituality helped them cope with their psychological pain. In contrast, only 11% of this sample reported their therapist asked them about their spiritual beliefs (d'Souza, 2002). Proctor (2011) similarly found that whilst almost half of the adolescent clients in her study endorsed some form of spirituality, only 5% of their therapists asked about it.

Both the adult and the adolescent literature on spirituality and mental health acknowledge the importance of the contribution of spirituality to an understanding of the whole person. When young people are facing significant problems in their lives, whether these problems are associated with loss, conflict with significant others, unwanted changes thrust on them that are outside their control, or a lack of resources to cope with the exigencies of life, young people have deep and wide-ranging needs. It is at these times that a biopsychosocial assessment may not be enough to fully uncover the complexities of the lived reality of the young person.

As one of his teaching strategies, Viktor Frankl showed his students an image similar to the one below:

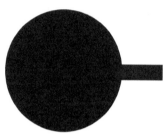

He then asked his students to describe the image as accurately as they could. Responses were many and varied but generally centred around the theme of an opaque black circle with a rectangular projection on the right-hand side, protruding from approximately halfway up and extending horizontally for a distance of approximately one-third of the diameter of the circle. Their descriptions were well thought out and, given the information, accurate. Then Frankl revealed that the image was a two dimensional projection from an overhead projector, on which was placed a cup: a hand painted seventeenth-century French tea cup, one of the first made—exquisite china, delicately designed—the cherished possession of the same family spanning several continents and two centuries. And the students saw a black circle with a horizontal protrusion. Whilst their descriptions were accurate, they were not enough. Their limited information prompted a description that missed the entire essence of the object.

In very much the same way, a biopsychosocial description of a young person may well provide an accurate description based on these variables, but unless it taps the essence of that young person, their *spiritus*, the things that give them life, that give them meaning, it may, like the black circle, be accurate but not enough. This essence may or may not have anything to do with religion, but in some cases it will have a lot to do with "meaning-making, feelings of connectedness to others, self, and/or a higher power and the openness to and search for self-transcendence" (Goldstein, 2010, p. 2). Some young people may find this in sport, in music, in drama, in their peer group, in religious beliefs and experience, in prayer or meditation, in their love of nature or animals, or even in their studies. Billy, at age 22, sought it in riding his motorbike.

---

**Box 2.1  Billy**

Riding down to the Island, Billy was feeling at one with the world. He was on board his Harley and was riding with a bunch of his best mates. He was on his annual pilgrimage to the Moto GP: good food, good beer, good company, and great racing; what could be better? Billy's heart sang. Setting up tents at San Remo worked up a pretty powerful thirst, so Billy and his mates adjourned to the pub, which was conveniently located only a short drunken walk from home base. But the first rehydration session was brief as the free bus to the track arrived and Billy and some of his mates took the opportunity to watch the Saturday practice sessions. The rest of his mates had not yet sufficiently dealt with their thirst and decided to stay at the pub to complete the job they had begun.

When Billy arrived at the track, Peter Brock's son was doing a couple of laps in the .05 Torana in memory of his dead father. Many Australians can remember where they were and what they were doing on the afternoon of 8 September 2006 when the news came that Peter Brock had died. "Peter Perfect", one of the best if not the best racing drivers Australia had ever produced, had died in a car accident. This fact in itself got Billy thinking because Brocky dying that way really challenged the natural order of the universe. If he was the best and the road got him, what hope was there for any of us? In anything?

As Brock Junior put his Dad's Torana through its paces, a palpable hush descended on Philip Island. The commentator was sure that Brocky would be looking down on the proceedings and that he would be chuffed, as would Barry Sheehan who was "up there" due to other circumstances, but "up there" nonetheless. Billy looked around at the silenced onlookers—some hardened old bikers with more metal and ink on their bodies than skin, tears shamelessly rolling down their faces. Men who by their colours would be mortal enemies now standing side by side, their differences dissolved. Then it suddenly occurred to Billy, we've got it all: the Creator and the afterlife. The commentator had invoked that, and we all believed him without question. We've come to the Island to respect and adore Mick Doohan, Wayne Gardiner, and the other high priests and to witness the miracles of the prophets like Casey Stoner and Valentino Rossi. Right around the track is the fellowship of believers, each of whom has gathered for communion, worship, and praise. And the sacraments: not bread and wine but transubstantiated pies and beer. For Billy, the Moto GP was a religious experience, a spiritual event.

The conversation about spirituality with a client begins by acknowledging that the young person is much more than a cluster of psychological symptoms occurring within a biological and social world. Understanding the client's spirituality begins with the therapist demonstrating a respectful curiosity about how she understands her world and, moreover, how she understands her symptoms within this world. And for the young person, this may be the only time in her life when an adult has sat with her, genuinely interested in how she understands the world, without an agenda of listening first, then telling her "how it really is". For the therapist, this provides an opportunity to access a deeper dimension of the complexities of the client's life experience and, in conveying a genuine interest in the young person's life, also represents an excellent opportunity to create a powerful therapeutic alliance.

What are some ways to begin a conversation about spirituality with a young person in therapy? Some examples include the following:

**Carl,** aged 16:

*Therapist:*  Some people find that when they are going through some tough times in life, they find some help in beliefs they have. Do you have any beliefs about life that help you out in these times?

**Alessia,** aged 14:

*Therapist:*  Alessia you told me that when you were little you used to go to church with your Mum and Dad. Have your beliefs about things changed from when you were little to now?

**Chris,** aged 13:

*Therapist:*  Some kids your age have conversations with each other about life and relationships and that sort of thing—I guess trying to work out what it all means. Do you and your friends have those kinds of conversations?

**Luke,** aged 15:

*Therapist:*  Last week you told me that you've been playing football since you were six and that you "live and breathe football". I guess by that you were letting me know just how huge this shoulder injury is for you. Luke, would you mind telling me about life with football? And, also, what life would be like without football?

**Millie,** aged 16:

The following part-conversation took place between a therapist and Millie, who presented with major depressive disorder and sub-threshold social anxiety.

Millie was sexually abused by a neighbour when she was ten years old and had not disclosed this event prior to the current clinical session.

*Therapist:* Millie it must have been so difficult telling me what happened with your neighbour. And you've kept it to yourself for all this time.
*Millie:* Yeah.... I couldn't bring myself to tell anyone. Especially Mum or Dad.
*Therapist:* Telling Mum and Dad would have been especially hard?
*Millie:* Yeah.... It's like it would bring shame on the family or something.
*Therapist:* How's that Millie?
*Millie:* It's like if their church friends found out, it would like make our family seem evil or something. Everyone would talk about it.
*Therapist:* Millie can I just check something out with you? I'm just wondering, the way you're talking it sounds to me like you're blaming yourself for what happened to you. Is that what it's like?
*Millie:* Yeah well since that happened everything's gone wrong in our family. My Nan died, Dad lost his job and can't get another one, Mum gets sick all the time, and now I'm just sad all the time and now I hate going to school. (Millie begins crying) It just sucks.
*Therapist:* And you feel responsible...
*Millie:* (Still crying) I just know God's punishing me.
*Therapist:* Tell me how that works Millie.
*Millie:* It's like with that neighbour, it was just so wrong, and now all this stuff's happening to my family...like God's blaming me for it all...and I try to pray about it but it's like my prayers just get stuck and don't go anywhere....
*Millie:* (Crying less now) God's supposed to be loving and forgiving and all that, but if that's true, then why's all this happening?

This excerpt provided some important information about Millie. First, she was sexually assaulted when she was 10; second, Millie has a sense of divine justice: wrong was done and she was being punished; third, Millie believes that some of the wrong was attributed to her, leaving her with a sense of guilt and shame; fourth, her past relationship with God has been compromised as part of this punishment (she can no longer pray); fifth, her depression has been compounded by the loss of her belief that God was loving and forgiving; and sixth (by inference) she believes she hasn't been forgiven by God for her (assumed) part in the sexual abuse.

This early stage of exploring the spiritual context of Millie's depression and social anxiety is providing the therapist with an added dimension to help understand the whole person. In addition, this understanding signals a possible complication in Millie's trajectory through therapy: if Millie sees her depression and anxiety as punishment from God, and at the same time she continues to believe she had some role in her sexual assault and harbours some guilt, then working on depressive symptoms alone without addressing the guilt and its consequences is fraught with the likelihood of significant resistance.[4]

**Eddy** was an 18-year-old Aboriginal Australian who described recent dreams that he was finding disturbing. In these dreams, his late brother (who died in a motor vehicle accident five years ago) and two friends who had also died within the last five years were making regular appearances over the past month or so. Eddy was finding this, in his words, "creepy" and was beginning to resist sleep to prevent the dreams from occurring. The therapist gave Eddy the opportunity to talk about these experiences as much as he was comfortable but conceded that this could be cultural business and it may help if Eddy discussed this with an Aboriginal elder. Eddy agreed to do so and together Eddy and the therapist identified a local elder, Lionel, whom Eddy felt happy about approaching. Eddy returned for a session two weeks later.

*Therapist:*   *Eddy, were you able to see Lionel about your dreams?*
*Eddy:*   *Yeah. Saw him Monday. Lionel said not to worry—they're from the Dreaming—they were just checking in on me. They were worried—I've been in a bit of trouble and they were just trying to straighten things out.*
*Therapist:*   *So is that okay for you?*
*Eddy:*   *Yeah. I talked to them a few times now. It's all right now. Lionel said they'll stay while I need them.*
*Therapist:*   *Are you going to talk to Lionel again?*
*Eddy:*   *No. He said it's okay, just listen...and he said to tell you it's okay.*
*Therapist:*   *Last session Eddy you said seeing these boys in your dreams was a worry, you were trying not to go to sleep because it was creepy. Sounds like it's okay now?*
*Eddy:*   *Yeah*
*Therapist:*   *Are they helping you straighten things out?*
*Eddy:*   *They will.*

It is not uncommon for Aboriginal Australian young people to report experiences like Eddy's. For some, these visitations can be nurturing, leaving them comforted and cared for, whilst for others, like Eddy, they can be quite disturbing. Conversations with elders or trusted people within the culture can provide a context to these experiences that transform the meaning of the experience for the young person. Similarly, young people from religious traditions can be assisted to find a trusted member from within their community who may be able to provide a helpful context to a spiritual problem. Millie, for example, with encouragement from the therapist was able to talk about her loss of faith with an adult friend from within her church community who was able to assure Millie that God did not blame her and was able to help her pray again, freeing her from the crippling belief that she had been abandoned by God because of her perceived role in the sexual abuse.

For many adolescents, their spirituality or meaning-making has altered significantly from its childhood construction. But although changes in the way young people understand the world are part of a normative process, these changes may leave some clients feeling vulnerable and exposed. The safety net they previously took for granted is now a safety net with many holes. Neglecting to adequately explore this domain risks missing vital information that may be, as many clients indicate, a necessary ingredient in their healing.

## Distress and impairment

The next key component of assessment appraises the level of distress and functional impairment associated with the current presentation. Some clients may endorse many symptoms of a disorder, but their index of distress may be low and they may still be able to function at school or within the family or their sport team, whereas other clients may endorse fewer symptoms but may not be able to function in any area of their lives.

In the previous classification system (DSM–IV), Axis V offered the Global Assessment of Functioning (GAF) scale for assessing symptom severity and the client's overall level of functioning. (APA, 2004, pp. 32–34). This scale provides therapists with a largely objective single measure that is divided into ten ranges of functioning from 1 (highly impaired) to 100 (superior functioning). Each ten-point range in the GAF has two components. The first covers symptom severity and the second covers functioning. For example, the first component within the range 41–50 describes "serious symptoms" (e.g., suicidal ideation, severe obsessional rituals, frequent shoplifting) and the second component includes "any serious impairment in social, occupational or school functioning" (e.g., no friends, not attending school).

GAF ratings give therapists an estimate of current functioning but can also be used to estimate premorbid functioning, which facilitates setting realistic clinical goals. GAF ratings are also a reasonable indicator of progress throughout therapy. Whilst they do not formally assess the presence of symptoms, they are sensitive to changes in levels of symptom severity and functional impairment.

Other less formalised measures of distress, such as rating scales, can also be useful in understanding the impact of distress or disorder on the young person and be informative in assessing movement through therapy.

Continuing the case of **Sarah**

*Therapist:* Sarah, I'd really like to get an idea of how difficult this is for you. So say 1 is as sad as you can possibly imagine being, feeling really low, no happiness at all and 10 is just the opposite—10 is feeling really good about life. On that 1–10 scale how sad have you been lately—say, when you woke up this morning? When you went to bed last night? How about right now?

A similar measure can be used for assessing changes in levels of distress:

*Therapist:* Sarah in our first session together about five weeks ago you said your average happiness was only about 2–3 out of 10. What would you say this average is now—say, over the last week?

## Readiness to change

Even though a young person may be experiencing significant symptoms of distress or disorder, we cannot automatically assume he wants to change. There may be many reasons why a client wants to continue experiencing distress, including these:

- it may attract care and attention from the family and others
- being comfortably numb may be preferable to alternatives
- it may be a means of getting out of unwanted social encounters
- it may attract special considerations at school
- it may be a badge of membership of a valued peer group
- other emotional states may be fear provoking
- the specific distress may be protective of trauma memories

If a young person is not ready to change, the therapist does not have a mandate for therapy. In fact, attempting to inflict therapy on a young person who does not want to change may be abusive. The therapy is unlikely to bring about positive change, and it can have negative effects on future help-seeking behaviour. Clinical Tool 2.4, Stages of Change, may assist the therapist in determining with the young person his current readiness to change and guide future decision making about subsequent sessions (Norcross and Goldfield, 2005; Prochaska and DiClemente, 1982).

Motivational interviewing techniques or supportive counselling may be appropriate interventions for clients who are at the first stage (Pre-Contemplation) or the beginning of the second stage (Contemplation). Once the young person indicates a willingness to move from the position of symptoms with accompanying distress and impairment towards comparative psychological health (late Stage 2 and Stage 3 Preparation), the standard evidence-based psychotherapies may become more appropriate.

## The formulation

"Case formulation is a central concept because it stands as the gatekeeper to treatment" (Page and McLean, 2008). "It includes descriptive information on which the hypothesis is based and prescriptive recommendations that flow from that hypothesis". (Eels, 1997).

The formulation is an interactive statement that summarises and interprets the client's current presentation in such a way as to convey understanding and to promote belief that the future can be better. The formulation must be developmentally informed. A case summary and interpretation will clearly be different linguistically and conceptually for a 12-year-old than it will for a 22-year-old and different again for the young person's parents. A case formulation will be sensitive to the young person's culture, values, and other characteristics such as gender and ethnicity.

However, the elements of a sound formulation will remain substantially the same: the formulation links the young person's presenting problems with information about

## Clinical Tool 2.4 Stages of change (adapted from Prochaska and di Clemente, 1982)

| Stage of Change | Stage of treatment | Clinical Focus |
|---|---|---|
| Pre-contemplation | Establish therapeutic alliance | Consider client's attachment style in establishing and maintaining therapeutic alliance (see Chapter 3 and Clinical Tool 3.2)<br>Validate client's needs and fears<br>Validate client's decisions<br>Encourage self-reflection, including exploration of ambivalence |
| Contemplation | Motivation | Validate lack of readiness<br>Clarify advantages and disadvantages of current behaviour<br>Re-visit ambivalence<br>Encourage client to identify new positive outcome expectations |
| Preparation | Planning changes | Identify supports<br>Address barriers<br>Identify or develop skills for behaviour change<br>Encourage small initial steps |
| Action | Active treatment | Plan changes that are desirable and achievable<br>Identify competencies and encourage confidence in managing barriers<br>Process feelings of loss<br>Revisit long-term benefits |
| Maintenance | Relapse prevention | Identify and plan for follow-up support<br>Reinforce internal rewards<br>Develop strategies for coping with future difficulties |

her gathered from discussion of the five domains. It provides a scientifically based explanation of how client characteristics and life experiences may predispose, precipitate, perpetuate, and/or protect from current symptoms in a developmentally accessible way. The formulation acknowledges the young person's current readiness to change. Finally, the formulation, in giving direction to treatment, provides the client with an evidence-based, believable pathway to improved psychological wellbeing.

Clinical Tool 2.5 The case formulation checklist is a self-evaluation tool that has been designed to assist therapists to reflect on their case formulations to ensure all salient aspects of the assessment and formulation have been addressed. This checklist comprises four steps:

### Clinical Tool 2.5  Case formulation checklist

#### (1) Presenting problems

3  Relevant presenting problems noted. Primary and secondary problems were recognised.
2  Most presenting problems noted. Primary and secondary issues were not adequately differentiated.
1  Some presenting problems noted but not distinguished from less relevant issues.
0  Presenting problems were not addressed.

#### (2) Holistic assessment

Circle numbers that approximately indicate the level at which the four Ps were addressed in each of the five domains:

(0 = The 4 Ps within the 5 domains were not addressed
1 = Little evidence of considering the 4 Ps within the 5 domains
2 = The 4 Ps within the 5 domains were considered but not linked to presenting problems
3 = The 4 Ps within the 5 domains were considered and linked to presenting problems)

|              | Biological | Psycho-logical | Social  | Cultural | Spiritual |
|--------------|------------|----------------|---------|----------|-----------|
| Predisposing | 0 1 2 3    | 0 1 2 3        | 0 1 2 3 | 0 1 2 3  | 0 1 2 3   |
| Precipitating| 0 1 2 3    | 0 1 2 3        | 0 1 2 3 | 0 1 2 3  | 0 1 2 3   |
| Perpetuating | 0 1 2 3    | 0 1 2 3        | 0 1 2 3 | 0 1 2 3  | 0 1 2 3   |
| Protective   | 0 1 2 3    | 0 1 2 3        | 0 1 2 3 | 0 1 2 3  | 0 1 2 3   |

#### (3) Readiness to change

Pre-Contemplation — Contemplation — Preparation to change — Action — Maintenance

#### (4) Provisional formulation

3  Well-integrated hypothesis that links the presenting problems with the five domains of the holistic assessment and presents a clear and accurate explanation of the client's presenting problems, noting client's readiness to change. The formulation also provides an evidence-based pathway to symptom improvement that is believable to the young person.
2  An hypothesis that provides a believable but incomplete explanation of the client's presenting problems, but nevertheless offers some hope of symptom improvement.
1  A poorly integrated explanation of the presenting problems that offers the client little understanding of symptoms and little reason to hope for symptom improvement.
0  The formulation was not presented.

© NSW Ministry of Health, 2012

*Step 1. Presenting problems*

In Step 1 the therapist notes the psychological and other problems the client presented with. A rating of 3 on this scale indicates the therapist is satisfied that they noted all presenting problems and distinguished between primary and secondary issues. A rating of 0 indicates the presenting problems were not addressed at all.

---

**Box 2.2**

3 Relevant presenting problems noted. Primary and secondary problems were recognised.
2 Most presenting problems noted. Primary and secondary issues were not adequately differentiated.
1 Some presenting problems noted but not distinguished from less relevant issues.
0 Presenting problems were not addressed.

© NSW Ministry of Health, 2012

---

*Step 2. Holistic assessment*

In Step 2 the therapist evaluates how effectively the four Ps (predisposing, precipitating, perpetuating, and protective factors) were assessed within the five domains (Biological, Psychological, Social, Cultural and Spiritual) of the holistic assessment. The therapist rates each on a 0–3 scale.

*Circle numbers that approximately indicate the level at which the factors were addressed as follows:*

1 The factor was not addressed.
2 Little evidence of considering these factors.
3 These factors noted but not linked to presenting problems.
4 All relevant factors noted and clearly linked to presenting problems.

---

**Box 2.3**

|  | Biological | Psychological | Social | Cultural | Spiritual |
|---|---|---|---|---|---|
| **Predisposing** | 0 1 2 3 | 0 1 2 3 | 0 1 2 3 | 0 1 2 3 | 0 1 2 3 |
| **Precipitating** | 0 1 2 3 | 0 1 2 3 | 0 1 2 3 | 0 1 2 3 | 0 1 2 3 |
| **Perpetuating** | 0 1 2 3 | 0 1 2 3 | 0 1 2 3 | 0 1 2 3 | 0 1 2 3 |
| **Protective** | 0 1 2 3 | 0 1 2 3 | 0 1 2 3 | 0 1 2 3 | 0 1 2 3 |

© NSW Ministry of Health, 2012

## Step 3. Readiness to change

In Step 3 the therapist makes a judgement about the young person's readiness to change. Clinical Tool 2.4 Stages of change may help the therapist decide if the young person is ready for a therapeutic input, such as Interpersonal Psychotherapy or if some other intervention such as motivational interviewing, supportive counselling, or psychoeducation would be more appropriate in order to move the client to a point where a therapeutic intervention would be indicated.

## Step 4. Provisional formulation

In Step 4 the therapist attempts to integrate the outcome of psychological assessment into a statement that relates the client's presenting problems with his or her life history and current experiences.

A rating of 3 indicates a well-integrated hypothesis that links presenting problems with the four Ps and within the five domains in an accessible statement that is sensitive to age, stage of development, values, and culture. For a rating of 3, this statement will be delivered in a way that is meaningful to the client, provides a new level of understanding, and instils a sense of hope of symptom resolution and increased enjoyment of life. A rating of 2 indicates a hypothesis that provides a plausible but incomplete explanation of the client's presenting problems but nevertheless offers some confidence that things might improve. A rating of 1 would indicate a poorly integrated explanation of the young person's presenting problems that conveys little reason for hope. A rating of 0 would indicate the formulation was not presented at all.

Clinical Tool 2.5 integrates the four steps of case formulation. This framework may also be useful within a supervision or peer supervision context in which supervisors can use the framework to encourage systematic analysis and

---

**Box 2.4**

3   Well-integrated hypothesis that links the presenting problems with the five domains of the holistic assessment and presents a clear and accurate explanation of the client's presenting problems, noting client's readiness to change. The formulation also provides an evidence-based pathway to symptom improvement that is believable to the young person.
2   An hypothesis that provides a believable but incomplete explanation of the client's presenting problems but nevertheless offers some hope of symptom improvement.
1   A poorly integrated explanation of the presenting problems that offers the client little understanding of symptoms and little reason to hope for symptom improvement.
0   The formulation was not presented.

© NSW Ministry of Health, 2012

reflection about assessment and formulation in their supervisees. Assessment and case formulation are core competencies in the therapeutic process; although many component skills can be taught in pre-service training, supervision can be a strategic step to moving from knowledge about assessment and formulation to the ability to conduct these processes in a way that increases understanding and hope in clients and ensures a science-informed therapeutic direction.

## Summary

There are two central purposes of assessment and formulation. The first is to help the young person and, if appropriate, their family, to make better sense of their current life experience and, with this increased understanding, develop some hope for a brighter future. The second purpose is to shape future intervention. The assessment and formulation will inform decisions about whether therapy is indicated and, if so, which intervention will be most appropriate and by whom it will be delivered. In other words, assessment and formulation will influence both client and therapist.

Once the holistic assessment has been completed and the formulation presented, the therapist will be in a position to decide if IPT-A will be the best-fit intervention for the young person, in which case therapy could proceed to the Initial Phase of IPT-A. The following two chapters focus on Attachment in young people (Chapter 3) and Clinical Techniques (Chapter 4). These provide material that will facilitate the clinical work to be negotiated in the Initial Phase (Chapter 5), the Middle Phase (Chapters 6–10), and the Consolidation Phase (Chapters 11 and 12).

## Notes

1 The use of the term "holistic" acknowledges that assessment is best informed by the belief that the parts of something are intimately interconnected and explicable only by reference to the whole, by the treatment of the whole person, taking into account multiple factors rather than just the symptoms.
2 We acknowledge the work of two of our colleagues, Tim Golding and Anthony Critchley, who developed this two-dimensional model.
3 Standard manuals such as DSM-5 (APA, 2013) and ICD-11-CR (WHO, in press) provide relevant information about psychiatric symptoms and syndromes, but it is of significance that, as these manuals were written to relate primarily to the adult population, some young people suffer considerable impairment and distress without actually reaching diagnostic criteria.
4 Giving Millie the strong message the abuse was not her fault is central to this intervention. However, words alone may not be enough. The abuse that occurred when Millie was 10 must be seen within the context of her whole life experience, including her belief set and the interpersonal consequences of keeping this event to herself for the past six years. Guilt and its psychosocial sequalae following sexual abuse (for example, shattered self-esteem, powerlessness, mistrust of others, fear of intimacy) usually do not remit by being told "it wasn't your fault" or "there's no need to feel guilty". Millie has had six years to process this event and most likely has spent countless hours

reliving it and trying to make sense of it. Telling her it wasn't her fault may not be enough. Understanding how Millie interprets the abuse in its holistic context will assist the therapist to lead Millie to a point where *she* reaches the conclusion that it was not her fault, at which point she may be in a position to begin rebuilding her sense of self and, integrally related to this, her interpersonal world.

## References

Anyan, F. & Hjemdal, O. (2016). Adolescent stress and symptoms of anxiety and depression: Resilience explains and differentiates the relationships. *Journal of Affective Disorders, 203*, 213–220.

APA. (2004). *Diagnostic and statistical manual of mental disorders: Fourth edition text revision*. Arlington VA: American Psychiatric Association.

APA. (2013). *Diagnostic and statistical manual for mental disorders: Fifth edition*. Washington, DC: American Psychiatric Association.

Bashir, M. (2000). Immigrant and refugee young people: Challenges in mental mealth. In M. Bashir, D. Bennett, & (Eds), *Deeper Dimensions - Culture, Youth and Mental Health*. Sydney: Transcultural Mental Health Centre.

Bowlby, J. (1988). *A secure base*. London: Routledge.

Cloninger, C., Svrakic, D. & Przybeck, T. (2006). Can personality assessment predict future depression? A twelve month follow-up of 631 subjects. *Journal of Affective Disorders, 92(1)*, 35–44.

Collishaw, S., Hammerton, D., Mahedy, L., Sellers, R., Owen, L., et al. (2016). Mental health resilience in the adolescent offspring of parents with depression: A prospective longitudinal study. *The Lancet, 3(1)*, 49–57.

d'Souza, R. (2002). Do patients expect psychiatrists to be interested in spiritual issues? *Australasian Psychiatry, 10(1)*, 44–47.

Eels, T. (1997). Psychotherapy case formulation: History and current status. In T. Eels, *Handbook of psychotherapy case formulation* (pp. 1–25). NY: Guildford Press.

Engel, G. (1977). The need for a new medical model: A challenge for biomedicine. *Science, 196*, 129–136.

Frydenberg, E. & Lewis, R. (2012). *Adolcescent coping scale—Second edition*. Camberwell, Vic: ACER.

Goldstein, S. (2010). The exploration of spirituality and identity status in *adolescence*. *Currents: New Scholarships in the Human Services, 9(1)*, 1–22.

Grotberg, E. (1996). The International Resilience Project: Findings from the research and the effectiveness of interventions. In B. Bain, *Psychology and Education in the 21st Century: Proceedings from the 54th Annual Convention of the International Council of Psychologists* (pp. 118–128). Edmonton: IC Press.

Hawton, K., Rodham, K. & Evans, E. (2006). *By their own hand: Deliberate self-harm and suicidal ideas in adolescents*. London: Jessica Kingsley.

Hillin, A. and McAlpine R. (2005). *Interpersonal psychotherapy for adolescents: Workshop handouts*. Sydney, Australia. Hillin and McAlpine.

Kessler, R., & Bromet, J. (2013). The epidemiology of depression across cultures. *Annual Review of Public Health, 34*, 119–138.

Kitano, H. (1989). A model for counselling Asian Americans. In P. Pedersen, J. Draguns, W. Lonner, J. Trimble, & (Eds), *Counselling across cultures (3rd edition)*. Honolulu: University of Hawaii Press.

Klimidas, S. & Minas, I. (1995). Migration, culture and mental health in young children and adolescents. In C. Guerra, R. White, & (Eds), *Ethnic minority youth in Australia: Challenging the myths* (pp. 85–99). Hobart, Aust: National Clearinghouse of Youth Studies.

Koenig, H. (2009). Research on religion, spirituality and mental health: A review. *The Canadian Journal of Psychiatry, 54*(5), 283–291.

Lawrence, D., Johnson, S., Hafekost, J., Boterhoven De Haan, K., Sawyer, M., Ainley, J. & Zubrick, S. (2015). *The Mental Health of Children and Adolescents. Report on the second Australian Child and Adolescent Survey of Mental Health and Wellbeing.* Department of Health, Canberra.

MacCulloch, A. (2004). Substance-related disorders in persons with mental retardation. *Journal of Substance Use, 9*(5), 253–254.

Manson, S. (1995). Culture and major depression: Current challenges in the diagnosis of mood disorders, *Psychiatric Clinics, 1*(1), 487–501.

Marsella, A. (2001). Cultural competence in assessing adolescents with mental health problems. *Developing cultural competence.* Sydney, Australia: Transcultural Mental Health Service.

Maston, A. (2008). Ordinary magic: Lessons from research on resilience in human development. *Education Canada, 49*(3), 28–32.

Matsumoto, D. (1996). *Culture and psychology.* Pacific Grove, CA: Thompson Brooks/Cole.

McAlpine, R. (1999). *Depression, anxiety and coping behaviours as correlates of stress: A study of senior secondary students.* Doctoral dissertation. Newcastle University, NSW, Australia.

Minas, H., & Lewis, M. (2017). *Mental health in Asia and the Pacific: historical and cultural perspectives.* New York: Springer.

National Institute for Health and Care Excellence (NICE). (2019). *Depression in children and young people: identification and management. NICE Guideline (NG134),* Published date 25 June 2019, www.nice.org.uk/guidance/ng134.

Nock, M. & Favazza, A. (2009). Nonsuicidal self-injury: Definition and classification. In M. Nock, *Understanding Nonsuicidal Self-Injury: Origins, Assessment and Treatment.* Washington: American Psychological Association.

Norcross, J. & Goldfield, M. (2005). *Handbook of psychotherapy integration, Second Edition.* NY: Oxford University Press.

NSW Ministry of Health, 2012, *NSW School-Link DVD Training Program,* Prod. A. Hillin & R. McAlpine. DVD. North Sydney: NSW Ministry of Health.

Page, A. & McLean, N. (2008). Toward science-informed supervision of clinical formulation: a training model and supervision method. *Australian Psychologist, 43,* 88–95.

Prochaska, J. & DiClemente, C. (1982). *Trans-theoretical therapy—toward a more integrative model of change. Psychotherapy: Theory, Research and Practice, 19*(3), 276–288.

Proctor, E. (2011). *The spiritual and religious beliefs of adolescents. Royal College of Psychiatrists,* Monograph. Available at https://www.rcpsych.ac.uk/docs/default-source/members/sigs/spirituality-spsig/elizabeth-procter-the-spiritual-and-religious-beliefs-of-adolescents-x.pdf?sfvrsn=211cd18a_2.

Rutter, M. (2008). Developing concepts in developmental psychopathology. In J. Hudziak, *Developmental Psychopathology and Wellness: Genetic and Envoronmental Influences* (pp. 3–22). Washington DC: American Psychiatric Publishing.

Salzman, M. (2018). *A psychology of culture.* New York: Springer.

Sowislo, J. & Orth, U. (2012). Does low self-esteem predict depression and anxiety? A meta-analysis of longitudinal studies. *Psychological Bulletin, 139(1)*, 213–240.

Stahl, S. (2011). *The prescriber's guide: Stahl's essential psychopharmacology, fourth edition.* New York: Cambridge University Press.

Stuart, S. & Robertson, M. (2012). *Interpersonal psychotherapy: A clinician's guide.* London: Arnold.

Tharper, A., Collinshaw, S., Pine, D. & Tharpar, A. K. (2012) Depression in adolescence. *Lancet, 379* (9820), 1056–1067.

Tonge, B., Gordon, M. & Melvin, G. (2009). Treating depression in the developmentally disabled: Intellectual disability and parvasive developmental disorders. In J. Rey, & B. Birmaher, *Treating child and adolescent depression* (pp. 310–320). London: Wolters Kluwer.

Torikka, A. (2017). *Depression and substance use in middle adolescence.* Academic Dissertation. University of Tampere, Faculty of Medicine and Life Sciences, Finland.

Vassoler, F., Byrnes, E. & Pierce, R. (2014). The impact of exposure to addictive drugs on future generations: Physiological and behavioural effects. *Neuropharmacology, 76*, 42–47.

World Health Organisation. (2010). *International classification of diseases, tenth revision, clinical modification (ICD-10-CM).* London: Centers for Disease Control and Prevention.

World Health Organisation. (In press). *International classification of diseases, eleventh revision, (ICD-11).* London: Centers for Disease Control and Prevention.

Zubrick, S. (2014). *School attendance: Equities and inequities in growth trajectories of academic performance.* The University of Western Australia Research Conference.

# 3 Attachment in young people

| Contents | |
|---|---|
| Introduction | 49 |
| Attachment theory | 50 |
| Attachment in adolescence | 51 |
| The three-dimensional model of attachment | 52 |
| The four-dimensional model of attachment | 53 |
| Assessment of attachment styles | 55 |
|     *The client's descriptions of past and current relationships* | 56 |
|     *The quality of the client's narrative* | 60 |
|     *The nature of the therapist-client relationship* | 62 |
| Clinical implications | 66 |
| Summary | 71 |
| References | 72 |

## Introduction

> *Attachment difficulties lie at the heart of many forms of mental disorder and substance use* (Flores, 2004), and at *the heart of the entire psychotherapeutic enterprise* (Fonagy, 2000).

Understanding attachment behaviour is an integral part of IPT-A. The principal reason for this is that much of the distress experienced by adolescents is related to their ineffective attempts to have their attachment needs met. Psychological problems occur and interpersonal relationships break down when a client's needs for attachment are not adequately met. In some other modalities, a therapeutic goal may be to change the young person's attachment style. In contrast, as IPT-A is a time-limited intervention, a key goal is to help clients develop interpersonal skills that will assist them to meet their attachment needs more effectively. Changes in the attachment behaviours of some clients may occur as a consequence (Gunlicks-Stoessel et al., 2018; Spence et al., 2016), but these changes are not an explicit goal of IPT-A.

The attachment style of a young person is a construct that helps clinicians understand the way their clients see and relate to the world. Attachment is a constellation of preferred ways clients have of interacting with their world. It is this constellation that clinicians are attempting to understand in assessment of the attachment process. And because assessment of this process is a work in progress during therapy, assumptions about attachment style should remain hypotheses that are continually shaped as new evidence emerges.

## Attachment theory

Attachment theory is based on the premise that humans have an instinctual motivation to form relationships with other humans. This drive is biologically grounded, and ethological research has demonstrated that the drive to form relationships is necessary to the survival of the individual and the species. Historically, the attachment of a dependent child to the mother, for example, ensured proximity to the mother and thus aided the offspring's biological survival by providing sustenance and protection from predators.

The continued presence of a secure attachment figure helps the child explore the physical environment, make peer contacts, achieve group membership, and eventually achieve independence. Humans function at their best when their attachment needs are met and develop problems, including psychological symptoms, when these needs are compromised.

Bowlby (1988) described attachment in the following way:

> "To say that a child (or older person) is attached to, or has attachment to, someone means that he is strongly disposed to seek proximity to and contact with that individual and to do so especially in certain specified conditions. This disposition to behave in this way is an attribute of the attached person, a persisting attribute that changes slowly over time and which is unaffected by the situation of the moment." (p. 28)

Bowlby described the behaviour that arises from this attribute as

> "[A]ny form of behaviour that results in a person attaining or maintaining proximity to some other clearly defined individual who is conceived as better able to cope with the world. It is most obvious whenever the person is frightened, fatigued or sick, and is assuaged by comforting and care giving. At other times the behaviour is less in evidence. Nevertheless, for a person to know that an attachment figure is available and responsive gives him a strong and pervasive feeling of security and so encourages him to value and continue the relationship." (p. 27)

Attachment organises the behaviour of interpersonal relationships and forms the basis for a relatively enduring pattern of the way people understand and interact with others. Attachment behaviour, while always present, is most noticeable in interactions in which individuals find their security threatened—usually when they are stressed, tired, or unwell—and drives the person to seek care.

Bowlby (1969) viewed the first five years of life as crucial in the development of attachment relationships, which are internalised as part of the child's sense of self in relation to others. This leads to the development of a "working model" of relationships, a template of the nature of relationships, based on actual relationship experiences during these formative years. This template informs expectations of what future relationships will be like. For example, a child who is born into a family in which the parents are able to care for and meet the physical and emotional needs of the child will develop a working model that includes others who are providers of love and care when care is needed. For them, the world is perceived as safe and good. The child's experiences of relationships will be characterised by their needs being met, and expectations of subsequent relationships will be reflective of that. This early template may not always be confirmed by subsequent relationships, but these early experiences can never be taken away from the child and will remain active in contributing to the current "working model".

On the other hand, a child who is born into a family that is unable to provide the love and care necessary to adequately meet the physical and emotional needs of him or her will develop a model that includes others who are not providers of love and care when care is needed. This child will carry into subsequent relationships expectations reflective of these experiences. All new experiences of relationships will be viewed by this child within a context of the amalgam of previous experiences. It would hardly be surprising for this child to approach new relationships with less optimism and trust than the child from the first family.

The objective accuracy of the expectations of both children in the examples above is far less important than their subjective experiences. It is these subjective experiences and the subsequent expectations derived from them that give shape to the way in which children view their world.

The working model of relationships allows both of these types of individuals to function interpersonally because it provides them with a template that they can use to predict how others will behave in relation to them. Children tend to carry this model with them into adolescence and adulthood. The working model of relationships is generally consistent both within and across relationships and coalesces to form a characteristic attachment style.

## Attachment in adolescence

Adolescence poses some specific difficulties related to understanding attachment. Erikson (1950) characterised adolescence as the phase of the human life cycle during which the individual must establish a sense of personal identity and avoid the dangers of role diffusion and identity confusion. In many Western cultures, the movement from early adolescence through middle to late adolescence is a period characterised by a movement towards independence and a firmer identity during which time the family plays less of a role as the primary source of nurture and belonging and during which the peer group takes up much of this role. "The adolescent individuation process helps establish a personal, social and sexual identity. It requires turning away from the parents and—because of still insufficient autonomy—a temporary turning toward the peer group culture" (Muus, 1982, p. 100). This process involves the young person disconnecting from the adult world in which they have been a child, connecting in a different manner with their peer group, before they can reconnect with the adult world as an adult.

During this disconnection and reconnection, the adolescent's body undergoes transformation. Associated hormonal changes contribute to a lability of affective experience: young adolescents begin to experience unfamiliar feelings that, for some, swing unpredictably. The adolescent's family, the group who previously provided nurture, acceptance, and belonging, suddenly seems unable to continue to meet those needs in the way its members had done. The young person seeks the peer group to fulfil these roles.

During the early years of life, the young child asked the question "is the world a good place, a bad place, or am I not sure"? The young adolescent finds himself or herself asking the same questions as exploration of the world begins again. But it's not exactly the same as it was a decade ago. The question about the world has already been answered once. This time around there's an expectation about how things will turn out, and this expectation is largely based on attachment experiences.

## The three-dimensional model of attachment

Bowlby (1969) and Ainsworth et al. (1978) described three basic styles of attachment: (1) secure, (2) anxious avoidant, and (3) anxious ambivalent. Securely attached individuals base their relationships on working models that are healthy and flexible. The classic securely attached young person generally trusts that others will be available when needed. They are, on the whole, able to explore the world and seek out new relationships with a sense of security. These young people generally manifest behaviours characteristic of good mental health. They are able to have their needs for belonging, security, and nurture effectively met by a supportive social network. The secure base that was developed in the first phase of their life is tested and not found wanting. These young people are able to ask for care from others when they need it and likewise are able to provide care to others when asked to do so.

Young people with anxious avoidant attachment often have had early life experiences in which care was inadequate. These young people develop working models of relationships in which care will never be sufficient, if it is provided at all. They believe their attachment needs will not be met. Due to those early life experiences, these young people approach adolescence with suspicion of the motives of others. They often demonstrate such behaviour as compulsive self-reliance, often forming only superficial relationships or avoiding closeness altogether. As a result, their social support networks tend to be insubstantial or, at best, transitory, and they have little in the way of psychosocial backup when things go wrong.

Young people with anxious ambivalent attachment styles are constantly preoccupied with ensuring that their attachment needs are being met. They bring from their childhood an uncertainty about whether their attachment needs will be met; as a result, during their adolescence, they constantly test others, particularly those who show some signs of caring, to see if they will be consistent with the care they have shown. However, this constant reassurance-seeking behaviour eventually fatigues even the most assiduous care provider, often resulting in rejection, or perceived rejection, compelling further reassurance-seeking behaviour, and so the cycle continues.

In contrast to avoidant young people, those with ambivalent attachment styles are able to form intimate relationships, but they tend to be unstable and are vulnerable to conflicts or losses that threaten a fragile attachment. These young people are usually so preoccupied with obtaining sufficient care within their relationships that they lack capacity to provide consistent care for others. As a result, they rarely develop mutually supportive relationships and so their social support network is often insubstantial.

(Main and Solomon (1986) identified a fourth variant of attachment, disorganised attachment, usually predicated by childhood traumatic events. This attachment is usually characterised by intrusive traumatic memories, dissociation, affect dysregulation, externalising behaviours, inability to tolerate closeness, and often severe depression. Young people with this attachment variant are usually not suitable candidates for IPT-A, at least until unresolved trauma has been sufficiently addressed.)

## The four-dimensional model of attachment

Bartholomew and Horowitz (1991) developed a four-dimensional model of attachment styles based on inner working models of the self and others. (See Figure 3.1.) Expanding on Bowlby and Ainsworth's model, they defined four prototypic attachment patterns using combinations of a person's self-image (positive or negative) and their image of others (positive or negative). Bartholomew and Horowitz retained the Secure dimension, the top left quadrant, identifying individuals in this quadrant as having a strong sense of self and a belief that others will be available for comfort, care, and assistance when they need them. The second quadrant of this model identifies individuals who have an insubstantial sense of self and need others to continually validate their existence. This quadrant is now labelled Preoccupied as these individuals seem to be preoccupied with having their fragile sense of self propped up by others. Bowlby and Ainsworth's descriptor of this quadrant, Ambivalent, also remains appropriate, as these individuals tend to polarise others as those who meet their attachment needs (these are often idealised) and those who do not (these tend to be devalued).

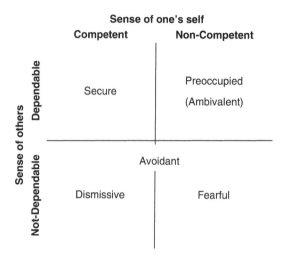

*Figure 3.1* The four-dimensional model of attachment (adapted from Bartholomew and Horowitz, 1991).

Bartholomew and Horowitz differentiated the avoidant attachment style into Avoidant Dismissive and Avoidant Fearful. Young people who endorse a positive model of themselves and who dismiss the importance of closeness to others (lower left quadrant) demonstrate a low level of dependence on others and often a high level of avoidance. They tend to convey a self-reliance and rarely self-refer for therapy as their belief is that they don't need help from others and probably wouldn't trust this help anyway. When these young people do present for therapy, it is usually because they have been referred by others, such as parents or school, or things have become so difficult that they are forced into the unfamiliar territory of not being able to manage alone.

A fearful avoidant style, on the other hand, is characterised by a conscious desire for social contact that is inhibited by fears of the consequences of relationship. These individuals have a negative view of themselves that drives a high level of dependence on others, but their negative view of others leads to a high level of avoidance. These conflicting motives of both wanting and fearing closeness are characteristic of individuals who tend to be insecure, hesitant, vulnerable, and self-conscious and have a low sense of self-worth.

Individuals who would have been identified as having Disorganised attachment according to Main and Solomon's model tend to fit into the lower right quadrant, Avoidant Fearful, of Bartholomew and Horowitz's model.

Young people with insecure attachment styles have two qualitatively different types of attachment-related difficulties. First, their working models of relationships leave them unsure whether others will be able to provide the connections or the care that they crave. Second, because these young people have not developed the social skills required to initiate and maintain mutually supportive relationships, their social networks are typically underdeveloped and unable to provide care and support when these are needed. In other words, young people with insecure attachment styles have neither the internal nor the external psychosocial resources to help them deal with interpersonal stress. Attachment theory would predict that insecurely attached young people are more likely to move from times of stress into symptomatology or mental disorder precisely because of the increased vulnerability associated with this low level of psychosocial resource.

However, securely attached young people can also develop psychiatric symptoms. But due to the nature of secure attachment—the buffering effect of a strong sense of self and a belief that others will be able and available to help in times of need—they may be less likely to progress from stress into symptomatology. Moreover, young people with a secure internal working model of relationships are more likely to effectively seek support when support is needed because their previous experience has established a positive set of expectations of others being available and caring.

## Assessment of attachment styles

Young people develop their relationship models on the basis of their lived experiences. They have no other way of seeing the world. Their relationship models reflect attempts to cope with early stressors and deprivations, which in most cases continue to trouble current and future relationships. Within this context, young people need understanding and compassion rather than labels to help them traverse what, for many, is a difficult journey.

There are at least three reasons why we should exercise care when considering the attachment style of young people. The first is that adolescence is a life stage characterised by changes and flux. It is this transitional nature of adolescence that confers work in progress status on the developmental tasks, including identity formation and, to a degree, attachment style. To be too rigid about the attachment style of the young person may be to ascribe to them attributes that are not a fixed part of their psychological makeup. Young peoples' attachment styles, though strongly influenced by their early life experiences, are not fixed by these experiences. They are continually modified by ongoing life encounters and are especially subject to modification during times of significant change, such as adolescence. And, in something of a parallel process, after the initial encounter with clients, we get to know them in increments during subsequent interactions with them. Our knowledge of their psychological makeup, including their attachment style, matures and develops as we progress through therapy. It would be surprising if our initial perceptions were the same as those we have after weeks of therapy with them.

The second reason care should be exercised in appraising attachment relates to difficulties inherent in any categorical classificatory system. Attachment style is a construct that helps clinicians understand the way clients see and relate to their world. In the four-dimensional model described above, Secure, Preoccupied, Avoidant Dismissive, and Avoidant Fearful are descriptions of archetypes that would rarely, if ever, be seen in their pure form. Perhaps a more useful way of thinking about attachment style would not be categorical but along the lines of a continuum. Descriptions of attachment style would in this case look more like "leaning towards preoccupied", "elements of dismissive style", or "a strong tendency towards a secure attachment". This way of describing attachment allows a more flexible and situational interpretation that more truly reflects young people's lived experiences.

The third reason concerns the nature of the client/clinician relationship. Given that many adolescents are in a perpetual state of partial disconnectedness from the adult world, it may be difficult for the clinician to distinguish this disconnectedness from elements of the client's attachment style. The clinician must ask the question "is this behaviour emblematic of a pervasive and persistent style of relating or is it specific to the relationship between my client and me today"?

Due to these complexities, assessment of adolescent attachment style must be multi-modal rather than relying on just one or two sources of information. In appraising the young person's attachment style, there are three main areas of enquiry:

1  The client's description of past and current relationships.
2  The quality of the client's narrative.
3  The nature of the therapist-client relationship.

## *The client's descriptions of past and current relationships*

The holistic assessment (see Chapter 2) and the Interpersonal Inventory (see Chapter 5) provide extended opportunity to explore the young person's attachment style, particularly when reflecting on the young person's care-seeking behaviours.

The Interpersonal Inventory provides a structure to discuss in detail the nature of the young person's past and current relationships. Although most of the focus in IPT-A is on current relationships, discussion of the young person's childhood can give some indication of whether or not current difficulties are adolescent or attachment specific.

**Britta**, aged 14, was referred by her parents over concerns about falling school grades. In the first two sessions, the therapist identified a longstanding pervasive depressive disorder. The following dialogue occurred during Session 3:

*Therapist:* Can you remember the last time you hurt yourself badly?
*Britta:* What do you mean?
*Therapist:* Well have you ever broken a bone or something?
*Britta:* Yeah, I broke my wrist at netball last winter.
*Therapist:* Broke your wrist? Was either of your folks at the match?
*Britta:* No—they'd never come to see me play. I wouldn't want them there anyway.
*Therapist:* Okay, so how did you get to the hospital?
*Britta:* My coach rang Dad and he came and got me.

*Attachment in young people* 57

| | |
|---|---|
| Therapist: | What did your Dad say when he saw you? |
| Britta: | (smiles) He looked really worried. He ran over to where I was and looked like he'd have a heart attack or something. I should have been more worried about him by the way he looked. |
| Therapist: | So is that like your Dad? I mean do you get the feeling he's pretty concerned about what happens to you? |
| Britta: | I dunno. He's more worried about his precious motor bikes than us. He's always working on his bikes or off riding. He wouldn't even know if we were home or not most of the time. |
| Therapist: | So if he was off riding when you broke your wrist and he got a call that you were hurt, do you think he would have come to get you? |
| Britta: | Yeah. |
| Therapist: | Yeah? What makes you think that? |

In the above interchange we see evidence of parent-child disconnection, but there is also evidence that Britta, despite her negativity about her parents, believes deep down that if she was hurt her father would drop everything to help and care for her. On the basis of this interchange, the therapist might develop an initial hypothesis that Britta's attachment style was more secure that anxious. This hypothesis would be continually tested and modified during the rest of the Initial Phase and also revisited in later stages of treatment.

In contrast, **Tracey**, aged 16, disclosed some of her working model quite differently:

| | |
|---|---|
| Therapist: | Can you remember the last time you hurt yourself badly? |
| Tracey: | What do you mean? |
| Therapist: | Have you ever broken a bone or something? |
| Tracey: | Yeah I broke my wrist at netball last winter. |
| Therapist: | Broke your wrist? Were either of your folks at the match? |
| Tracey: | You've gotta be joking. They don't even know I play netball. |
| Therapist: | So how did you get to the hospital? |
| Tracey: | They called my parents but they were busy. My coach called the ambulance and Jason came in with me. His brother picked me up after they finished and took me home. |
| Therapist: | What did your parents say when you got home? |
| Tracey: | They were cool. Dad drew a picture of a feather on my plaster. |
| Therapist: | A feather? |
| Tracey: | Yeah, it's sort of the logo of his printing company. |
| Therapist: | Do you think your Mum and Dad were worried about your wrist? |
| Tracey: | Oh yeah. They let me have tea in front of telly. |
| Therapist: | Can you think of any other ways your folks show their concern for you? |

Tracey, in contrast to Britta, appears to be less sure about her parents' care for her. The above dialogue suggests there may be some denial and some ambivalence about her parents' capacity or willingness to care for her:

58  Introduction

"You've gotta be joking. They don't even know I play netball", "They were cool. Dad drew a picture of a feather on my plaster" and

"Oh yeah. They let me have tea in front of telly".

Tracey's therapist might develop a tentative hypothesis that Tracey may have some difficulties with attachment. The therapist would continue to explore this by eliciting further real-life examples from Tracey that would illuminate her beliefs about her expectations of care and nurture. Tracey's views about how others regard her may also indicate a belief Tracey holds about herself, that she is unworthy of the care of others.

Obtaining information from the young person about relationships is usually not difficult. Most adolescents quite enjoy talking about their relationships and respond well to open-ended as well as closed-ended questioning. While the primary focus of this enquiry remains on current relationships, past relationships may also provide a rich source of information, especially if the therapist is having difficulty distinguishing characteristics of the attachment style from characteristics of adolescence:

*Therapist:* So, Tracey, since you broke up with Jason, you say most of your friends have deserted you?
*Tracey:* Not most, ALL of them.
*Therapist:* All of them?
*Tracey:* They're all siding with him. No one believes what I say anymore. Even my best friend Jodi takes his side. There was a party last weekend and I didn't even know about it until yesterday.
*Therapist:* (Pause) How did that make you feel Tracey?
*Tracey:* Pissed off at first, but they're not worth it—I couldn't care.
*Therapist:* Your best friend, Jodi, how long have you known her?
*Tracey:* Ever since primary school. We live near each other, we play netball, my mum knows her mum, our brothers play football together, that sort of stuff.
*Therapist:* When you were little kids together, can you remember what it was like? Did you get on okay then?
*Tracey:* Yeah, we've always been best friends.
*Therapist:* Can you remember any times when you've had a disagreement with her, like a major fight or something?
*Tracey:* Yeah like all the time. She can be a real bitch—just like her mum—but I'm kinda stuck with her.
*Therapist:* Can you remember the last time you had a major fight with Jodi? I mean can you remember the details of what it was about, where it was, what you said—that sort of stuff?

In this dialogue, the therapist explores if Tracey's current feelings of rejection and isolation are specific to her current circumstances or are more general. When the earlier relationship with Jodi was explored, Tracey indicated that although she is her best friend, Jodi's central role in life was not to provide a constant source of nurture and comfort. The therapist's last line paved the way for further exploration of a specific incident between Tracey and Jodi. This strategy of exploring interpersonal incidents may be useful not only in highlighting to our clients elements of miscommunication between them and their significant others but also as a strategy to elicit information about the young person's attachment. Tracey responded to the above question in the following way:

*Therapist:* Can you remember the last time you had a major fight with Jodi? I mean can you remember the details of what it was about, where it was, what you said—that sort of stuff?
*Tracey:* Yeah—last week. She wanted to go to see her boyfriend play football and I just wanted to stay home—watch a movie or something.
*Therapist:* What happened?
*Tracey:* We went to the football didn't we.
*Therapist:* So how did the conversation go? What did Jodi say?
*Tracey:* I dunno. She just said, "I want to go and see Troy play footie".
*Therapist:* And what did you say?
*Tracey:* I said you can go if you want—I'm watching a movie.
*Therapist:* How did you feel as you said that, Tracey?
*Tracey:* I knew I'd be the one to give in. It always happens that way—whatever Jodi wants, Jodi gets. She can be such a bitch.
*Therapist:* So what did Jodi say?
*Tracey:* Jodi says, "Well stay here then—I'm going to the footie".
*Therapist:* And?
*Tracey:* I told you she always gets what she wants—we went to the footie.

In the interchange with Jodi, Tracey showed that she was not expecting to have things go her way. This is consistent with her expectations about her parents coming to her aid after being injured at netball and also consistent with her belief about all her friends abandoning her after her breakup with Jason. The therapist would feel a little more confident that Tracey's attachment style had more anxious than secure characteristics. Tracey has shown evidence of having a set of expectations that people are more likely to let her down than to be supportive of her. In addition, this interchange showed the therapist that Tracey may not have well-developed techniques for meeting her attachment needs. Instead of talking to Jodi about not wanting to go to the football, Tracey, in line with her expectations about how things would turn out, acceded to Jodi's wishes without any discussion, adding weight to Tracey's conviction that others will not meet her needs.

In assessing the client's descriptions of their relationships, a range of questions such as the following can be helpful:

- How do things change between you and your parents when you're hurt or sad?
- How do things change between you and your parents when they are angry?

- Can you think of how your parents reacted one time when you were hurt or upset?
- How are things different between you and your parents now compared with when you were younger?
- How do you get on with your brothers and sisters?
- When you were younger, how did you go about asking for help?
- How do you ask for help now?
- How is it different with your friends compared with you parents?
- If you were really hurt or upset, who would you ask for help?
- Tell me a story about....

Questions such as these help the therapist gain an understanding of the "Others" dimension in the Bartholomew and Horowitz model, specifically whether the young person has a positive or negative sense of the helpfulness, reliability, and availability of others.

To explore the "Self" dimension in this model, the therapist may ascertain the way the young person views his or her traits, beliefs, values, and purpose in the world. A salient characteristic of self is the client's self-worth. A consideration of Lerner's (2005) 6 Cs, for example, from Positive Youth Development (competence, confidence, character, connectedness, compassion, and contribution) will help the therapist gauge characteristics of the client's self and her attitude towards herself. High self-worth will register on the high end of Bartholomew and Horowitz's Sense of self dimension, (Figure 3.1), whereas young people with feelings worthlessness will typically fall at the low end. It is these low feelings of self-worth that characterise Preoccupied and Fearful-Avoidant young people.

### The quality of the client's narrative

In addition to clients' descriptions of their relationships and detailed accounts of interpersonal incidents, the therapist can glean significant information about the nature of the clients' attachment style by examining the quality of their narratives. Important inferences can be made about the young persons' attachment style based on the way they tell their stories. Young people who have secure attachment styles usually have a rich history of relationships on which they are able to draw when relating stories about their present circumstances. On the contrary, young people who have a history of preoccupied or avoidant relationship patterns are usually only loosely connected to the world of others. Young people with a preoccupied style are usually so engrossed with having their own attachment needs met that they seem unable to relate stories about their world that connect well with the world of others. For young people with avoidant attachment styles, others have not figured substantially in the way they construct their world, and, as a consequence, they haven't paid much attention to the world of others.

Stuart and Robertson (2012) have proposed that securely attached individuals are generally able to describe others in three dimensional terms. They are able to describe others realistically, with positive as well as negative characteristics, and the shades of grey in between. Individuals with a preoccupied attachment style, on the other hand, often describe others in two dimensional terms. They are so preoccupied with having their attachment needs met that they are hesitant to be critical of others who might provide them with care. Since they may have already decided that some people will not or cannot meet their attachment needs, these people are devalued. These young people tend to either idealise or devalue the others in their lives—there is very little middle ground—and the decision as to whether the other is idealised or devalued may depend on how the young person is seeing them at that moment. Young people with preoccupied attachment tend not to see others as complete people—they only see the good and the bad parts. Tracey, for example, stated her parents wouldn't have even known she was playing netball and were too busy to take her to the hospital when she was hurt. She also reported, however, that they were so worried about her injury that they "let me have tea in front of telly".

If young people with secure attachment styles tend to describe others in three-dimensional terms, and individuals whose attachment style tends towards preoccupied talk about others in their lives in two-dimensional terms, then young people with the avoidant attachment styles usually describe others in one-dimensional terms. Their descriptions contain little detail. Therapists may find it difficult to develop hypotheses about the nature of these clients' relationships because they offer no firm material on which to form clinical opinion. This emptiness is a clear reflection of the interpersonal world of these young people in which relationships carry much less meaning than they do for others.

**Jeff**, aged 16, has been referred to the school psychologist by a teacher who has become concerned about falling grades. Jeff is a lad of above average ability in his last year of secondary school. Until recently Jeff has been a quiet and conscientious student who did well in all subjects and excelled in computer studies. Lately his marks have deteriorated, and his teachers are concerned he may have burned himself out.

The school psychologist suspects Jeff may be experiencing a depressive episode and is in the process of exploring whether Jeff would be a suitable candidate for IPT-A. During the initial sessions, the school psychologist formed a tentative hypothesis that Jeff's attachment style could best be described as avoidant. The following segment from the Interpersonal Inventory illustrates how the quality of the Jeff's narrative helped the school psychologist form this opinion.

*Therapist:* *Jeff last week we talked about how things have been going for you lately at school and at home. This week I'd like us to talk about your relationships with some of the important people in your life. Is that okay?*

*Jeff:* Okay.
*Therapist:* So first off, (referring to the Closeness Circles—see Chapter 5—constructed in a previous session) let's talk about some of the people in your inner circle, say some of the people you spend a fair bit of time with.
*Jeff:* I don't know. (Pause). Probably some of my friends ... maybe my family.
*Therapist:* Okay—friends and family—so pick someone you want to begin with. Someone we'll talk about first.
*Jeff:* (Pause.) Well we could start with Alex if you want.
*Therapist:* Alex? A friend?
*Jeff:* Yeah, she's a friend.
*Therapist:* Is she a special friend? Like a girlfriend?
*Jeff:* No, not really.
*Therapist:* Okay.... Tell me a bit about Alex.
*Jeff:* Well she's kinda nice—I don't know, she's just kinda nice—that's all.
*Therapist:* What is it you like about her?
*Jeff:* I don't know—she's a good person. We get on pretty well.
*Therapist:* What sort of things do you do together?
*Jeff:* Oh, not much. (Pause).

In this segment Jeff was unable to provide much meaningful information about Alex. Not only is the information Jeff provided of poor quality, it also appears that he has an inability to convey his inner experiences and perceptions to others. These responses are fairly typical of the responses one would expect from a young person with avoidant attachment. However, the therapist would investigate whether his responses were indicative of Jeff's working model of relationships rather than reflective of the dynamic between a depressed adolescent and an adult therapist. The therapist would explore other relationships Jeff has, enquiring about basic details, expectations in relationships, whether relationships are satisfying to Jeff, and changes Jeff would like to see in his relationships. The therapist would use this information to inform the developing hypothesis about Jeff's attachment style. Jeff's sense of self would also be explored to determine whether his attachment was Avoidant Dismissive (strong sense of self) or Avoidant Fearful (fragile sense of self).

### *The nature of the therapist-client relationship*

A major difference between IPT-A and more psychoanalytically oriented therapies is seen clearly in the manner in which these approaches deal with the transference relationship. In psychodynamic therapies, the transference relationship is directly addressed by the therapist during treatment. Transference is an unconscious process and therefore occurs outside the awareness of the client. In the transference relationship, early patterns of interpersonal relatedness are repeated in the relationship with the therapist and the manifestations of these patterns are examined in detail. For example, the therapist would assume that many of the young person's feelings towards him or her would be re-enactments of feelings associated with early significant relationships in the client's life. The therapist would focus on these feelings "under the microscope of therapy" to explore the hidden forces of the client's unconscious world that drive current affect, cognitions, and interpersonal behaviours.

IPT-A is largely based on Bowlby's model of attachment. Bowlby argued his working model of relationships was based on real experiences and reflects an accurate appraisal of an individual's previous relationships. IPT-A recognises that unconscious processes may strongly influence an individual's interpersonal world but focuses on those elements that are accessible to the young person. The young person's working model of interpersonal relationships is imposed onto the therapist as much as onto any other relationship. However, a therapist using IPT-A, in contrast to a therapist using a psychodynamic approach, does not utilise the transference relationship to analyse and understand the transferential processes or dysfunctional working models of relationships. In IPT-A, the therapist can help the young person better understand and subsequently change problematic aspects of his or her relationship behaviour without the need to interpret the underlying unconscious determinants. In this way, the focus of IPT-A is on symptom relief and improvements in interpersonal functioning rather than on intrapsychic insight.

However, despite not directly utilising the transference in therapy, consideration of the client/therapist relationship remains an essential tool for increasing the therapist's understanding of the client's interpersonal world. The relationship between the client and the therapist does not develop within a vacuum but parallels the attachment and communication style used by the young person outside therapy, for example, with family and friends. This relationship, therefore, provides fundamental information about the young person's attachment style and communication style. The client/therapist relationship is subject to the same working model of attachment as other relationships. It informs the therapist about potential problems that may arise in therapy, about the potential for a successful therapeutic outcome, and about specific relationship difficulties the young person may be having outside the therapy.

For example, in the case of Jeff (above), the therapist had to work fairly hard to get any response at all. While the content and quality of Jeff's narrative presents information relevant to the assessment of attachment, the therapist's experience of this client provides a different type of information. What was the therapist's *experience* of Jeff? What responses in the therapist were elicited by this client? What did these elicited responses tell the therapist about Jeff's attachment style? Did the therapist, by his or her reaction to Jeff, gain any insight into problems Jeff might be having in other relationships in his life?

To assist clinicians in the process of using the client/therapist relationship as a source of information about the client's attachment style, McAlpine and Hillin (2007) have developed the Clinician's Response Scale (CRS). Drawing on a technique utilised by Sheard et al. (2000), the CRS uses therapists' responses to their clients as significant clinical data. The CRS consists of a series of responses therapists may have to their clients and uses these responses to draw inferences about the client's attachment style. Responses contained in the CRS were gleaned from more than 220 clinicians who work with adolescent clients. These clinicians were first presented with a description of a securely attached adolescent, derived from the literature, and asked to reflect on what responses this young person would elicit in them. This process was then repeated with descriptions of preoccupied and avoidant adolescents. The responses were analysed, repeat items culled, and then cluster analyses performed to derive three scales, Secure, Preoccupied, and Avoidant, of five items each. These fifteen items were then randomly placed throughout the scale. The therapist completes the scale after an early session with the client and rates his or her response to each item on the Likert scale described in Clinical Tool 3.1.

In developing this tool, the authors found from multiple trials with clinicians who were working with adolescent clients that

Items 3, 4, 8, 9, and 10 are responses likely to be elicited by a securely attached young person.

Items 1, 7, 11, 12, and 13 are responses likely to be elicited by a young person whose attachment style is preoccupied.

Items 2, 5, 6, 14, and 15 are responses likely to be elicited by an avoidant client.

---

**Clinical Tool 3.1    The Clinicians Response Scale (research edition)**

| # | Item | Scale |
|---|------|-------|
| 1 | In today's session I feel I have been walking on eggshells | 0 1 2 3 |
| 2 | This person doesn't need me—they don't need anyone | 0 1 2 3 |
| 3 | This client is going to be easy to help | 0 1 2 3 |
| 4 | I feel optimistic about the outcome of this intervention | 0 1 2 3 |
| 5 | No one can help this client | 0 1 2 3 |
| 6 | I just couldn't get through to this client | 0 1 2 3 |
| 7 | I feel if I push too hard, this client will fall over | 0 1 2 3 |
| 8 | This client took me in to their confidence | 0 1 2 3 |
| 9 | I felt trusted by this client | 0 1 2 3 |
| 10 | I felt I could make a difference with this client | 0 1 2 3 |
| 11 | I feel drained and used up | 0 1 2 3 |
| 12 | I did so much caring that I now need care | 0 1 2 3 |
| 13 | I felt engulfed by this client but suspicious it was fake | 0 1 2 3 |
| 14 | After today's session, I felt I had done a lot of work for no result | 0 1 2 3 |
| 15 | I feel this client is never going to trust me | 0 1 2 3 |

Therapists rate each item on the 4-point Likert-type scale:
   0 = I didn't notice this response at all
   1 = I noticed this response, but it was weak
   2 = This response was moderate
   3 = This response was strong

Attachment in young people 65

Therapists sum items for each attachment style, as indicated above.
Secure attachment comprises scores obtained in items 3 + 4 + 8 + 9 + 10.
Preoccupied attachment comprises items 1 + 7 + 11 + 12 + 13.
Avoidant attachment comprises items 2 + 5 + 6 + 14 + 15.

The highest total score represents the therapist's response to the client's attachment-related behaviours apparent in that session.

The CRS for Tracey, the young woman we met previously, appears in Figure 3.2.

The therapist's response to Tracey is indicative of avoidant attachment, and this is supported by the therapist's observation that Tracey was somewhat difficult to engage. To determine if Tracey's avoidant attachment is Dismissive or Fearful, the therapist would assess Tracey's sense of self. If sense of self was assessed as positive, this would be indicative of an Avoidant Dismissive style and if negative, of Avoidant Fearful.

As attachment styles are generally consistent across relationships, there is a good chance that the attachment behaviour manifested by Tracey on this occasion would be her preferred attachment style in other circumstances with other people at this time of her life.

| 1. | In today's session, I feel I have been walking on eggshells | 0 **(1)** 2 3 |
| 2. | This person doesn't need me – they don't need anyone | 0 **(1)** 2 3 |
| 3. | This client is going to be easy to help | **(0)** 1 2 3 |
| 4. | I feel optimistic about the outcome of this intervention | 0 **(1)** 2 3 |
| 5. | No one can help this client | 0 1 **(2)** 3 |
| 6. | I just couldn't get through to this client | 0 1 **(2)** 3 |
| 7. | I feel if I push too hard, this client will fall over | 0 1 **(2)** 3 |
| 8. | This client took me into his confidence | 0 **(1)** 2 3 |
| 9. | I felt trusted by this client | 0 **(1)** 2 3 |
| 10. | I felt I could make a difference with this client | 0 **(1)** 2 3 |
| 11. | I feel drained and used up | 0 1 **(2)** 3 |
| 12. | I did so much caring that I now need care | 0 **(1)** 2 3 |
| 13. | I felt engulfed by this client, but suspicious it was fake | **(0)** 1 2 3 |
| 14. | After today's session, I felt I had done a lot of work for no result | 0 1 2 **(3)** |
| 15. | I feel this client is never going to trust me | 0 1 **(2)** 3 |

0= I didn't notice this response at all   1= I noticed this response but it was weak
2= This response was moderate   3= This response was strong

| Secure attachment: | Items 3,4,8,9, and 10: | 0+1+1+1+1 | Total: 4 |
| Preoccupied: | Items 1,7,11,12, and 13 | 1+2+2+1+0 | Total: 6 |
| Avoidant: | Items 2,5,6,14, and 15 | 1+2+2+3+2 | Total:10 |

*Figure 3.2* Clinicians Response Scale: Tracey.

Importantly, this scale is only one of the many pieces of information the therapist uses to develop hypotheses about the young person's attachment style. Within this context, the outcome of this scale should not be given undue weight.

## Clinical implications

Understanding the young person's attachment will influence therapy in a number of ways:

First, the therapist will hold two general clinical questions in his or her mind during the intervention:

(1) How will the young person's attachment style influence the way this client relates to me? For example, what will he/she expect of therapy? What will he/she expect of me? How difficult will it be for this young person to trust me? How will his/her attachment style influence their commitment to therapy? How difficult will it be for this young person to complete interpersonal homework?
(2) How will the young person's attachment style influence my response to this client? For example, how will this young person's attachment style influence my construction of the therapeutic alliance? What do I need to do to increase the trust this client has in me? What boundaries do I need to set for this client? What will be my expectations regarding speed of recovery? What therapeutic strategies will I employ?

Clinical Tool 3.2 provides some examples of typical behaviours clients with the various attachment styles may exhibit in the therapy room. This tool also provides some suggestions that may be appropriate for therapists to utilise to address these attachment-related behaviours.

The second way attachment style will influence therapy is by the therapist recognising that the young person's symptoms or distress may be related to her ineffective attempts to meet attachment needs. The therapist will need to consider which therapeutic strategies will be best employed to assist this client to meet her attachment needs more effectively.

Third, an understanding of the young person's attachment will assist the therapist to avoid collusion with the client's possibly rigid and habitual relationship patterns. Once the therapist can identify the young person's attachment behaviours, he or she can be vigilant for habitual relationship patterns that appear in the therapy room. The therapist is then in a better position to respond in ways that would not collude with or reinforce these dysfunctional patterns. For example, Mif, an 18-year-old with avoidant attachment, sought to avoid closeness with the therapist by telling engaging and entertaining stories. If the therapist had responded as Mif expected, that is, by being entertained and thus being kept at arm's length, this avoidant behaviour is reinforced. If the therapist, on the other hand, was aware of this avoidant strategy, he or she may respond in a less predictable way, thus interrupting habitual patterns. The therapist, in this case, may respond in the following way:

*Therapist:* *I've really enjoyed listening to your stories, Mif, but I'm beginning to think those stories are getting in the way of dealing with some of your difficult feelings. And those feelings are the reason you're here.*

Fourth, the attachment style of the young person will be related to how well this person will progress in therapy. Due to internal psychological strength and robust social support, young people with secure attachment tend to have better therapeutic outcomes than those with insecure attachment.

Finally, understanding the young person's attachment behaviours will assist the clinician to position herself or himself in the role of *transitory attachment figure*. This role is by definition transitional and, as described later in this text, paves the way for identifying who in the young person's life can fulfil the varied roles the clinician has undertaken as therapy moves towards its conclusion.

These and other clinical implications for the client's attachment are addressed in the chapters that follow.

---

**Clinical Tool 3.2   Working with the young person's attachment style Adapted from Hillin and McAlpine (2015)**

This clinical tool summarises behaviours commonly shown by young people with different attachment styles. Strategies are identified to assist therapists to work effectively with these clients. The client behaviours are examples only and the therapist strategies are by no means prescriptive.

**Avoidant attachment styles**

Young people with avoidant attachment styles usually have had life experiences in which the care provided was not adequate for their needs and have developed working models of current and future relationships that reflect this. Typically, these clients approach relationships with a suspicion of the motives of others, find trust difficult, form superficial relationships, and avoid closeness and intimacy. Their social support networks are often insubstantial and offer limited psychosocial support when things go wrong.

Young people with dismissive avoidant attachment will usually be supported by a robust sense of self whilst minimising the potential support offered by others. Young people with fearful avoidant attachment lack the protective factor of ego strength and simultaneously lack trust and confidence in others.

The left-hand column in the following table provides examples of behaviours commonly exhibited by young people with avoidant attachment. The right-hand column offers suggestions for working with these clients.

Table 3.1 Avoidant attachment: Client behaviours and therapist responses

| Behaviours towards the therapist | Strategies for working with avoidant attachment |
|---|---|
| These clients may | The therapist may |
| 1. Avoid relationships and closeness. | Hand power to the client by giving explicit choice. List options of what is available in therapy. Adjust expectations and timeframes for progress. Identify practical and concrete issues the client is motivated to address. |
| 2. Miss appointments. | Provide respectful proactive outreach, e.g., between-session reminders of appointments. (This lets the young person know the therapist is thinking about her even when she is not there.) Identify self-help strategies including manualised and online treatment protocols. Send handouts for missed appointments. |
| 3. Be noncommunicative. | Acknowledge possible discomfort with therapy. Reframe attendance as an achievement. Model being comfortable with silence, while checking on young person's level of comfort. Consider having tactile distractors (stress balls, etc.) available. |
| 4. Be more interested in things than people. | Relate issues to their interests (see 6 below). |
| 5. Be charming or entertaining as a way of deflecting from emotional content. | Be aware of your responses (e.g., "am I missing something here?"). Gradually build engagement to create safety. |
| 6. Show discomfort, irritation, or aggression. | Model non-rejection. Acknowledge feelings and behaviours. Distinguish the behaviour from the person. |
| 7. Be more willing to communicate about a problem by externalising it. | Consider music, art, or craft as part of therapy. Prepare metaphors or analogies related to their interests. |
| 8. Appreciate instrumental help, such as filling in forms, assisting with a nuisance teacher, aid with financial problems. | Assist with issues that will help with their day to day irritants and problems. |

### Preoccupied attachment style

Young people with preoccupied attachment have developed a working model of relationships in which they are unsure if others will be there for them when they need support. Their fragile sense of self equates to low self-worth ("am I worthy of help?") and their experience of others indicates that others will sometimes be available—leading to those being idealised—or will sometimes not be available—leading to those being devalued. These young people, in their constant need for reassurance, relentlessly test the availability and capacity of others to care.

The left-hand column in the following table provides some examples of behaviours commonly exhibited by young people with preoccupied attachment in the therapy room. The right-hand column offers suggestions for working with these clients.

*Table 3.2* Preoccupied attachment: Client behaviours and therapist responses

| *Behaviours towards the therapist* | *Strategies for working with preoccupied attachment* |
|---|---|
| These clients may<br>1. Have little confidence in their ability to manage distress. | The therapist may<br>Identify strengths and develop interpersonal coping skills. Demonstrate belief in the young person's capacities. |
| 2. Have little confidence in others meeting their attachment needs. They may<br>• continually test you<br>• break boundaries<br>• present in dramatic crises | Provide consistency and predictability. Provide clear written boundaries. Model belief in the young person's ability to manage distress. Briefly (only) deal with current crisis, providing perspective by relating it back to current structured intervention and therapeutic goals. |
| 3. Seek friendship with therapist. They may<br>• not be as interested in solving problems as in maintaining the relationship with the therapist<br>• continually present in crisis in order to keep the therapist engaged<br>• not understand professional boundaries | Reinforce and explain the boundaries of the therapeutic relationship as needed. Explain the difference between the therapeutic relationship and friendship. Revisit this as needed. Add value to relationships outside of therapy. |
| 4. Either idealise or devalue the therapist based on their perception of whether you are meeting their needs. | Model consistency and trustworthiness to reduce the perception of the young person either being favoured or neglected. If the young person tends to idealise, increase the formality of the therapeutic relationship. If the young person devalues, remind him or her of the parameters of the therapeutic relationship. |

(*Continued*)

70  Introduction

**Table 3.2** (continued)

| Behaviours towards the therapist | Strategies for working with preoccupied attachment |
|---|---|
| 5. Use "manipulative" behaviour (driven by 1 above) to elicit caring responses from the therapist, e.g., "doorknob" disclosures: disclosing important information just prior to the session ending. | If appropriate, use this behaviour as an educational tool about the unintentional interpersonal impact this type of behaviour has on others, e.g., "I'm glad you told me that, but I'm annoyed you left it until now. Our session is almost over. Now I'm not sure you meant for me to get annoyed, and I'm wondering if this happens a bit in your life: you annoy other people without really meaning to. We'll pick this up next week". |

### Secure attachment style

Young people with secure attachment base their relationship expectations on working models that are healthy and flexible. Constructed on the basis of real relationship experiences, the securely attached young person
generally trusts others to meet his or her attachment needs. Securely attached young people have a sound sense of self and a belief that others will be available for care and nurture when needed. It should be noted though that these young people can also experience difficult times and develop significant symptomatology. But due to their expectations of others being available and their sound sense of self, they are likely to have developed a robust social support network that will assist them when necessary.

The left-hand column in the following table provides some examples of behaviours commonly exhibited by young people with secure attachment in the therapy room. The right-hand column offers suggestions for working with these clients.

*Table 3.3* Secure attachment: Client behaviours and therapist responses

| Behaviours towards the therapist | Strategies for working with secure attachment |
|---|---|
| These clients may<br>1. Readily believe the therapist is trustworthy. They may test you a little but then settle down to work. | The therapist may<br>Capitalise on relatively straightforward engagement. Once the therapeutic alliance has been established, progress towards symptom resolution may be relatively straightforward. |

(Continued)

**Table 3.3** (*continued*)

| Behaviours towards the therapist | Strategies for working with secure attachment |
| --- | --- |
| 2. Be motivated to work on the identified problems and initiate progress between sessions. | Take advantage of the young person's motivation to get well. This means homework, such as interpersonal tasks and self-help strategies will often be well tolerated. |
| 3. Understand and respect boundaries, including the parameters of the therapeutic relationship, once explained, and not confuse it with friendship. | Not have to spend inordinate time addressing the therapeutic relationship. The therapist can provide feedback on the client's relationship behaviour observed within therapy without too much concern about damaging the therapeutic alliance. |
| 4. Have underlying resilience and interpersonal capacity. This may currently be camouflaged by distress or symptomatology. | Expect these clients may have well developed coping skills and strategies that do not have to be developed, just uncovered. In addition, these clients will mostly likely have a supportive social network that the young person may need reminding of. He or she may need some additional skills and encouragement in reconnecting with supports, especially if the depression or distress has existed for some time. |
| 5. Be highly distressed by their current inability to cope. This level of distress may be unfamiliar territory to securely attached young people. | Tend to minimise the young person's distress. The therapist must remain aware that although the client appears to be securely attached and the prognosis for recovery is good, his or her current distress is real and, for some, life threatening. The therapist must strive for an appropriate balance between understanding and reflecting the level of distress and remaining hopeful of a positive outcome. |

## Summary

IPT-A is predicated on the attachment style and behaviours of the young person. Attachment theory predicts that all individuals are programmed to seek relationship with others. This programming, defined as the "working model" of self and others, strongly influences mental health due to the link between mental wellness and successful relationship outcomes. A secure attachment in adolescence is characterised by the ability to seek comfort and support from meaningful relationships when the young person is going through difficulties.

Preoccupied and avoidant attachment styles are usually associated with a greater likelihood that stress will progress into disorder, without the buffering effects of secure relationships.

Understanding the attachment style of adolescents is a complex process and is best accomplished utilising a variety of sources, comprising an exploration of the young person's interpersonal world and her description of past and current relationships, exploring the quality of the young person's narrative, and attending to the nature of the client-therapist relationship.

Although an appraisal of the young person's attachment style remains an hypothesis during the therapeutic process, this hypothesis provides significant clinical guidance that shapes many aspects of the IPT-A intervention.

## References

Ainsworth, M., Blehar, M. C., Waters, E. & Wall, S. (1978). *Patterns of attachment. A psychological study of the strange situation*. Hillsdale, NJ: Erlbaum.

Bartholomew, K. & Horowitz, L. M. (1991). Attachment styles among young adults: A test of a four-category model. *Journal of Personality and Social Psychology*, 61(2), 226–244.

Bowlby, J. (1969). *Attachment and loss*. New York: Basic Books.

Bowlby, J. (1988). *A secure base: Parent-child attachment and healthy human development*. New York: Basic Books.

Erikson, E. H. (1950). *Childhood and society*. New York: Norton.

Flores, P. (2004). *Addiction as an attachment disorder*. New York: Jason Aronson.

Fonagy, P., Target, M. & Gergely, G. (2000). Attachment and borderline personality disorder: A theory and some evidence. *Borderline Personality Disorder*, 23(1), 103–122.

Gunlicks-Stoessel, M., Westervelt, A., Reigstad, K., Mufson, L. & Lee, S. (2018). The role of attachment style in interpersonal psychotherapy for depressed adolescents. *Psychotherapy Research*, 29(1), 1–8.

Hillin, A. & McAlpine R. (2015). *Interpersonal psychotherapy for adolescents: Workshop participant handbook*. Sydney: Hillin and McAlpine.

Lerner, R., Almerigi, J. & Theokas, C. (2005). Positive youth development: A view of the issues. *Journal of Early Adolescence*, 25(1), 10–16.

Lerner, R. (2007). *The good teen*. New York: Crown.

McAlpine, R. & Hillin, A. (2007). The clinicians response scale (research edition). *Interpersonal psychotherapy for adolescents: Workshop participant handbook*, Sydney: McAlpine and Hillin.

Main, M. & Solomon, J. (1986). Discovery of a new, insecure-disorganized/disoriented attachment pattern. In M. Yogman & T. B. Brazelton (Eds.), *Affective development in infancy* (pp. 95–124). Norwood, NJ: Ablex.

Muus, R. (1982). *Theories of adolescence*. NY: Random House.

Sheard, T., Evans, J., Cash, D., Hicks, D. et al. (2000). A CAT-derived one to three session intervention for repeated deliberate self-harm: A description of the model and initial experience of trainee psychiatrists in using it. *Psychology and Psychotherapy: Theory and Research*, 73(2), 179–196.

Spence, S., O'Shea, G. & Donovan, C. (2016). Improvements in interpersonal functioning following interpersonal psychotherapy (IPT) with adolescents and their association with change in depression. *Behavioural and Cognitive Psychology, 44*(3), 257–272.

Stuart, S. & Robertson, M. (2012). *Interpersonal psychotherapy: A clinician's guide* (2nd Edition). London: Arnold.

# 4 Clinical techniques

**Contents**

| | |
|---|---|
| Introduction | 74 |
| The therapeutic relationship | 75 |
|    *Setting relationship boundaries* | 75 |
|    *Monitoring communication patterns* | 76 |
|    *The interpersonal laboratory* | 79 |
| Encouragement of affect | 82 |
|    *Content and process affect* | 86 |
| Exploration and clarification | 90 |
| Interpersonal incidents | 90 |
|    *Collecting information about a specific Interpersonal Incident* | 92 |
|    *Analysing the Interpersonal Incident* | 95 |
|    *Changing communication* | 98 |
| Conflict-solving styles | 102 |
| Role play | 105 |
| Empty chair technique | 108 |
| Interpersonal mindfulness | 111 |
| Summary | 114 |
| References | 115 |

## Introduction

The Greek language, particularly ancient Greek, distinguishes at least four words for the word defined in the English language as "love". The therapeutic relationship comprises several key features, including a characteristic proposed by Yalom (2002): "let the client matter". When our clients matter to us, and they know they matter, they potentially feel loved by us. But traditionally, in nearly all forms of psychotherapy, the idea of love between the therapist and client has been actively discouraged. Interpersonal Psychotherapy is, by definition, about relationships—the relationships our clients have with significant others in their lives and with the therapist. The nature of the client/therapist relationship, the therapeutic alliance, provides the context for therapy. In establishing this context, the therapist strives to develop a relationship that includes parameters such as trust; honesty; openness; acceptance; positive regard; hope; care; nurture; and, where appropriate, comfort. In other words, the therapist strives to establish a loving relationship. The four primary Greek words for love are *philia, eros, storge,* and *agape*. The fourth of these, *agape*, best describes the loving relationship the therapist strives to develop with the young person. *Agape* denotes an unconditional love that wishes, above all, for the good of another. In the words of Thomas Aquinas "to will the good of another" (Hause and Pasnow, 2014). *Agape* conveys the original meaning of charity, a pure love in which things are given with no expectation of getting anything back in return, striving only for the recipient to benefit. In "letting our clients matter", and our clients knowing they matter, *agape* love will drive the therapeutic alliance "to will the good of another".

Yalom (2002) notes that in time-limited therapies, which are necessarily favoured by insurance companies and government agencies who often foot the bill for therapy, therapists run the risk of focussing so much on evidence-based practice that they lose their human-ness, jeopardising the authenticity of the person-person interaction, becoming more psychological technicians than humans who happen to be therapists. But when the therapeutic alliance is characterised by *agape*, this risk diminishes and the life and needs of the client take centre stage in the therapeutic process, rather than this stage being occupied by the specific techniques of whichever therapeutic model the therapist is currently employing.

In this chapter on clinical techniques of IPT-A, we discuss the use of the therapeutic relationship before any of the other techniques. The techniques that follow will be utilised within the context of this therapeutic relationship and this relationship remains central to the therapeutic process.

## The therapeutic relationship

> "*Every event or intervention that occurs within psychotherapy does so with some aspect of the relationship serving either as its direct mechanism or its immediate context*"
>
> (Kiesler, 1996, p. 217).

### Setting relationship boundaries

The client-therapist relationship in IPT-A is complex. Adolescent clients are involved in the normative process of individuation: attaining personal independence from adults via connectedness with members of their peer group. A complicating factor in the therapeutic process is that therapists are adults and often perceived by young minds as aligned with other adults in their lives. It is incumbent on the therapist to establish a relationship that assumes neither the role of friend nor the role of authoritarian adult. The therapeutic role is a unique one characterised by three primary considerations: acknowledging the expertise of the young person in their life story; communicating that the client matters to the therapist; and by openness: attempting to create a therapeutic environment where the client feels comfortable talking about anything.

When two humans meet socially for the first time, a process identified by Sullivan (1954) as "strategic positioning" occurs. That is, initial communications are aimed generally at identifying how the other fits in relation to self and, specifically, what is appropriate to talk about. In other words, what are the rules that will govern this relationship? For example, in an initial conversation with someone met at a party, one may conclude early in the encounter that politics, religion, sexuality, personal income, or social status are off limits. As topics are intuitively identified as off limits, boundaries are established regarding what may be comfortably discussed. Transgression of these unspoken boundaries, once established, creates discomfort ranging from mild tension through to overt hostility. This is sometimes referred to as *moving outside the comfort zone*. If the relationship develops beyond this first encounter, these boundaries may be gradually broadened to the point that, within friendships that have stood the test of time, these boundaries bear very little resemblance to those established during that first encounter. Time-limited therapy does not afford this luxury. One unique characteristic of time-limited psychotherapy is that in early sessions, the therapist takes charge of positioning these boundaries, using a communication style characterised by respectful curiosity, by setting these limits as widely as possible. The holistic assessment provides multiple opportunities to discuss topics such as fear, love, hate, anger, bullying, grief, belief, extremes of mood, sexuality, death, suicide, self-harm, drug and alcohol use, trauma and abuse, etc. Although young people may not be totally forthcoming with their responses initially, the therapist has nonetheless communicated to the young person that those topics are safe to discuss in therapy. Conversely, failure to do this may mean that subsequent attempts to introduce these necessary topics after boundaries have been set will create that experience of moving outside the comfort zone, thus increasing the possibility of unhelpful defensive behaviour. It may also communicate to the young person that the therapist is uncomfortable with certain material, once again fostering a reluctance in the client to introduce salient emotional responses or difficult experiences.

### *Monitoring communication patterns*

Whilst establishing these broad relationship parameters, the IPT-A therapist will also be attempting to develop a therapeutic alliance in which the three dimensions of communication identified by Kiesler and Watkins (1989) can be monitored. Kiesler and Watkins suggest that three aspects of relationship operate in every dyad: Affiliation, Inclusion, and Dominance. Reflecting on the therapeutic relationship guided by these dimensions will assist the therapist to monitor how the therapeutic alliance is progressing.

Affiliation is a dimension that describes the degree to which the therapist and client have positive or negative feelings toward one another. It identifies where the relationship is situated along the friendliness—hostility continuum. Affiliation is an estimate of how much the client and therapist are liking each other.

This dimension is particularly significant when considering the attachment styles of clients. For clients with relatively secure attachments, the dimension of Affiliation will usually be relatively easy to negotiate. Therapists can monitor where the relationship currently lies along the friendliness—hostility dimension and make adjustments where necessary: either by increasing personal warmth, for example, to move in the direction of friendliness, or by increasing the level of formality if the therapist perceives the therapeutic dyad is moving from a therapist—client model towards friendship.

Young people with preoccupied attachments, however, being focussed on others providing validity for a fragile sense of self, will often strive to engage the therapist as friend, confidante, and ally. With these clients, the therapist must tread the fine line between an appropriate degree of warmth to provide a level of connectedness, balanced with a constant eye on relationship boundaries so that the client is less likely to cling to the therapist as rescuer. A complicating factor is that another characteristic of young people with a preoccupied attachment style is their propensity to categorise others as givers or withholders and to idealise givers and devalue withholders. The idealised therapist will be regarded by these clients as a solver of all of life's problems whilst the devalued therapist will often be relegated to the list of failed helpers. It would not be unusual for this young person to terminate therapy and resume his ongoing quest for someone who can meet his constant need for affirmation.

One characteristic of avoidant dismissive and avoidant fearful clients, due to their general perception of others as being unhelpful and difficult to trust, is to be suspicious of the ability of the therapist (and of therapy) to be useful to them. Whilst it is not necessary for clients to like their therapist a lot, in order to continue the therapeutic process, the clients must remain engaged enough to return for future sessions. For avoidant clients, a key goal of the therapist will be to create a therapeutic environment where the young person feels less uncomfortable with closeness. Strategies that may be useful to accomplish this will include the therapist showing an interest in the instrumentals of the young person's life—for example, in their sports, cars, interests, conflicts with teachers, financial difficulties, and problems with welfare agencies—and taking time during sessions to demonstrate this interest. For young people with avoidant attachment, it is strategic for the therapist to demonstrate trustworthiness by remaining reliable and scrupulous in following up on undertakings made in session. For example, after agreeing to talk to the young person's parole officer, the therapist would be certain to do so prior to the next session.

Whereas Affiliation is about the feelings therapists and clients have about each other, Inclusion is about the degree to which the therapeutic relationship stands as important to both therapist and client. As mentioned above, it is not always necessary for clients to like their therapists, but it is necessary for clients to see the therapeutic relationship as holding some importance and value for them. For some, parents, the courts, or insurance companies may have mandated attendance at therapy, and this may hold enough value in itself. For most, however, the importance of therapy lies in a client's experience of therapy and in her expectations of its role for potential change towards a better life. Therapists strive to construct a therapeutic alliance in which the young person sees value in coming to therapy because she expects the therapy will provide a vehicle to achieve a more positive life experience, including the resolution of symptoms.

Dominance refers to the degree to which one person or the other is in charge of decisions about the relationship. It is an index of power in a relationship and a measure of how the power balance may shift over time. In IPT-A, it would be expected that the therapist would exercise more power in the relationship in the Initial Phase of therapy and would gradually relinquish this power as therapy progressed. By the Consolidation Phase, the power balance would have shifted in favour of the client as the client prepares to leave therapy and resume normal functioning in his or her world. This predicted trajectory in the power balance however does not always play out in therapy. Anxious attachment styles, for example, may distort the manner in which Dominance manifests in the therapeutic relationship. Kiesler and Watkins (1989) note that interpersonal difficulties may arise when clients unintentionally elicit negative responses from others. These are reflected on a micro level as specific interactions that elicit responses that do not effectively meet their attachment needs. The accumulation of these communications then establishes a relationship reflective of the attachment style of the young person. For example, a young person with an avoidant style will typically expect that the therapist, like others, will be unable to meet her attachment needs and may, as a consequence, seek to retain power in the relationship to either protect her self-reliance (avoidant dismissive) or to protect herself from the consequences of vulnerability (avoidant fearful). Young people with a preoccupied style, on the other hand, may resist any attempt by the therapist to shift the power balance in favour of the client, due to their belief that only others can provide validity to their fragile sense of self, and accepting more power in the relationship reduces the capacity of the therapist to provide this validation.

Affiliation, Inclusion, and Dominance exist on a moment-by-moment or statement-by-statement basis, but it is the cumulative effect of these patterns that determine the nature of relationship as patterns become set between individuals. By monitoring each of these variables, therapists can regulate the nature of the emerging therapeutic relationship so that the balances within each of Affiliation, Inclusion, and Dominance remain optimal for the therapeutic process to be maximally effective. One way to assist this process is to complete the following chart (Figure 4.1) at the conclusion of each session, according to the therapist's perceptions of the balances in each of these dimensions. For the dimension of Affiliation, the therapist estimates the level of positive or negative feelings that have been evidenced during that session; for the dimension of Inclusion, the

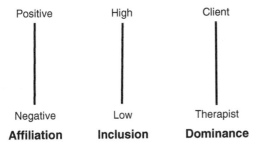

*Figure 4.1* Monitoring communication patterns.

therapist estimates the degree of importance or value the young person derived; for Dominance, the therapist estimates the power balance. The therapist can then plan in subsequent sessions to maintain current balances or alter them as required.

## *The interpersonal laboratory*

It is acknowledged in IPT-A that healing occurs within the context of the therapeutic relationship. However, whilst the therapeutic alliance remains central to the therapeutic process, it never becomes a focus of treatment. Perhaps the best way to regard the client/therapist relationship in IPT-A is as an interpersonal laboratory. The therapist strives to create an environment where the young person feels safe enough to accept feedback from the therapist about potential maladaptive relationship patterns that emerge either directly during therapy or indirectly as young people report interpersonal experiences external to therapy and safe enough to experiment with new ways of relating. Clients' maladaptive communication patterns that emerge during therapy will reflect relationship patterns that exist in their interpersonal world outside of therapy as well. These patterns become a rich source of data for the therapist, and the therapy sessions become an interpersonal laboratory when the therapist tentatively reveals these patterns to the client and collaboratively explores alternative interpersonal patterns that might help meet his attachment needs more effectively. Prior to this, the therapist would have a conversation with the young person to establish that this type of interaction is acceptable to him:

*Therapist:* *If I notice some things about our conversations in these sessions that might help us better understand what happens between you and others, is it okay if I point these things out?*

Then the therapist can say the following:

*Therapist:* *I also want you to take notice of any thoughts or feelings you may have during our time together. I'd really like you to be able to talk about these because I'm sure that if you have them in here, you're also going to have*

> them with others in your life. We can learn a lot by noticing these thoughts and feelings and by trying to work out where they come from and how they affect the way you get on with others. Does that sound okay to you?

The style and language in comments such as these will be influenced by the age and stage of clients, their attachment style as well as by the therapist's perception of the readiness of the young person to process these comments. The therapist's goal for the therapeutic relationship is to provide opportunities for young people to reflect on their interpersonal experiences in order to enhance their communication skills in other significant relationships.

There are a number of ways that this attention to the therapeutic relationship can assist therapy in IPT-A. First, the interactions that occur in therapy provide an immediate and reliable source of information. What the client reports about his or her relationships outside therapy, while valuable, are subject to distortions of memory and may include attempts to preserve Affiliation with the therapist.

Second, some young people are very good at telling stories, but the affect associated with these stories may be camouflaged or supressed when relating them. Attending to affect that arises between the client and therapist provides an immediacy that may counter intellectual resistance. When therapists draw attention to affect that arises, significant insights may occur, as the following example illustrates. **Gemma**, aged 16, was in therapy for depression. In the fifth session, the conversation turned to her boyfriend's move interstate.

*Therapist:* Gemma I noticed you sighed heavily and looked away when I asked you to tell me about your boyfriend's new job. I can't help thinking that my question brought up some fairly strong feelings for you. Can we talk about those feelings for a bit?

*Gemma:* It's just that you bring my boyfriend up all the time. This isn't about him you know.

*Therapist:* So you're annoyed at me for wasting our time together? And maybe for taking the focus away from you for a bit. Gemma can you remember the last time you had this annoyed feeling with one of the people in your inner circle?

*Gemma:* Like I'm pissed off with Luke all the time. He's the one moving away and I'm only going to get to see him once a month.

*Therapist:* Just then when you were annoyed with me you sighed and looked away. I'm wondering what you do when you're pissed off with Luke.

*Gemma:* I dunno. I want to tell him but it's his life and I don't want him to think I'm a bitching girlfriend. I say nothing, I guess. (Gemma smiles.) Maybe just sigh and look away.

*Therapist:* What would you like to say to Luke?

Third, by attending to affective changes in the relationship within session, the therapist can provide the young person with immediate feedback about how she is currently impacting on another human being. **Ali**, for example a highly intelligent 19-year-old, characteristically intellectualised most of her interpersonal interactions. The Problem Area was Interpersonal Gaps. Ali had no trouble initiating relationships but had difficulty developing closeness. Ali would frighten off potential friends of both genders by her analytical thinking and acid wit, creating an aura of unapproachability. The following interchange occurred after six sessions, when Ali surprisingly cried whilst relating an Interpersonal Incident that brought home to her the lack of closeness in her relationships outside her immediate family.

*Therapist:* *Ali you know for the time we've been together, I've really struggled to get close to you. We both know you're really smart, and in therapy so far, I've felt that you've been one step ahead of me all the way. I've felt I've had not much to offer you because you were always that one step ahead. And that's created a distance. I feel you've been keeping me away—maybe not meaning to but stopping me from getting to know you. But you know just now when you cried, I suddenly felt closer, like a wall between us had collapsed.*
*Ali:* *I hate showing my emotions—it sucks, it's a sign of weakness.*
*Therapist:* *I'm wondering if there is anyone you do show your emotions to Ali?*
*Ali:* *Nup—only at home*
*Therapist:* *(Looking at Ali's Closeness Circle). So you do show your emotions to those in your inner circle. And it's those people you do feel close to.*
*Ali:* *Yeah but it's okay to show feelings at home—they don't reject you for being a jerk.*
*Therapist:* *And what about now? You've just shown a strong emotion—and I feel closer to you. That's pretty much the opposite of rejection. Are you surprised by that?*
*Ali:* *(Laughs) But you're paid not to reject me.*
*Therapist:* *I'm wondering about your friends—the ones in your outer circle who you want to bring in a bit. Can we talk about that connection between showing your feelings and expecting to be rejected?*

In subsequent sessions in the Middle Phase, the therapist explored Ali's fear of vulnerability and collaboratively developed a hierarchy of vulnerability, beginning with examples of relatively low-grade display of emotion, ("D'you know I cried in that movie!") gradually increasing to a more open expression ("I was so hurt when Bree said that stuff about me"). Ali then identified a safe person with whom she could experiment and proceeded to gradually increase the level of disclosure with this friend. It surprised Ali when her friend called her at home, and Ali reported feeling closer to her as well. As Ali's attachment behaviours were consistent with an avoidant dismissive style, the pace of change had to be realistically regulated, but by the Consolidation Phase, Ali had moved two friends from her outer circle to the middle circle. Although she remained guarded about revealing her emotions to others, Ali did acknowledge feeling more hopeful about closeness.

Fourth, addressing interpersonal issues in the therapeutic relationship provides an opportunity to model ways of relating that may challenge the young person's belief that expressing affect can have a damaging effect. For example, in the above vignettes, Gemma discovered there were direct ways of conveying her annoyance that were more likely to be understood than her usual oblique, indirect, and unsatisfactory sighing and looking away. Ali experienced that expressing emotion doesn't always lead to rejection. Directing the young person's attention to these experience within therapy implicitly conveys that it is possible to reflect on these interactions and express these feelings without negative consequences.

Finally, interpersonal matters that occur within therapy can increase mentalization. These reflections provide an avenue for the young person to think about his state of mind and that of the therapist. This process encourages the young person to reflect on how he thinks and feels about himself and others; how this may influence unhelpful responses; and, with this new insight, how to make more adaptive communication choices. The therapist's role is to guide the discovery process, moving from the therapy room to relationships outside of therapy and how to improve communication within these other relationships.

In summary, in IPT-A the therapeutic relationship is never a focus in itself, but this relationship provides a context for therapy. The therapist first, sets wide boundaries about the subject matter of therapy; second, monitors communications patterns through attention to Affiliation, Inclusion, and Dominance; and third, establishes the therapeutic relationship as a laboratory in which young people can reflect on interpersonal processes. This learning is then generalised to relationships outside of therapy.

The following clinical techniques, although not specific to IPT-A, are adapted for application within an interpersonal intervention.

## Encouragement of affect

IPT-A usually does not encourage the expression of affect without clear end goals. These goals are symptom reduction through (1) helping the client recognise and better understand his or her experienced emotions, (2) helping the client communicate feelings and emotions more effectively to significant others, and (3) assisting clients to deal with suppressed affect.

The centrality of interpersonal processes to IPT-A suggests that a young person's emotions and their interpersonal interactions are closely linked. Helping the client understand his or her emotional world then becomes a priority. Emotional swings in adolescence are, for many, normative; because of this, many young people believe that the lability of their emotions is largely outside their control. Young people may believe they are victims of their emotions and have very little influence in when, where, why, how, and with whom these uncontrollable feelings surface. Therapeutic techniques, for example, the feelings diary commonly used in cognitive behaviour therapy (CBT), assist young people to see some degree of structure or order in their affective world; potentially challenge this belief; and open up the possibility that they do, in fact, have some agency in their emotional world.

Other techniques to address the encouragement of affect include the Personal Diagram (adapted from Sheard et al., 2000). This technique articulates a causal pathway centred on negative affectivity such as depression or anxiety. Together, the therapist and young person develop a schematic representation of the connection between events in relationships and the client's affective experience. The Personal Diagram begins with exploring a recent event in which the client had experienced a significant negative emotion, for example, depression. The antecedents and the consequences of this event are discussed and exit strategies explored as seen in the following example.

**Steph**, a 17-year-old student, was referred by her family doctor after she disclosed to him that she had been self-harming. She had been cutting herself for about three months. In the initial session, the therapist identified significant depressive mood, but without enough symptomatology to warrant a diagnosis of major depressive disorder. During the Interpersonal Inventory, the therapist hypothesised an avoidant dismissive attachment style. Collaboratively, the therapist and Steph agreed that the Problem Area most closely associated with her current state is Interpersonal Disputes. During session 4, the therapist used a Personal Diagram to help Steph understand the affect surrounding her self-harm and to assist her to develop more appropriate affect regulation skills.

Construction of the Personal Diagram began with a discussion of the last time Steph harmed herself, which was during the previous week. Steph had difficulty labelling the feelings that preceded her self-harm, but after discussion of some possibilities recognised her affective state as *angry out of control feelings*. The second step was to identify the antecedent to these feelings. Steph clearly remembered coming home from school, feeling "miserable", and finding a note from her mother requesting her to do the weekly shop that evening. Steph's immediate response was to feel extremely annoyed at her mother as Steph had already made plans to meet up with some friends that night. As she could not contact her mother, Steph decided to phone her friends to tell them she could not make it. During this phone call, Steph formed an impression that her friends were glad she couldn't go out with them and believed she could hear some of them in the background laughing about the dilemma with her mother. Steph's irritation at her mother suddenly turned into a spiralling frustration fuelled by anger and feelings of abandonment—in her words, "angry and out of control".

The third step in constructing the Personal Diagram was to explore the thoughts and feelings that Steph experienced as she contemplated what to do next. At this point, the therapist encouraged Steph to recall in detail the events on this night, requesting a description of the factual events and also of her affective response to these events:

*Therapist:*   *Steph after you got off the phone with your friends what was going through your mind?*
*Steph:*   *What do you mean?*
*Therapist:*   *Well to begin, can you remember exactly what you did after you hung up?*
*Steph:*   *I don't know—I think I swore a few times, put my music on. Loud.*
*Therapist:*   *And do you remember what you were thinking about?*

84  Introduction

*Steph:* Just what a lot of bitches they are. I don't need them anyway.
*Therapist:* So you swore a bit, turned up the music, and you were thinking that you can get by without them. Did that make you feel any better?
*Steph:* Nope. I got angrier and angrier. The more I thought about it, the more pissed off I got. I was pissed off at Mum, at them, at everyone....
*Therapist:* And....?
*Steph:* Well I had some of mum's vodka and went to my room. Turned the music up more, sat on my bed for about ten minutes and then got the razor.

At this point the therapist showed Steph how to construct a Personal Diagram. As the diagram (Figure 4.2, Part 1) was taking shape, the therapist explained to Steph how the events were linked to the feelings.

After construction of the first part of the diagram, the therapist and Steph continued the discussion of the events of that night.

*Therapist:* Steph after you cut yourself, how did things change?
*Steph:* I felt heaps better—I was so angry before, but after, it was more under control.
*Therapist:* And what happened next?
*Steph:* I cleaned up a bit and then went and got some dinner.
*Therapist:* So it seems the cutting worked—you felt better after and you were able to calm down.
*Steph:* Suppose so.
*Therapist:* So there were some good things about cutting—it helped you manage difficult feelings. Were there any not so good things as well?

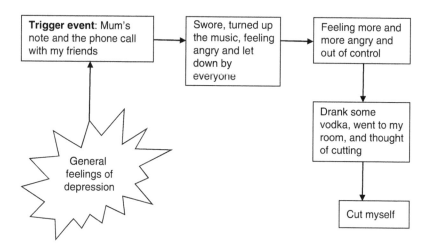

Figure 4.2 Personal Diagram (Part 1).

*Steph:* None I can think of.
*Therapist:* Okay. So Steph when you were cooking dinner, what was going through your mind?
*Steph:* Nothing. I was just cooking dinner—I wasn't thinking about anything.
*Therapist:* And afterwards that night—like just after you got into bed, before you went off to sleep?
*Steph:* I suppose I felt a bit sad really—like that it has all come to this.
*Therapist:* Okay.... Let's finish the diagram.

The therapist encouraged Steph to complete the diagram (Figure 4.3. Personal Diagram, Part 2), using her words to describe the events and the affect that preceded and followed these events.

The Personal Diagram identifies the link between event and affect, thereby challenging a common adolescent belief that feelings occur randomly. Seeing this pattern also helped Steph understand her emotional world a little better and helped her begin to see the association between interpersonal relationships and affectivity. Steph was frustrated and angered by the actions of her mother and she felt abandoned by the actions of her friends. She responded to these negative emotions by an affect regulation strategy that proved effective: Steph's cutting helped her manage her intolerable affect. But it had some negative sequelae. These consequences fed her feelings of depression, thus

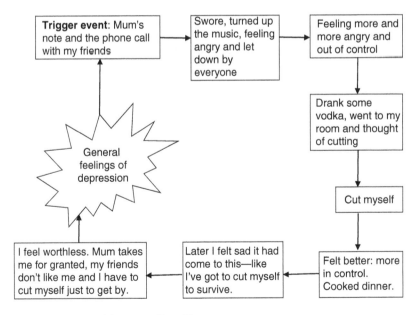

*Figure 4.3* Personal Diagram (Part 2).

setting the scene for another trigger event in her interpersonal relationships to precipitate another episode of self-harm, and so the cycle continues.

The Personal Diagram also provides the opportunity to explore exit strategies: strategies that interrupt the habitual sequence of event—emotion—action, enabling the choice of other behaviours that potentially break the self-defeating cycle. In Figure 4.3 possible exit points could occur at a number of places. For example, at the point of the actual trigger event, Steph reacted to an interpersonal event in an habitual, nonconstructive manner. Her emotion-focussed response predicted the spiralling negative affectivity that followed. The therapist discussed some differences between problem-focussed and emotion-focussed responses and how each can lead to different outcomes. Following this psychoeducation, the therapist invited Steph to suggest possible problem-focussed responses to her triggers and speculate how things may have turned out differently. In the next session the therapist repeated this process for different potential exit points until Steph demonstrated she was familiar enough with the process to approach it independently. The therapist then asked Steph if she would construct another Personal Diagram about an Interpersonal Incident during the following week, for discussion at the next session.

The goal of the Personal Diagram was to help Steph more fully understand the link between interpersonal events and her emotional, cognitive, and behavioural responses to these events and to demonstrate that there were alternative options for her other than the habitual, self-defeating responses she was accustomed to.

### Content and process affect

Process affect is the set of feelings the client displays during the therapeutic session, while content affect is the set of feelings the client reports having experienced during real-life events. For example, when Steph was describing her affective state after the phone call with her friends she said: "I got angrier and angrier. The more I thought about it the more pissed off I got. I was pissed off at Mum, at them, at everyone …".

Steph was reporting the content affect related to a recent real-life event. As she was describing this event, the therapist noticed Steph's voice was louder and, for the first time during the interview, Steph looked directly at the therapist. The therapist hypothesised that Steph's process affect was fairly consistent with her content affect. That is, as Steph was describing feeling angry in a real-life event, she was re-experiencing some of that anger in the therapeutic session.

Content affect and process affect can be congruent, as in the above example, or they may be incongruent.

**John** was a 13-year-old, the oldest child from a farming family. On returning from school, John found his seriously injured father under a farm implement that had fallen on him during repairs. John called the emergency number, but his father died soon after. John's attachment style appeared to be secure and his

Problem Area was Complex Grief. He met criteria for major depressive disorder but not for PTSD.

During discussion of the timeline in the Interpersonal Inventory, John related the story of finding his injured father. His recount of the story was flat and monotonous, delivered without any noticeable emotion. The therapist noted that John's mother reported that John and his father were close, spending a lot of time together on the farm and also away on fishing trips.

When process affect and content affect are incongruent, as in John's case above, it is a sign to the therapist that something in the psychological world of the client may be operating to defend him from the consequences of congruence. For example, in John's case, the therapist might have hypothesised that John's lack of congruence was protecting him from re-experiencing painful emotions and this defence may be blocking him from processing this affect.

With young people, the decision to point out incongruity must be considered carefully. Adolescence can be a time of emotional lability when the young person feels that their affect is not completely under their control. If the client interprets the enquiry of the therapist as critical of their affective responses, the therapist may unwittingly pathologise their difficult and unpredictable feelings. That is, if the therapist pointed out the lack of congruence between the distress caused by the farm accident and the relative unemotional way he recounted the events of that day, John may construe this enquiry as a criticism of his response to an event that caused him enormous distress. In addition, John may infer disapproval of his affective life, about which he is feeling uncertain, fragile, and vulnerable.

Therefore, it is usually a safer practice to assist young people to monitor their feelings (for example, through a Feelings Diary) and assist them to draw their own conclusions about these feelings rather than risk confirming their suspicions that their feelings are in some way abnormal and outside of their control. Alongside this, it is good practice to routinely offer adolescents strategies to develop their affect regulation skills. Some of these strategies will be discussed in some detail later in this chapter.

*Therapist:* John that must have been an unbelievably difficult time for you. And I can understand how things have been tough since then. Major things like that can affect every part of our lives—our thoughts, our feelings, some of the things we do ... but it can be especially tough on our feelings.
*John:* (no response).
*Therapist:* I was wondering if we could look at how things have changed for you since the accident. Is that okay?
*John:* Yeah okay.
*Therapist:* I'd like to start if it's all right with you by thinking about how you've been feeling lately. Sometimes our feelings really take us by surprise, especially after something major, like you've had.

The therapist then introduced a Feelings Diary. This tool in itself challenges possible beliefs that feelings occur randomly. In addition, the Feelings Diary

---

**Clinical Tool 4.1   Feelings Diary**

Date:

**Scale,** for example:

5. Unbelievably happy
4. Content
3. Just even
2. Miserable
1. Devastated

**Best I felt all day:**

1   2   3   4   5

What was happening interpersonally?

**Worst I felt all day:**

1   2   3   4   5

What was happening interpersonally?

**Average for the day:**

1   2   3   4   5

---

demonstrates that feelings are, in some cases at least, related to specific daily events or circumstances. Clinical Tool 4.1 provides a Feelings Diary that invites clients to consider links between their emotions and interpersonal dynamics.

In the following session, the therapist followed up John's responses to the Feelings Diary, remaining mindful of the incongruity between process and content affect that occurred in the previous session.

*Therapist:* John, it seems your worst time is at night just before you go off to sleep.
*John:* (Pause) Yeah.
*Therapist:* Can you recall what's going on in your thoughts at those times?
*John:* It's usually about the accident … about Dad.
*Therapist:* Thinking about the accident…and your Dad…. And that's when you feel worst.
*John:* But I think about the accident all the time … sometimes I just couldn't care…I feel nothing.
*Therapist:* So some of the time when you think of your Dad you feel so incredibly sad, but other times you just feel numb…. What do you make of that?

The therapist has guided John to the point where John introduced the fact that there are times when he feels sad about the accident and times he feels numb.

The therapist normalised and validated these responses and helped John to understand that as he acknowledged his sadness and loss, although his sadness would remain for quite a while, many of his depressive symptoms would begin to resolve and he would again be able to engage more fully in life.

Encouragement of affect is a clinical technique employed in all Problem Areas. Some adolescents split off their feelings from their cognitions, especially when conflict arises with a significant other, particularly an attachment figure. An example of how this technique may be utilized in the Problem Area Interpersonal Disputes follows:

> **Tanya** was a mature 14-year-old girl living at home with her mother, a single parent, and her twin younger siblings. Tanya reported that most of her friends were allowed out at least one night on the weekend, having to be home by midnight. Tanya's mother insisted on a 10:00 pm curfew. Tanya presented for therapy after a suicide attempt which she attributed to not having any friends and not having any life. She felt sad and hopeless. During initial sessions, Tanya revealed that prior to the last three or four weeks things were good for her. She was doing well at school, she was singing in a school rock band, and she was happy with her friends. Things started to fall apart two weeks ago when her band was asked to play at an eighteenth birthday party. Tanya was nervous but excited, but her mother refused to let her go, explaining she believed Tanya was growing up too quickly and she would be able to go to these parties when she was older. Tanya seemed to accept her mother's decision without much difficulty. In fact, Tanya's mother commented on how pleased she was with the way Tanya responded.

When Tanya related to the therapist the conversation in which her mother refused to let her go to the party, her affect was flat, and she described feeling "just nothing" after the conversation with her mother. The therapist asked Tanya how this conversation would go if it occurred between one of her friends and their mother. Not surprisingly, Tanya was more animated during this description, expressing an appropriate amount of indignation. When this was pointed out, Tanya acknowledged she never felt angry towards her mother, even when she stopped her doing things her friends were able to do. She just felt "sad and defeated", not motivated to do or say anything that might change the situation.

Tanya endorsed the symptoms for major depressive disorder and the Problem Area Interpersonal Disputes was collaboratively identified. She felt "stuck" in her relationship with her mother who made many decisions about Tanya's life without input from Tanya.

A therapeutic goal may be to encourage Tanya to get in touch with appropriate affect to empower her to seek solutions to the conflict with her mother that address both their needs. Too much anger can get in the way of resolution of conflict, but appropriate anger can help provide the motivation for change. Encouragement of affect is a technique that may assist Tanya discover that unlocking her feelings will not destroy her attachment figure and that there are appropriate ways to express angry feelings that can lead to better outcomes for both her and her mother. We will return to Tanya later in this chapter.

## Exploration and clarification

Many adolescents report that adults often pay only token attention to young people and are all too ready with advice without taking the time to find out what is really going on in their inner world. That is one of the reasons therapy with young people can be difficult: some young people approach adults with the expectation that they are not going to be listened to let alone taken seriously. The course of therapy is enhanced when therapists listen and provide evidence to young clients that we are listening and are vitally interested in their story.

In IPT-A the dual aims of the clinical techniques are (1) decrease the troublesome symptomatology and (2) improve the client's ability to communicate effectively in relationships that matter. Within exploration and clarification, IPT-A utilises both directive and nondirective questioning. The goal of both questioning styles remains symptom reduction and improving communication. In time-limited interventions, therapists are not afforded the luxury of exploration for exploration's sake. The end goal must be that the client has moved in a direction that will facilitate improvement in one or both of these two goals. Generally, as the IPT-A intervention progresses and the therapeutic alliance is deepened, the questioning profile changes. At the beginning of the intervention, direct questions are usually over-represented, while towards the end of the intervention, one would expect to find more open-ended questions.

## Interpersonal incidents

Interpersonal Incidents are specific episodes in which a communication occurs between the client and a significant other. Examples include a conversation with a friend, an argument with a parent, or an exchange between the young person and a teacher. The relaying of Interpersonal Incidents helps the therapist understand how the young person is using language and other forms of communication to meet his or her interpersonal needs. The use of Interpersonal Incidents allows the therapist to gain a more thorough understanding of the communication patterns the young person is employing and is helpful in assisting the young person to begin to understand how the message he or she intends to send to others may not always be the message the other receives. It is a description by the client of a specific encounter, not a description of a relationship pattern or a story about how things usually are. To elicit reports of Interpersonal Incidents, the therapist asks questions about a specific event. For example, in the case of Tanya, introduced earlier in this chapter, the therapist may decide to explore in some detail how Tanya communicated her disappointment about not being allowed to attend the party. The therapist would ask Tanya to accurately describe the details of the communication that occurred with her mother:

*Therapist:* Tanya, when your Mum said you weren't allowed to go to the party what did you say?
*Tanya:* I didn't say much really.... I think I just said, "Why not?".
*Therapist:* And what did Mum say then?
*Tanya:* Just that I'm growing up too quickly and I'll be able to go to those parties when I'm older.
*Therapist:* What happened next?
*Tanya:* Well, not much. There's no point in arguing with her.
*Therapist:* How were you feeling inside then, Tanya?
*Tanya:* I don't know.... Nothing.... What can you do?
*Therapist:* So what did you do?
*Tanya:* Went outside. I just wanted to be by myself. I felt bad that the others were going and I'd be letting them down 'cos I'm the singer.
*Therapist:* How do you think your Mum was feeling then Tanya?
*Tanya:* I dunno. She won again.
*Therapist:* When did you see Mum again?
*Tanya:* She called me soon after to bath the twins.
*Therapist:* And did you and Mum talk about the party again?
*Tanya:* Not really...it's like it's over then.... There's no point in arguing.... She'll never change her mind.

There are several reasons for eliciting this information. The first is to better understand the communication styles of the young person and to shed some light on any miscommunication that may routinely be occurring. Even given the different attachment styles and behaviours of young people, most can still learn that some forms of communication are more effective than others. Understanding that some patterns of communication don't work well is often a first step in unlearning ineffective behaviour before more effective patterns can be incorporated into the communication repertoire. The technique of looking in detail at Interpersonal Incidents can reveal these patterns effectively and, if used sensitively by the therapist, should not contribute to a sense of social failure felt by some adolescents. Information about miscommunication is useful in all the Problem Areas.

Secondly, Interpersonal Incidents can help the young person see his current problem from a different perspective. Many adolescents describe their interactions with significant others in very general terms, such as "Mum never lets me go out on Sundays", "my maths teacher is always picking on me", or "I can never be friends with them again". These statements, although rarely accurate, derive from core beliefs and shape future expectations of others. In the above interchange, Tanya made it quite clear that she believed it was no use talking to her mother about her dilemma because, in Tanya's words, "She'll never change her mind". The actual words or cognitions used by clients in their reports of Interpersonal Incidents give valuable information about how they see the world and, consequently, valuable information about the cognitive errors that reflect their beliefs about the world. Managing cognitive errors that occur within relationships with significant others through challenging their accuracy (disputing) and challenging their potency (decatastrophising) can provide a useful platform for interpersonal growth within the parameters of IPT-A.

Stuart and Robertson (2012)[1] identify three processes for working with Interpersonal Incidents that clarify the nature of the communication patterns used by clients:

1  Collecting information about a specific Interpersonal Incident.
2  Analysing the Interpersonal Incident.
3  Changing communication.

These authors suggest a grid, which can be completed collaboratively with the young person and can be used to graphically display the exploration of an Interpersonal Incident (Figure 4.4a). The young person's communication (Content) can be categorised as General statements and Specific incidents and the emotional description of the event (Affect) can also be described as General and Specific.

|  | Specific incident | General statement |
| --- | --- | --- |
| Content |  |  |
| Affect |  |  |

*Figure 4.4a* Interpersonal Incidents grid.

### Collecting information about a specific Interpersonal Incident

As noted above, an Interpersonal Incident is a specific episode in which a communication occurs between the client and a significant other. It is not a description of patterns of interaction. The therapist requests the young person to relate specific details of a communication with as much accuracy as possible, noting what was said by both parties, the manner in which it was said, and any affect that was connected to the incident. The therapist will focus on the manner in which the young person communicates attachment needs, being alert for maladaptive communication styles.

The first step in utilising the Interpersonal Incidents grid is to record the young person's General statement about communication with the significant other. In Tanya's case, her General statement is "Mum won't listen to me". (Figure 4.4b)

|         | Specific incident | General statement |
|---------|-------------------|-------------------|
| Content |                   | Mum won't listen to me |
| Affect  |                   |                   |

*Figure 4.4b* Interpersonal Incidents: General statements.

The second step is to record the young person's affective responses to the General statement and to the relationship more broadly.

Tanya reported feeling sad, hopeless, and defeated. (Figure 4.4c)

|         | Specific incident | General statement |
|---------|-------------------|-------------------|
| Content |                   | Mum won't listen to me |
| Affect  |                   | Sad, hopeless, defeated |

*Figure 4.4c* Interpersonal Incidents: General affect.

The third step is to ask the young person to describe a specific Interpersonal Incident. The therapist requests a detailed description of a recent event, not a typical pattern of interaction, as this would reinforce the link between the general statement and the affective response.

For example, the therapist could ask the following:

*Therapist:* Tanya, when your Mum said you weren't allowed to go to the party, what did you say?

The therapist continues to encourage the young person to relate the precise details of the dialogue and also to attend to the emotional content. The goal here is to re-create in as much detail as possible a precise description of the interactions that occurred: the words used; tone of voice; body language; any behaviours such as hitting, punching walls, slamming doors, storming out in the middle of an argument, quietly withdrawing; and so on.

94  *Introduction*

*Tanya:* I didn't say much really.... I think I just said, "Why not?".
*Therapist:* And what did Mum say then?
*Tanya:* Just that I'm growing up too quickly and I'll be able to go to those parties when I'm older.
*Therapist:* What happened next?
*Tanya:* Well, not much. There's no point in arguing with her.

The therapist should also pay particular attention to how the interchange ended, as often young people run out of communication options towards the end of conflict situations and may demonstrate self-defeating or aggressive behaviours in the absence of any alternative.

*Therapist:* So what did you do?
*Tanya:* Went outside—I just wanted to be by myself. I felt bad that the others were going and I'd be letting them down 'cos I'm the singer.
*Therapist:* When did you see Mum again?
*Tanya:* She called me soon after to bath the twins.
*Therapist:* And did you and Mum talk about the party again?
*Tanya:* Not really ... it's like it's over then.... There's no point in arguing.... She'll never change her mind.

Asking about a specific incident allowed the therapist to clearly examine the communication that was occurring and to observe Tanya's response in detail, providing more accurate conclusions about what was driving the interaction and what might be done to resolve it. Tanya's response is recorded in Figure 4.4d.

|  | Specific incident | General statement |
|---|---|---|
| Content | Mum refused to let me go out | Mum won't listen to me |
| Affect |  | Sad, hopeless, defeated |

*Figure 4.4d* Interpersonal Incidents: Specific incident.

The fourth step is to connect emotional responses to the specific incident. The therapist asks questions about what emotions were conveyed, how the young person felt during and after the incident, and about the young person thought the other was responding emotionally.

Therapist: How were you feeling inside then, Tanya?
Tanya: I don't know.... Nothing.... What can you do?
Therapist: How do you think your mum was feeling then Tanya?
Tanya: I dunno. She won again.

From Tanya's response, her feeling state would be characterised as numb and helpless and defeated, which are recorded in Figure 4.4e.

|  | Specific incident | General statement |
|---|---|---|
| Content | Mum refused to let me go out | Mum won't listen to me |
| Affect | Numb, helpless, defeated | Sad, hopeless, defeated |

*Figure 4.4e* Interpersonal Incidents: Specific affect.

The purpose in clarifying the specific communication and the associated affect is to examine the ways in which the young person may be ineffectively communicating attachment needs. In the above dialogue, Tanya, in not communicating with her mother, left her with a sense of helplessness and defeat ("What can you do?"; "She won again"), which would then reinforce her general statement (and belief) that "Mum won't listen to me". This then promotes noncommunication in future interchanges, completing this maladaptive circle. This clarification assists the therapist and young person to identify some specific problems in communication and suggest some strategies that may help the young person communicate more effectively.

## Analysing the Interpersonal Incident

The aim of this analysis is to help the young person understand how his or her ineffective communication contributes to distress and symptoms. When the therapeutic alliance is strong, particularly with securely attached young people, this process can be fairly direct, but with clients who are avoidant or preoccupied, the feedback to the young person must be more circumspect.

After the Interpersonal Incident has been established and clarified, the therapist and young person go through the dialogue once more in detail, with the focus being on what the young person was trying to communicate. Asking Tanya what she was trying to communicate and what her mother may have heard, in contrast to what was actually spoken or communicated, can make these discrepancies transparent for both young person and therapist to consider in further analysis.

96  Introduction

*Therapist:* So Tanya, we've just worked out at the end of that conversation with your mother you felt nothing inside, just numb, but also I think the word you used was "helpless"—and you felt also that Mum had won.
*Tanya:* Well, she had. I didn't get to go to the party, so she won.
*Therapist:* Do you think your mum would have known how you felt about it?
*Tanya:* Well, she did when I ended up in hospital.
*Therapist:* But what about then ... when you were having that conversation. Do you think she knew how you were feeling about not going?
*Tanya:* Probably not.

At this point the therapist asks the young person one of the key questions of IPT-A: "How well did you feel understood?" This is a central question because at the heart of IPT-A is the premise that clients' distress and symptoms are being perpetuated (and often precipitated) by the ineffective communications clients are using in attempt to have attachment needs met.

When the therapist asks, "How well do you feel understood?" it may be the first time any adult has ever shown that level of interest in the young person's interpersonal world and in this respect provides an opportunity for deepening the therapeutic alliance. Most clients will answer that they don't feel very well understood at all. They have not discovered how to communicate with others in such a way that their attachment needs are being met, and as a consequence of unmet attachment needs, particularly at a time of interpersonal crisis, respond with feelings of being misunderstood and feeling alone. The therapist's response to the young person's disclosure of not feeling understood will be something like "Well that's what we can work on—helping you communicate with people who are important to you, so that you begin to feel better understood by them". This is precisely the brief of IPT-A: to help young people communicate their attachment needs and needs for support more clearly and to develop and utilise a social support system that can respond to those needs. Once the young person has disclosed his or her sense of being misunderstood and alone, the therapist will explain that the next phase of therapy is designed to address that very problem—to identify communication strategies that are ineffective and to develop some alternative strategies that will facilitate their communication with significant others.

In analysing the Interpersonal Incidents, the therapist attempts to collect more data and to generate insight in the young person. The goal is to move the client from the feelings of helplessness, sadness, hopelessness, and emptiness to the feeling of being misunderstood. This reframes the situation into one that the therapist and young person can do something about, including assisting the client to understand what the other in the dyad is experiencing. (Understanding "the other" in the dyad is explored in Chapter 8.)

*Therapist:* Tanya, I'd like to go back through that conversation you had with your mum to see if there may have been any other way that it could have gone that would have worked out better for you. Is that okay?

| | |
|---|---|
| Tanya: | I still couldn't have gone though. |
| Therapist: | See, Tanya, when we look back at that table we just drew up, I can't help but think that your mum got the wrong message. She thought you didn't care too much about not going. She even said she was pleased with how well you took it. |
| Tanya: | Well, that way we don't fight. |
| Therapist: | So at that moment, how well do you think your mum understood you? |
| Tanya: | She didn't get it at all. |
| Therapist: | And what about you. What was it like for you, to feel Mum didn't understand you? |
| Tanya: | Guess I'm used to it now. |
| Therapist: | "Used to it now".... And you don't like to fight with your mum. Maybe that feeling of being misunderstood is easier to take than fighting, Tanya? |
| Tanya: | Maybe. Except look where it got me. (Referring to her suicide attempt.) |
| Therapist: | You know, I was just thinking that. Maybe easier than fighting in the short term, but in the long term it sort of adds up. |
| Tanya: | Misunderstood. It's kinda like a tug-o-war, you know. I don't think Mum's ever understood about my friends. She seems interested sometimes, but I think it's fake—just so she thinks she's being a good mum. Especially about the band. She thinks it's something I'll grow out of. She just doesn't get it. |
| Therapist: | Tug-o-war? |
| Tanya: | Yeah, like fighting with Mum about what I want to do is on one side and just keeping the peace on the other side. And it's always about keeping the peace. |
| Therapist: | So keeping the peace wins, but then you feel your mum doesn't get you. |
| Tanya: | Yeah—I think that's right—you can't feel misunderstood all your life. It adds up. |

In the above interchange, the therapist and Tanya shifted the affective focus from "numb, helpless, defeated" towards the direction of "misunderstood" recorded in Figure 4.4f.

| | Specific incident | General statement |
|---|---|---|
| Content | Mum refused to let me go out | Mum won't listen to me |
| Affect | Numb, helpless, defeated, *Misunderstood* | Sad, hopeless, defeated |

*Figure 4.4f* Interpersonal Incidents: Identifying misunderstandings.

### Changing communication

Once the original affective responses to the Interpersonal Incident have been reframed to include "being misunderstood", the therapist and client together explore alternative strategies that would contribute to communicating differently. More of the same communication strategies will produce more of the same results. Young people usually respond well to this concept, and stories such as this adaptation of a story told by Glasser (1976) often reinforce this critical point in a meaningful way:

> *I was on a picnic with some friends and family a little while ago. We were relaxing in a park by the water, and right next to the park was a boat ramp, where people launch their boats before their day out on the water, then retrieve them when they come back. This guy brought his boat in and while his mate was holding it steady in the shallow water, he went to get his car. He reversed down the concrete ramp, hooked the boat up, then proceeded up the ramp a bit to drain the boat, tie it onto the trailer properly, and connect the electrics to his car. Although the trailer was still on the concrete ramp the car itself was just off the concrete—on some sand. When the guy tried towing the boat up the ramp, the back wheels of his car started spinning in the sand. I was watching the action and wondered what the guy would do. He had lots of options—there were palm fronds around—he could have jammed some of them under his back wheels for more traction; he possibly could have reversed back a bit until his car wheels were also on the concrete and tried again. But no—he must have liked the sound of spinning wheels because he just put his foot down further on the throttle. The wheels spun more—digging quite a hole in the sand. He stopped for a little while, but then more throttle—a deeper hole—until the whole chassis of the car was sitting on the sand and he had to ask another driver for a tow.*

Stories last longer in memory than facts and information. The moral of this story of course is "if something is not working it's probably best not to do more of the same, but to try something else". Young people will, if given the opportunity, often tell the therapist a story of their own that illustrates the same point. It is well worth the time reinforcing this point, because in interpersonal communication, if something is not working (that is, not effectively meeting attachment needs), it is good practice to try something else.

*Tanya:* So you think I'm like that guy with the boat. What I'm doing isn't working, but I keep doing it anyway.
*Therapist:* What do you think?
*Tanya:* In some ways, maybe. But what else am I supposed to do? Whatever I do I'm still stuck. Remember that tug-o-war?
*Therapist:* Yeah, I do. Can we just look at that table again? When you look at the bottom left box it's got "numb, helpless, defeated", but it's also got "misunderstood" now. And you were telling me that in the long term

|  | *being misunderstood is a pretty powerful experience.* |
|---|---|
| Tanya: | *So what do you think I should do about it then?* |
| Therapist: | *I'm hoping we can work something out together. So can we focus on being misunderstood for a bit...got any ideas?* |
| Tanya: | *It's just that if I tell Mum stuff, she still won't let me do what I want, then I'm back where I started but I've wasted the energy telling her.* |
| Therapist: | *Okay I get that. Plus there's the possibility of an argument, and I know you want to avoid them. I'm just wondering if there's a way your mum could understand you better. Like now, with you not saying much, she just doesn't get you.... Do you want her to get you better, Tanya?* |
| Tanya: | *Yeah, I do. I suppose I could start with the band. Like my music teacher says, I've got heaps of talent, and the others in the band are all older and they love my singing—I just want Mum to see that. That it's not just a passing thing. I do get that she doesn't want me to go to gigs where there's heaps of grog and weed. And anyway I'm not even allowed into pubs yet—I'm only 15.* |
| Therapist: | *Can we go back to that table? So if you were somehow able to talk to your mum about that and then you felt she did understand you better, would those feelings—numb, defeated, helpless—change?* |
| Tanya: | *If she understood about the band, I'd still be pissed off that I can't go, so I guess I'd be more angry than numb. But if she did understand, it wouldn't seem like a battle so much—so not so much helpless and defeated. More just pissed off.* |
| Therapist: | *Okay. Let's think about how you could get your mum to understand you better.* |

At the end of the discussion of this Interpersonal Incident, Tanya had a slightly different understanding of the nature of the relationship between herself and her mother. Tanya was able to predict that if she told her mother more about what she valued and what she wanted, even in a single area—her band—then her mother would understand her more. She still may not always get what she wants, but her feelings would move from the paralysing tryptic of "numb, helpless, defeated" as well as "misunderstood" to the more "call-to-action" response of "pissed off". This response is consistent with the normative adolescent process of disagreeing with parents as part of the larger goal of creating a separate and independent identity.

This change is depicted graphically in Figure 4.4g, which also summarises this process of utilising Interpersonal Incidents. Tanya's General statement began with the assertion "Mum won't listen to me" and the associated affect was "sad, hopeless, defeated". When discussing the Interpersonal Incident, Tanya initially described her affect as "numb, helpless, defeated". As the incident was discussed in detail and as "being misunderstood" was introduced, Tanya came to see that the feeling of being misunderstood was prominent. Tanya also identified that her tendency not to communicate how she was feeling with her mother precipitated then perpetuated her feeling of being misunderstood. She eventually envisaged the possibility that if she did communicate with her mother a bit

|         | Specific incident | General statement |
|---------|-------------------|-------------------|
| Content | Mum refused to let me go out, but she didn't know how important it was to me. | Mum won't listen to me, but I don't tell her much |
| Affect  | Pissed off but not so *misunderstood* | A bit suspicious but more hopeful than before |

*Figure 4.4g* Interpersonal Incidents: Affective shift.

more, her mother might begin to understand her. Tanya freely acknowledged she still wouldn't get everything she wanted and that she would remain angry about that, but at least she would feel that her mother was understanding her better. We will return to Tanya later.

Having attachment needs met doesn't always mean getting what you want, but it does have a lot to do with feeling understood by significant others.

Interpersonal Incidents in many ways form the foundation of the clinical techniques used in IPT-A. Discussing these incidents is one of the most powerful means of gathering information about clients' relational world. It is this information therapists use to assist clients to make the changes that will ensure their attachment needs are more effectively addressed.

Interpersonal Incidents are often associated with key moments in therapy. Lemma et al. (2011) identify five steps that facilitate the use of Interpersonal Incidents.

First, mark a moment in the interpersonal exchange by inviting the client to pause and reflect on the exchange. For example,

*Therapist:* I'd like to stop for a moment and think about what's happening here.

Second, explore the feelings that are not directly communicated.

*Therapist:* I'm getting the feeling that you're not happy about having to be here today, but for some reason you're not too comfortable talking to me about that.

Third, empathise with the client and begin to explore what may underlie the current interaction.

*Therapist:* You're just very quiet today and you're not looking at me or saying much at all really. I do understand how hard it is for you. You're struggling with pretty strong feelings about things right now—you're angry, but instead of telling me how you're feeling, you've just kind of shut down.

Fourth, link the interaction with the therapist with other interpersonal issues that are the focus of therapy.

*Therapist:* We worked out earlier that your Problem Area is Interpersonal Disputes, right? I'm wondering if what is happening here today is pretty much what happens when you have a problem with your parents. Instead of being able to let them know what is going on for you, you tend to withdraw. And then you feel even more alone because they just don't understand you.

Fifth, return to an Interpersonal Incident outside the therapy room, use this new information to assist the client to recognise the maladaptive nature of his or her response, and then collaboratively develop a better alternative.

Continuing the case of **Steph:**

*Therapist:* So can we think for a moment about that? Maybe there's a pattern there for you. You get angry with something your mum says and then withdraw into yourself. But then no one understands what's going on for you, and you get even angrier and still no one gets it. I remember your mum said she's proud of the way you handle arguments at home. When you go quiet, she thinks it's all over but for you that's when you're stewing about stuff and getting more and more quietly angry. But because no one knows, there's no opportunity to do anything about it. And sometimes you get so frustrated—that's when you cut yourself.
*Steph:* It's always like that. No one listens. I just feel like screaming or something, but I just can't.
*Therapist:* You were telling me last session about the last time you cut. I think it was that same pattern wasn't it?
*Steph:* Pretty much.
*Therapist:* Let's just return to that scene you told me about. Your mum said you had to do the shopping, but you had made plans with your friends. I remember you said you just went up to your room and got angrier and angrier. After a while you cut yourself to get rid of those feelings, and it worked for a while. But then you still had to deal with the problem that caused your anger. So let's see if there might have been a different way of doing things that night. Any thoughts?

The conversation that followed explored options Steph had, other than to go quiet, ruminate, and get angrier. Collaboratively, the therapist and Steph identified ways to break this pattern, for example, by talking to her mother about the plans she had to go out with her friends and telling her mother about her disappointment. Whilst probably not changing the outcome, new patterns such as this would provide Steph with an opportunity to communicate her feelings and thus feel, in her words, "less unheard".

## Conflict-solving styles

Conflict is a part of the life experience of most adolescents and if not well managed can exacerbate distress or symptomatology. Building capacity around resolving conflicts between the young person and significant others in their lives can have a role in each of the four Problem Areas identified in IPT-A. In IPT-A, young people learn a lot about their mental distress or disorder, but equally importantly, a lot about themselves. Young people are often surprised to learn about their habitual responses to conflict situations. They are often equally surprised to learn that there may be other ways of responding to conflict. Once they have learned about these other ways, they are able to choose if they want to respond in their habitual way and, if not, to do something different. Fisher, Ury, and Patton's (1991) approach to conflict styles is particularly suited for young people. They propose five habitual responses to interpersonal conflict: Withdrawal, Suppression, Compromise, Win/Lose, and Win/Win. These responses are described in Figure 4.5.

The key issue is not so much the end point but the goals or motivations that underlie the methods of dealing with the conflict. One can approach an interpersonal conflict with the goal of Win/Win, but the Win/Win outcome is not guaranteed. However, the behaviours, cognitions, and affect involved in the process will be distinctly different from those employed by a client who was more used to dealing with conflict through, for example, Suppression. Young people are often fascinated to discover their habitual style of dealing with conflict and are, on the most part, keen to experiment with new possibilities. This fascination drives the development of new interpersonal learning that can contribute significantly to positive therapeutic outcome, particularly for young people whose identified Problem Area is Interpersonal Disputes.

**Tanya**, after learning about the five conflict-solving styles had little trouble identifying her default position as Suppression. This style was demonstrated in dialogue reported above, but Tanya also saw it as characteristic of several other interactions she had recently had with her mother, friends, and some teachers. She also recognised this style as characteristic of her interactions before she became depressed.

*Therapist:* So you think the second style, Suppression, most closely fits what you do when you're having an argument with someone?

*Tanya:* (Pause) Yeah, nearly always, come to think of it.... It's like it's better to pretend everything's okay. That way there'll be less fights.

*Therapist:* Less fights are important for you Tanya, I remember the tug-o-war, but I'm wondering what the downside of this style might be.

*Tanya:* I just don't like conflict. This way keeps conflict low ... but it never really changes anything.

*Therapist:* And in the end, you feel defeated.... So how do you think that conversation with your mum about the party would have gone if you had used one of the other styles....say if you had used "Win/Lose"?

| Style for addressing conflict: | **Withdrawal** |
|---|---|
| Strategies employed: | Sulk. Refuse to talk. Walk away. Punish with silence. Often a passive aggressive attitude. |
| Attitude to the relationship: | No relationship: no direct communication. |
| People vs problem: | Hard on the people, ineffectual on the problem. |
| Who wins? | No one, the issue is not addressed. |
| **Style for addressing conflict:** | **Suppression** |
| Strategies employed: | Stay cheerful or resigned and treat the problem as if it doesn't exist. Sometimes the "martyr complex" is apparent. |
| Attitude to the relationship: | Preserve the status quo at all costs. |
| People vs problem: | Easy on the people, ineffectual on the problem. |
| Who wins? | On the surface win/win, but someone is losing. |
| **Style for addressing conflict:** | **Compromise** |
| Strategies employed: | Make concessions to preserve the relationship. |
| Attitude to the relationship: | Non-assertive, but participants are cooperating. |
| People vs problem: | Easy on the people, sometimes soft on the problem. |
| Who wins? | Because both give a bit, neither is totally satisfied. |
| **Style for addressing conflict:** | **Win/lose** |
| Strategies employed: | Demand concessions, using power over the other to achieve the outcome. |
| Attitude to the relationship: | Aggressive. |
| People vs problem: | Hard on the people and tough on the problem. |
| Who wins? | One wins, one loses. (But often the winner's outcome is sabotaged by the dissatisfied loser.) |
| **Style for addressing conflict:** | **Win/win** |
| Strategies employed: | Negotiate a mutually acceptable solution. |
| Attitude to the relationship: | Assertive. Participants are the problem-solvers. |
| People vs problem: | Easy on the people and tough on the problem. |
| Who wins? | Both get what they want. |

*Figure 4.5* Identification of Conflict-Solving Styles (Adapted from Fisher, Ury, and Patton, 1991).

Tanya:     I dunno (smiles).... Maybe I would have yelled at her and just gone. I win, she loses.
Therapist: I notice you're smiling.
Tanya:     I'm just thinking of Mum's face....

Young people often have quite a bit of fun exploring the different styles of dealing with conflict in relationships. Tanya, whose default style was Suppression, quite enjoyed exploring other styles and proposing how things would have ended differently had she employed an alternative style. The clear message to Tanya was that there is more than one way of doing things.

The therapist encourages clients to reflect on any interpersonal consequences that may occur as a result of using the different styles. The therapist may discuss with young clients that they can choose a style of conflict to match a situation, that some styles may be better than others for different situations, and that they don't have to use one style all the time. For example, for low level conflict, Withdrawal and Suppression may buy a bit of time and allow the conflict to resolve by itself, without drawing unnecessary attention to the issue. But for conflict that is more intense or has been around for some time, the young person perhaps should consider Compromise or Win/Win. It may also be helpful to ask the young person to see if she can come up with a situation where Win/Lose may be the most appropriate style. Whilst exploring these styles with the young person, it is important for the clinician to remain mindful of the link between the client's depression and the dysfunctional relationship patterns of which the conflict style is just one example. Empathically drawing the client's attention to this link may be another reminder to the young person that her depression or distress is not random but is an integral part of their interpersonal world, over which she is gaining an increasing level of control.

*Therapist:* *Tanya let's just think about Win/Win for a moment. Going back to the conversations you and your mum had about going to that party, how do you think that would have gone if you had gone for Win/Win rather than used Suppression?*

*Tanya:* *Win/Win? So we both get what we want. I dunno, Mum didn't want me to go—I did want to go. How can we both get what we want?*

*Therapist:* *What do you think is behind your mum not wanting you to go?*

*Tanya:* *She doesn't want me to get raped that's all. Nah, it's more than that—that's part of it but she thinks I'm doing stuff now that 18-year-olds are doing.*

*Therapist:* *Just wondering if your mum knew beforehand how important the band was to you, maybe you could both have given a little bit. What style would that be?*

*Tanya:* *Compromise?*

*Therapist:* *How do you think the conversation would have gone then?*

*Tanya:* *Maybe work out a deal—like just go until 11:00 or something? At least I'd get to do some of the band stuff then. Or maybe Mum could come along for a while. She knows Jay's mum and they could hang out in the kitchen or something.*

*Therapist:* *So Tanya, I've just noticed a shift in two areas. First, you're thinking about letting your mum know a bit more about what's important to you—communicating with her more—and second, you now know you can use more problem solving styles than just Suppression, the one you're most used to using.*

Analysing and using these strategies for addressing conflict situations is an exercise most clients find intrinsically engaging and easily leads to other strategies for effectively communicating feelings and opinions accurately and empathically. The therapist's continuing role is to demonstrate to clients how these skills, strategies, and attitudes will significantly contribute to the resolution of their symptoms by improving the degree of agency they are developing within their interpersonal world.

## Role play

In IPT-A, therapists help young people to learn to identify their own maladaptive communication styles, mainly through the analysis of communication patterns observed during the reporting of Interpersonal Incidents. Once these patterns are identified, the young person learns new ways of relating that are more likely to lead to their attachment needs being met. Role play is used to model and practice interactions between the young person and significant others. The use of role play is usually indicated when there is a strong therapeutic alliance such that the young person can tolerate a degree of confrontation by the therapist. Role play can be utilised in all of the Problem Areas and is particularly useful in the areas of Interpersonal Disputes and Interpersonal Gaps.

Stuart and Robertson (2012) note five goals when using role play:

1   To gather information about the client's style of communication.
2   To help the client develop new insights into his or her interpersonal behaviour.
3   To help the client to better understand the reactions of others to his or her communications.
4   To allow the therapist to model new modes of interpersonal behaviour and communication.
5   To allow the client to practice new interpersonal communication skills.

Role play adds to the information already gathered about the young person's communication styles by providing the opportunity to observe him or her, as it were, in the real world. When the young person is playing himself, the therapist can observe the words communicated and also the tone of voice, intensity, body language, eye contact, the displayed affect, and congruence between affect and verbal message as well as speculate about the young person's internal emotions. Role play importantly offers the therapist the opportunity to observe how the young person communicates affect and emotion to others and can use her own experience of the young person's communication style to either reinforce adaptive communications or provide feedback to the young person about communication behaviours that were less adaptive.

For example,

*Therapist:* Jane, I really got a sense of your frustration then. I think you're getting that message across to your mum really clearly.

Or, for example,

*Therapist:* Jorge, you were telling Karen that you were feeling sad about her going away. But somehow it came across to me as you being just kinda bored. And if Karen thought you were bored, maybe she'd respond differently to you than if she thought you were sad.

In role play activities, clients can alternate between playing themselves (and the therapist playing the other) and playing the other (with the therapist playing the young person). When the young person is playing the other, it gives him a unique opportunity to feel what it's like to be "in the other's shoes" for a few minutes and to experience what it is like to be on the other side of his own communications. This can be a powerful learning opportunity for some clients as, for perhaps the first time, they may see a side of themselves that was quite invisible to themselves, albeit visible to others. In the above example, when roles were reversed and the therapist played **Jorge** and Jorge played Karen, Jorge was quite surprised at how emotionally flat he came across when he thought he was displaying appropriate sadness. This helped Jorge better understand Karen's response to him (Jorge was upset that Karen just shrugged off his comments about her leaving) and paved the way for learning and rehearsing communication patterns in which there was more consistency between felt emotion and displayed affect.

There are several steps involved when using role playing as a tool for implementing changes. First, the therapist explains to the young person that the exercise is about looking for new ways of communicating when the existing ways aren't working all that well. The exercise is not about criticism, but about exploring patterns of communication.

Second, the therapist and young person should select a manageable Interpersonal Incident that is relevant to the Problem Area and symptomatology.

Third, the incident will be discussed, and a rough transcript developed that preserves with as much accuracy as possible the details of the actual event.

Fourth, the young person and therapist role play the incident with the young person playing himself or herself and the therapist the other. This step may be repeated several times until the young person is satisfied that it is an accurate portrayal of the actual event.

Fifth, the therapist and young person discuss the details, particularly whether or not the other actually got the correct message from the young person.

Questions that may be helpful include the following:

- *What did you do that was good?*
- *Did you think you got your message across?*
- *What feelings did you recognise in yourself?*
- *What new things did you learn?*
- *How do you think Karen might have been feeling?*
- *Is there anything you would want to change?*

Sixth, if there is anything the young person would like to change, or if the therapist would like to suggest some alternatives, the therapist and young person collaboratively propose alternative communication strategies, which are then incorporated into the new version of the role play. The goal of this step is to explore other ways of communicating in order to convey more accurately the client's attachment needs. Once these new strategies have been discussed, the therapist may suggest a role change, so the therapist can model existing and alternative communication behaviours. For example,

*Therapist:* Jorge, you were telling Karen that you were feeling very sad about her going away. But somehow it came across to me as you being just kinda bored. And if Karen thought you were bored, maybe she'd respond differently to you than if she thought you were sad. Can you understand how Karen may have misunderstood you?

*Jorge:* I didn't want to be all needy and stuff. But I wasn't trying to seem bored.... And I am sad she's going.

*Therapist:* So how do you think you could have shown her that—without being all needy?

*Jorge:* I dunno—maybe used different words or something?

*Therapist:* Let's just swap for a minute—I'll be you and you be Karen. Okay?

*Jorge:* Okay.

*Therapist:* We'll just do that bit from where you asked her when she was going.

*Therapist:* (as Jorge) (Soft voice, mumbling a bit and looking at his feet) So how long are you going for?

*Jorge:* (as Karen) About four years; Dad's got a transfer to London.

*Therapist:* (as Jorge) When are you going?

*Jorge:* (as Karen) In about three weeks.

*Therapist:* (as Jorge) Oh, okay—have a good time.

*Jorge:* (as Karen) Okay. See ya.

*Therapist:* We'll just stop there for a minute Jorge. So you were Karen then—how do you think she was feeling during that?

*Jorge:* Not sure. Probably she thought I didn't care.

*Therapist:* Okay. Let's just try something. You're still Karen and I'm still you.

*Therapist:* (as Jorge) (Slightly louder voice, speaking a little more clearly, looking directly at Jorge playing Karen). So how long are you going for?

*Jorge:* (as Karen) About four years, Dad's got a transfer to London.

*Therapist:* (as Jorge) When are you going?

108  Introduction

| | |
|---|---|
| Jorge: | (as Karen) In about three weeks. |
| Therapist: | (as Jorge) Four years is a long time. I'm gonna miss you. |
| Jorge: | (as Karen) (spontaneously) Yeah? |
| Therapist: | (as Jorge) Wanna have coffee before you go? |
| Jorge: | Laughs. |
| Therapist: | So Jorge, what differences did you notice? |
| Jorge: | Your words, you said "I'm gonna miss you". |
| Therapist: | I did say that, but nearly all the other words were yours. Notice anything else? |
| Jorge: | Not really—except the bit about "a long time". |
| Therapist: | Let me point out a difference to you. It's not so much to do with the words, but how you deliver them. Did you notice where I was looking when I was talking to Karen? |
| Jorge: | You were looking at me. |
| Therapist: | So when you noticed I was looking at you, how did that make you feel? |
| Jorge: | Like you were interested? |
| Therapist: | Not bored? |
| Jorge: | Not bored. |
| Therapist: | Needy? |
| Jorge: | Not needy. |
| Therapist: | Okay so let's change again—you be you and I'll be Karen. This time, look at me, clear voice, and use your words. Maybe add that bit about "I'm gonna miss you" if you want to. |

The therapist and Jorge replay the role play. This time Jorge looks directly at the therapist and speaks more clearly. He does add "I'm gonna miss you".

| | |
|---|---|
| Therapist: | So how was that Jorge? |
| Jorge: | Yeah better, I think. It made a big difference looking at her. And it helped me say "I'm gonna miss you"—I am gonna miss her. |
| Therapist: | So let's just spend a bit of time going over that. First, what do you think you did well? |

The therapist continued to draw out Jorge's response to the new role play, focussing particularly on the communication of feelings and on the specific things Jorge learnt from the experience. By the conclusion of the session, Jorge believed he had worked out how to show Karen he would miss her without appearing to her to be needy. Jorge also commented he now understood how Karen would have thought he was uninterested in her going away. He suggested he could approach Karen again before the next session to try to correct things.

### Empty chair technique

Not all young people, nor all therapists, will be comfortable with using role play. The empty chair technique is a slight variation on role play and provides an alternative for some young people. This method was pioneered by Fritz Perls, the founder of Gestalt Therapy, (1973), and has also been used more widely by therapists from other theoretical orientations (Elliott et al., 2004). The empty chair approach when used in IPT-A is a form of self-dialogue in which the young person speaks to an empty chair as if a significant other were sitting in it. Similarly to role play, the young person can also play the role of the significant other by swapping chairs. The therapist has the role of observer and director, calling the young person's attention to what has been said and how it was said and directing the young person's attention to affect or emotions in either himself or herself or perceived in the other. The goals of the empty chair in IPT-A are to help clients (1) be more aware of their own thoughts and feelings towards others; (2) understand how their words and actions affect others; (3) develop an awareness of the feelings of others; and (4) modify their communication with others, based on information gathered from (1) to (3) above.

The empty chair approach can be effectively used with all the Problem Areas in IPT-A. For example, in Complex Grief, many young people report difficulty communicating with close others following their loss. Clients report a distance develops between themselves and people in their lives who, prior to the loss were close, maybe even in their inner circle. The empty chair technique can be used to help clients reconnect with these significant others, enabling a more productive communication that will assist meeting the young person's attachment needs.

**Erin**, aged 16, who is discussed further in Chapter 5, developed depressive disorder following significant losses, including feeling disconnected from her friend and confidante, Dallas. Erin indicated she would like to see Dallas again and that she really missed him, but because they had not spoken for a while Erin felt uncomfortable about reconnecting with him.

*Therapist:* *Erin, a couple of sessions ago you told me that you really missed Dallas but still couldn't bring yourself to talk to him yet. Has that changed at all?*
*Erin:* *Not really. I still see him at school, but we just don't talk. Not like we used to. We talk shit at lunch and stuff but that's all—nothing meaningful.*
*Therapist:* *And you said you'd probably want him back in your inner circle in the future?*
*Erin:* *Yeah, I suppose.*
*Therapist:* *I want to try something today. It's called the empty chair—for good reason that you'll get in a minute. I just want to check out that it's okay with you. So we're going to use this empty chair here and, to begin, imagine that Dallas is sitting in it—and you're sitting opposite him, here in your chair. And then I'm going to ask you and Dallas to have a conversation. I don't want to say too much more about it now Erin—we'll talk about what happens later. Any questions?*
*Erin:* *No—sounds weird though.*
*Therapist:* *It does a bit. Okay to give it a go?*
*Erin:* *Okay.*

| | |
|---|---|
| Therapist: | Well to begin with can you picture Dallas sitting in that chair opposite? Tell me what he's wearing? |
| Erin: | Okay so he's wearing grey shorts, trainers, that red Alice Cooper t-shirt he always wears. |
| Therapist: | And how is he sitting? |
| Erin: | (Erin adjusts how she is sitting to mimic how she imagines Dallas sitting). |
| Therapist: | What expression does he have on his face Erin? |
| Erin: | He looks kinda confused and a bit sarcastic. But he always looks like that. |
| Therapist: | Erin would you change chairs for a bit and be Dallas? I'd like to meet him and you know him really well so you can help me get to know him.[2] |
| Erin: | Okay (Erin changes chairs). |
| Therapist: | Dallas thanks for being here. I like your t-shirt! Can you tell me how long you've known Erin? |
| Erin: | (As Dallas) Since we started high school. |
| Therapist: | And where did you meet? |
| Erin: | (As Dallas) We met on the bus on the way to school. |
| Therapist: | So you've known her for over four years and you met on the bus. What do you like most about her? |
| Erin: | (As Dallas) I don't know. Maybe what she used to be like. |
| Therapist: | So Dallas you've noticed a change in Erin lately. Do you understand what's been going on for her? |
| Erin: | (As Dallas) I know she found out she was colour-blind and couldn't be in the Air Force anymore. Plus her dog died. I know she needed to be by herself for a while. |
| Therapist: | Is that it? |
| Erin: | (As Dallas) Yeah pretty much. |
| Therapist: | Erin could you change chairs. You're Erin again now. I guess lots of thoughts crossed your mind while you were being Dallas. So what do want to say to Dallas? He's sitting opposite you. |
| Erin: | It was more than that Dallas. You know that. It wasn't just about the Air Force, it was my whole life. It was like I died. Then Pepe. And it just got worse. (Erin cries) |
| Therapist: | (Pause) Change chairs again now Erin. So now you're Dallas again. Just focus for a minute on how Dallas may be feeling. Can you do that? |
| Erin: | Yes. I guess he's just getting how serious this is for me. I think he's a bit surprised because I'm usually the strong one. |
| Therapist: | What does Dallas want to do now that he gets it more? |
| Erin: | Not much—he never does much. But just knowing he understands.... |
| Therapist: | Dallas was really close to you and up to now you've felt he hasn't understood just how sad you've been. You haven't been able to tell him. And there's been a real distance between you. But telling him just now what it has been like for you and him getting it, that makes a difference. |
| Erin: | I really do miss him. I just miss him knowing how I'm feeling and him calling me to check up. And me calling him at 2:00 in the morning if I want to. |

During this interchange and the discussion that followed, Erin learned at least five things about her current relationship with Dallas: (1) Erin had concluded Dallas did not grasp the significance of her losses; (2) he had not grasped this because Erin hadn't told him; (3) if Erin did talk to Dallas, she was sure he would understand; (4) if they continued their relationship as it had been prior to Erin's losses, she would at least experience the understanding and support she was used to; and (5) within the context of this supportive relationship, Erin suggested that at least some of her symptoms of depression, isolation and loneliness, anger and irritability, anhedonia and self-doubt, would begin to resolve.

The next step with Erin was to plan and rehearse an interaction with Dallas. The empty chair technique would again be employed, giving Erin the opportunity to experiment with language and to monitor feelings in both herself and in playing Dallas. Erin would then organise to meet Dallas prior to the next session of therapy. The outcome of this interaction would be explored including what went well, what could be improved, and the affect and emotions that Erin noticed during the interaction with Dallas. The therapist would guide the conversation to assist Erin to extract learning of a more general nature that may help her to meet her attachment needs more effectively in other relationships.

## Interpersonal mindfulness

Mindfulness is the awareness of one's thoughts, feelings, and body sensations at that moment while striving not to judge them (Kabat-Zinn, 1994; 2005). Mindfulness has been included in a number of mental health interventions for example, Mindfulness-Based Cognitive Therapy (e.g., Segal et al., 2002), Acceptance and Commitment Therapy (e.g., Hayes et al., 2011), and Dialectical Behaviour Therapy (e.g., Linehan, 2014; Mazza et al., 2016; Rathus and Miller, 2014). Mindfulness has not previously been incorporated into the IPT literature and research but may be a helpful technique for addressing the aims of IPT-A by

- helping the young person to recognise responses in themselves that may undermine their efforts to communicate effectively with others
- increasing the young person's distress tolerance, including discomfort in interpersonal encounters

These benefits may help the young person to approach relationships in adaptive ways that are more likely to meet his or her attachment needs.

The characteristics of mindfulness are appealing to some young people because it is gentle, self-respectful, and noncoercive. Mindfulness is often taught by initially focussing attention on a particular body sensation, such as the breath, to cultivate calmness and stability. Awareness can then be broadened to noticing other body sensations, thoughts, or feelings. The aim is to observe without reacting. As the young person practices mindfulness, however, she notices that she inevitably does react. For example, she may analyse, evaluate, avoid, suppress, or judge what she observes. Cultivating an attitude of

112  *Introduction*

nonjudgment is key. When the young person notices that she is judging, then the idea is to take a step back and not judge the fact that she is judging but rather continue to observe and notice. As the young person becomes more conscious of her responses, she may become less entangled in them and gain a new perspective. This, in turn, can place her in a better position to choose to respond adaptively.

The young person may have tried unsuccessfully to change an unhelpful relationship pattern, only to find that their best efforts are counterproductive. The therapist might suggest that, instead of trying to change the dynamic, the client pays attention to see what he can learn, including the early signs that this behaviour is emerging. If the young person is able to do this, mindfulness may bring about adaptive changes.

For example, in the case of **Troy**, aged 19, his depression was related to Interpersonal Gaps (see Chapter 10). Troy was overly sensitive to negative feedback and often assumed he was being negatively judged by others. His habitual pattern of dealing with this was to withdraw from social interactions. He became increasingly isolated in his last year of high school and struggled to make friends at university. The therapist used a combination of role play and mindfulness to assist him to deepen his existing relationships and to establish new ones. Mindfulness helped Troy recognise when he was beginning to withdraw, which allowed him to question this response and to choose different ways of behaving. The therapist introduced mindfulness at the end of the sixth session.

*Therapist:*    *I'd like to sum up and suggest where we go from here. You've done brilliantly with our role plays. You recognise that you are prone to thinking other people are judging you negatively even when they may not be, and you've identified some alternative ways you could respond when you're feeling judged. Afterwards you realise that you might be overreacting, but when you're in the middle of it, it's hard to think like that. It's very uncomfortable and you want to get away. Understandably this makes it hard for you to remember the alternative strategies we've talked about.*

*Troy:*    *It's like I've already reacted before I realise what I'm doing.*

*Therapist:*    *Exactly, and there are some things we can do to help with that. Have you heard of mindfulness?*

*Troy:*    *Not sure.*

*Therapist:*    *It's similar to meditation. You mentioned you did some meditation in your yoga. (Troy nods.) It's about noticing what's going on internally. That might include body sensations, thoughts, and feelings. It can help us be more aware of our responses, and sometimes just by observing them without reacting they may shift and change. I'm going to suggest you start by letting go of trying to change this pattern of withdrawing for the time being. Sometimes when we struggle to change part of ourselves, it can be counterproductive. Would you be willing to pay attention to when you start to feel that others are judging you or that you're getting*

|            | the urge to pull away? See what you can notice, and we will discuss next week. |
|---|---|
| Troy: | Yes, but are you saying you want me to walk away if that's what I feel like doing? |
| Therapist: | I'm asking you to observe what you can about the urge to withdraw from people. For example, it might be you notice something like this going on in your mind: "I'm feeling uncomfortable. I'm noticing I'm thinking the guy I'm sitting next to in biology thinks I am a jerk. He probably thinks what I just said is stupid. They're making plans to go for a coffee after the tutorial. I'm feeling really uncomfortable. I want to get away. I will make an excuse". That might not be exactly what you notice but does that sound familiar? |
| Troy: | Yeah. |
| Therapist: | I'm suggesting you stop trying to change for now and just notice what you are actually experiencing. The ironic thing is that, as we observe a sensation, such as feeling uncomfortable or wanting to get away, we may notice it does begin to change. For example, you might not find it as overwhelming or automatic as it was. The discomfort might shift a little or you might find you can delay moving away from the situation but that's jumping ahead. Is this making sense to you? |
| Troy: | Yeah. It would be good if it wasn't so automatic. I don't realise I'm doing it. |
| Therapist: | I'll be interested in what you can report back next week. All you need to do is to be alert to when it's starting to happen and see what you can notice. |

Troy found that the therapist's suggestion that he stop trying to change was helpful. His urge to pull away from people when he felt uncomfortable became less automatic and he was able to respond in ways he had rehearsed in therapy, including talking with people he could trust about his discomfort.

There is more to mindfulness than can be addressed within IPT-A. Due to the time-limited nature of IPT-A, mindfulness instruction, along with the other clinical techniques, is restricted to directly addressing the aims of therapy. When appropriate, the therapist might suggest regular mindfulness practice as an adjunct to therapy to foster the young person's capacity for awareness in the present moment, as in the case of Troy. As Troy's interest grew, the therapist provided encouragement by suggesting he try adding a daily mindfulness practice to his yoga and discuss this with his yoga teacher. The therapist recommended a website and app that included guided mindfulness practice.

The cases of Ava, Kylie, and Caleb further illustrate ways that mindfulness can be used within IPT-A. Mindfulness is also discussed in Chapter 7 Complex Grief, Loss activity number 7.3: Body oriented approaches to grief and loss.

**Ava**, aged 14, (discussed in Chapter 10 Interpersonal Gaps) had difficulty controlling her anger, and this contributed to her being socially isolated. The therapist taught Ava anger management strategies. Ava was involved in a mindfulness program at her school and found this helpful in recognising her early warning signs of anger. This early recognition created opportunities for her to utilise strategies to prevent her anger escalating, such as briefly walking away from an encounter to get a drink of water. Additionally, the therapist encouraged Ava to be mindful of the physiological sensations of drinking water, which helped her to relax, and this increased the effectiveness of this strategy.

**Kylie**, aged 21, (see Chapter 7 Complex Grief) was uncomfortable with sharing her emotions about her mother dying. She avoided talking with others about her grief. This prevented her accessing the psychological and social support she needed and was a key factor in maintaining her depression. Mindfulness increased Kylie's capacity to tolerate her distress, which made it easier for her to share her feelings with others. As she did so, she felt closer to her significant others, and as the important people in her life came to understand more about her grief, they were able to respond in ways that were more attuned to her attachment needs.

**Caleb**, aged 19, (see Chapter 10 Interpersonal Gaps) experienced depression due to gaps in his nonverbal communication skills, which made it hard for him to initiate and maintain friendships. He had difficulty making eye contact and generally looked more severe and sombre than he intended. Mindfulness was key in helping Caleb to discover a new relationship with the discomfort he experienced during eye contact. By attending to his experience of eye contact, he learnt that he could endure his discomfort. Caleb was then able to develop more effective ways of communicating through discussion and role play with the therapist.

Mindfulness will not be appropriate for all young people. Contraindications may include severe depression, unresolved trauma, dissociation, or psychosis, where the ability to concentrate can be severely compromised (Britton, 2019). Even if the young person is able to concentrate, he or she may become increasingly focussed on the negative outlook of depression or the alternative reality of psychosis. It is good practice to monitor these in young people who are using mindfulness.

## Summary

The therapeutic relationship is central to an IPT-A intervention. The therapist strives to develop a relationship with the client best described as that of a transitory attachment figure, before strategically stepping back from this stance as therapy concludes. This relationship provides the context for the clinical techniques described above to be deployed within a therapeutic environment characterised by trust and safety. Towards the end of the intervention, the therapist and the young person will identify others in the client's interpersonal world who will be able to meet the client's ongoing attachment needs, focussing on how and with whom this may best occur.

This chapter describes some of the clinical techniques that may facilitate this process. The use of Interpersonal Incidents—the day-to-day relationship events that take place within the young person's life—remains a primary tool to explore the association between relationship difficulties and psychological distress. Techniques such as exploration of affect, role play, empty chair, interpersonal mindfulness, and strategies for managing conflict provide mechanisms to identify dysfunctional relationship patterns that contribute to psychological distress, replacing those patterns with relationship behaviours that are more likely to assist the young person to meet his or her attachment needs more effectively.

The list of clinical techniques described in this chapter is by no means exhaustive. Experienced clinicians will no doubt bring to IPT-A other strategies that they have found to be effective in their work with young people. However, to stay true to an IPT-A intervention, these strategies should focus on the identified Problem Area(s), within the negotiated timeframe and remain consistent with the three primary aims of IPT-A: (1) decrease symptomatology; (2) improve interpersonal functioning by enhancing communication skills in significant relationships and (3) strengthen social networks.

IPT-A offers clinicians a structure within which a range of clinical tools may be used to achieve these aims. The tools described in this chapter have been found to be demonstrably engaging for young people and effective in challenging habitual relationship patterns that contribute to distress and symptomatology.

## Notes

1 We acknowledge Scott Stuart and Michael Robertson, who developed the Interpersonal Incidents grid, and thank them for their permission to modify the grid for this text.
2 This strategy of suggesting the client begin the empty chair session by being "the other" was suggested by J. Moreno (1969) for two reasons. First, the therapist potentially gains valuable information about the other, and second, the other becomes "existentially present". That is, the empty chair is no longer empty, the other now occupies it, enabling the young person to experience the other as present in the moment.

## References

Britton, W. (2019). Can mindfulness be too much of a good thing? The value of a middle way. *Current Opinion in Psychology, 28*, 159–165.

Elliott, R., Watson, J., Goldman, R., & Greenberg, L. (2004). Empty chair work for for unfinished interpersonal issues. In R. Elliott, J. Watson, R. Goldman, & L. Greenberg, *Learning emotion-focused therapy: the process-experiential approach to change* (pp. 243–265). American Psychological Association.

Fisher, W., Ury, R., & B. Patton (1991). *Getting to yes: Negotiating an agreement without giving in (2nd Edition)*. Sydney: Century Business.

Glasser, W. (1976). *Ten-step discipline program (Video tape)*. Conference Presentation, NSW Department of Education, Sydney, August 1982.

Hause, J., & Pasnow, R. (Eds). (2014). *Thomas Aquinas: Basic works*. Indianapolis: Hackett Publishing Co.

Hayes, S., Strosahl, K., & Wilson, K. (2011). *Acceptance and Commitment Therapy: The Process and Practice of Mindful Change (2nd Edition)*. New York: Guilford Press.

Kabat-Zinn, J. (1994). *Wherever you go, there you are: Mindfulness meditation in everyday life*. New York: Hyperion.

Kiesler, D. J. (1996). *Contemporary interpersonal theory and research: Personality, psychopathology, and psychotherapy*. New York: Wiley.

Kiesler, D. J., & Watkins, L. M. (1989). Interpersonal complementarity and the therapeutic alliance: A study of relationship in psychotherapy. *Psychotherapy: Theory, Research, Practice, Training, 26*(2), 183–194.

Lemma, A., Target, M., & Fonagy, P. (2011). *Brief dynamic interpersonal psychotherapy. A clinician's guide*. Oxford: Oxford UP.

Linehan, M. (2014). *DBT (R) skills training manual (2nd Edition)*. New York: Guilford Press.

Mazza, J., Dexter-Mazza, E., Miller, A., Rathus, J., Murphy, H., & Linehan, M. (2016). *The Guilford practical intervention in the schools series. DBT (R) skills in schools: Skills training for emotional problem solving for adolescents (DBT STEPS-A)*. New York: Guilford Press.

Moreno, J. L. (1969). *Psychodrama volume 3: Action therapy and principles of practice*. New York: Beacon House.

Perls, F. (1973). *The gestalt approach and eye witness to therapy*. New York: Bantam Books.

Rathus, J., & Miller, A. (2014). *DBT(R) skills manual for adolescents*. New York: Guilford Press.

Segal, Z., Teasdale, J., & Williams, M. (2002). *Mindfulness-based cognitive therapy for depression*. New York: Guilford Press.

Sheard, T., Evans, J., Cash, R., Hicks, D., et al. (2000). A CAT-derived one to three session intervention for repeated deliberate self-harm: A description of the model and initial experience of trainee psychiatrists in using it. *Psychology and Psychotherapy: Theory and Research, 73*(2), 179–196.

Stuart, S., & Robertson, M. (2012). *Interpersonal psychotherapy: A clinician's guide (2nd Edition)*. London: Arnold.

Sullivan, H. S. (1954). *The psychiatric interview*. New York: Norton.

Yalom, I. (2002). *The gift of therapy: An open letter to a new generation of therapists and their patients*. New York: HarperCollins.

# Part II
# The Initial Phase of IPT-A

# 5 The Initial Phase of IPT-A

**Contents**

| | |
|---|---|
| Introduction | 119 |
| Client suitability | 120 |
| Psychoeducation | 120 |
| The Interpersonal Inventory | 125 |
|    1  *Developing an Interpersonal Map* | 126 |
|    2  *Linking life events to the presenting problem* | 130 |
|    3  *Identifying the Problem Area(s)* | 134 |
|    4  *Linking symptoms to the Problem Area* | 143 |
|    5  *Exploring attachment* | 145 |
| The Interpersonal Formulation | 147 |
| The Treatment Agreement | 148 |
| Orientation to the Middle Phase of treatment | 154 |
| Summary | 155 |
| References | 156 |

## Introduction

The Initial Phase of IPT-A usually comprises two to three sessions. The aim of these sessions is to explore the links between the young person's interpersonal world and their presenting problems. Although the Initial Phase is primarily a continuation of assessment, albeit with an interpersonal focus, the new insights gained during this phase and the developing therapeutic alliance suggest that therapy has already begun.

This chapter addresses client suitability for IPT-A, the continuing role of psychoeducation, the Interpersonal Inventory, the Interpersonal Formulation and the Treatment Agreement prior to beginning the Middle Phase of treatment.

## Client suitability

Determining if IPT-A is the best-fit intervention for the young person will depend on several factors, some of which will have been established during the holistic assessment. For example, the young person's willingness to be involved in therapy and his or her readiness to change will already have been canvassed. Further, the young person's ability to establish a relationship with the therapist and his or her willingness and availability to commit to therapy are also necessary components.

A recent meta-analysis of IPT-A studies concluded the following:

> "The results indicate that IPT-A was significantly effective at reducing depressive symptoms in adolescents and significantly more effective than control or treatment-as-usual groups in treating depression in adolescents. IPT-A yielded an overall effect size (Hedges' g corrected effect size) of 1.19, while the aggregate effect size for control/placebo groups was 0.58. Overall, the results of this review suggest that IPT-A holds similar promise for improving adolescent depression as the original version does for adults".
> (Mychailyszyn and Elson, 2018, p. 123)

Although IPT-A was initially designed for non-psychotic adolescents with unipolar depression who were not actively suicidal, and whose parents or caregivers were prepared to be involved in the therapeutic process (Mufson et al., 1993), with additional research its effectiveness and efficacy with a wider population of young people have been demonstrated. For example IPT-A has demonstrated efficacy with adolescents with bipolar presentation (Hlastala, 2010), depressed adolescents with suicidal risk (Tang et al., 2009), depressed young people with coexisting anxiety (Young et al., 2006), some adolescents with eating disorders (Tanofsky-Kraff, 2010), and for adolescents who engaged in non-suicidal self-injury (Jacobson and Mufson, 2012). Family-based IPT has also demonstrated efficacy for depressed pre-adolescents, from 9 to 12 years old, and directly involves other family members (Deitz et al., 2008). In addition, IPT-A delivered in a group format has shown positive results (O'Shea et al., 2015).

In summary, IPT-A may be a best-fit intervention for young people with a range of psychological difficulties who are ready to make some changes in these difficulties and who are willing and able to commit to a therapeutic intervention involving several sessions over several weeks. In addition, therapy will be facilitated if the young person's parents or caregivers are supportive of the intervention and will enable attendance at sessions and be prepared to be involved at some stage of the therapeutic process if necessary.

## Psychoeducation

Education about the presenting problems and the therapeutic process acknowledges clients' core interest in their life experience. Learning about the genesis of their current depression and how this depression makes sense within the context of recent life events and relationships will reinforce to clients that they are the focus of the therapeutic process. Understanding how changes in their relationships contribute to and maintain depressive experiences and also offer a pathway to healing will assist in keeping them engaged in therapy. Once clients *understand* how they became depressed and begin to see a plausible pathway forward, they will be more likely to *believe* in the therapeutic process. These two consequences of psychoeducation, understanding and believing, together enhance the prospect of optimal clinical outcome.

**Erin**, aged 16 (introduced in Chapter 4)
Erin was referred to a psychological service provider by her general practitioner who had tentatively diagnosed depression and requested psychotherapy prior to considering medication. Erin, who initially presented with her mother, was in the second last year of secondary school. She lived with her mother; father; and younger brother, Liam, aged 13. Both parents were in full-time employment, Jane a teacher and Jim a manager at an auto repair shop.

Erin was initially given the opportunity to see the therapist alone or with her mother. She elected to begin with her mother present. She appeared average for height and weight, dressed in school uniform but with her own flare, dyed red-brown shoulder length hair, and wearing silver jewellery including a pierced eyebrow. Erin responded only when directly addressed, allowing her mother to do most of the talking. From this discussion, it appeared that Erin's mood and behaviour had deteriorated significantly over recent months. According to her mother, Erin was previously mostly happy and compliant, did well at school, and had lots of friends. Recently, she had become generally surly, aggressive towards her younger brother, and defiant and rude to her father. She had begun spending much more time in her room, coming out only for meals and sometimes refusing to do even that. Erin's mother was becoming increasingly concerned about the amount of time Erin was spending on the internet, to the detriment of her school studies. Her mother also expressed concern that Erin was spending virtually no time with her friends anymore, particularly her best friend Dallas, with whom she had previously been very close. Although Erin sat in silence during most of this discussion, she was not disengaged, nodding from time to time and arguing with her mother about the amount of time she spent on the internet. Erin's mother could not identify any possible trigger events that occurred prior to Erin's mood change, but thinks the change was most likely due to "being 16". Before Erin's mother left the session, she noted that Erin's father had difficulties with depression for most of his adult life and was currently taking prescription antidepressant medication. Erin's mother left the session after about 30 minutes.

The therapist reminded Erin of the confidential nature of therapy (and the limitations to the confidentiality) and asked if there was anything she wanted to add to the information her mother had already furnished. After an initial hesitation, Erin described in detail, almost it seemed, with relief, her current life experience. Her symptoms included pervasive sadness and irritability (about which she experienced some guilt) as well as a recent inability to enjoy things she previously enjoyed. She described her current internet usage as excessive (she had denied this when her mother was in the room); however, it had lost some of its original attraction. She regarded her internet usage now almost as a chore but maintained it was the only thing "keeping her sane" at present. She described difficulties concentrating at school and major difficulties getting motivated to begin homework tasks, although she acknowledged these tasks were important. Erin reported no appetite disturbance (despite her mother's claims that she would not eat some meals); she described significant difficulty waking in the morning and remaining tired all day despite, at times, getting 12 to 14 hours of sleep. While Erin claimed not to be having suicidal thoughts, she did admit to wishing she'd wake up one day to find she had a terminal illness. When asked if she had recently hurt herself in any way, Erin commented that whilst some of her friends had done so she had never considered self-harm as an option for herself.

Erin's mood and behaviour in session were consistent with depression. Her speech was a little slow and her thoughts seemed to wander on at least three occasions. Although Erin did lose concentration on these occasions, her thought processes remained intact without any sign of delusion or thought disturbance. Erin demonstrated age-appropriate insight into her current mood and behaviour.

By the conclusion of the first session, it appeared Erin was experiencing a significant depressive episode.

Following this session, with Erin's permission, her school psychologist was contacted. She confirmed Erin's school performance had been discussed amongst her teachers, mainly due to late or nil submission of assessment tasks, which was atypical for her. Erin's teachers also reported uncharacteristic surliness, similar to that reported by her mother.

At the beginning of this session, Erin's current life experience was further explored. In addition to the symptoms described above, Erin's faith in the divine had been challenged, and she currently reported a sense of profound meaninglessness. Her symptoms were associated with significant distress and impairment in social, school, and family functioning. Erin reported little anxiety, no psychotic-like features; she reported no previous manic or hypomanic episodes. Her recent history had not included bereavement and she reported no substance use, with the exception of infrequent age-consistent binge drinking and some low-level cannabis use, both of which had ceased during recent months. She reported no previous episodes of depression and only minimal anxiety during early schooling. This anxiety appeared to be related to perfectionistic characteristics.

Exploration of Erin's pre-morbid functioning revealed significant social and academic strengths. She had chosen advanced levels of study at school and was performing at a high level—usually in the top three or four in her classes. In addition to comments made by her mother, reports from her teachers (via the school psychologist) described her as an extremely capable student, sociable, and popular amongst staff and students. Figure 5.1 provides a summary of Erin's holistic assessment.

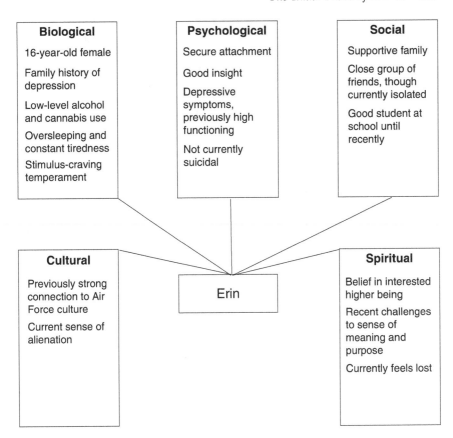

*Figure 5.1* Erin—holistic assessment summary.

The following dialogue occurred during session 2. It begins with a summary of recent history—first, to check out the therapist's accuracy of understanding and, second, to demonstrate to Erin that the therapist was listening and interested. The dialogue proceeds to confirm the diagnosis of major depressive disorder, then to provide some psychoeducation about Erin's depression and about how IPT-A may help. The therapist remains mindful of establishing a trusting, caring, empathic relationship.

*Therapist:* Erin thanks for telling me all that. Can I just try to summarise where we're up to—mainly to make sure I've got it right?
*Erin:* Yeah, okay.
*Therapist:* So it looks like that before the last few months or so, things were pretty good for you. You were doing well in school, had lots of friends, and home was okay as well. Then things changed for you. Now you're sad a lot of the time, you get mad easily, and then you feel pretty bad about that, especially towards your dad. Yeah?

Erin: Yeah.
Therapist: And also you've pulled away from lots of people in your life. You're spending a lot more time in your room at home, not seeing nearly as much of your friends. Plus, you can't seem to find enjoyment in things you used to like doing—like being online, being with your friends, and even going to school. And also you're tired all the time, got no motivation to do anything much, and not going well at school because you can't seem to get started with your homework. I know you're really over all this and you said you sometimes even wish you were dead just to get away from it all. Anything I've left out?
Erin: That's about it.
Therapist: I do agree with your doctor Erin. I'm pretty sure you're depressed at the moment. Do you know much about depression?
Erin: Yeah a bit. I looked it up on Wiki and some other sites. I think I've got depression, too. I tick all the boxes.
Therapist: Depression is a really horrible experience, as you've found out. Sometimes it seems to come out of the blue, and some people get depressed after some of the circumstances of life change. All those things you've been telling me points to you being really depressed lately, and I've got a pretty good idea it's related to some of the things that have happened in your life. We'll talk more about that later. One thing I'd like to talk about now, though, is how to start feeling better again. See when we get depressed, it affects lots of things, but one of the things it affects most is our relationships with others. You were telling me you've crashed out in your relationships with your mum and dad, your brother, also with your friends. And this is making your depression worse, like it's feeding your depression and you just can't seem to do anything about it. Right?
Erin: Yeah, the loneliness is the worst, but I still just want to be by myself. Like I've got no energy to be around people and when I am I arc up at the smallest thing.
Therapist: At this stage I think our best way forward is called Interpersonal Psychotherapy. So you can guess by the name this therapy has got a lot to do with our relationships. Interpersonal Psychotherapy, we call it IPT. Now, IPT tells us that depression and relationships are really closely linked. And I think you've been telling me that's your experience: as you've got depressed, the most important relationships in your life have all changed for the worse. Plus it's really confusing because you hate the loneliness but just don't want to be around people.
Erin: More than confusing, it's annoying and frustrating.
Therapist: Annoying and frustrating. You were such a sociable person before you got depressed and now it seems that's all so different. One of the things IPT shows is that depression and relationships are linked. So maybe if we can figure out some ways to improve those important relationships in your life you'll start to feel better. IPT tells us that as that happens, slowly at first, your depression will gradually begin to dissolve. Now I know that might

|  |  |
|---|---|
|  | seem a bit hard to believe. But just try this: try to imagine sitting in a room with your friend Dallas. Just picture sitting there with him and he's really listening to you and you are able to tell him stuff you haven't been able to tell him over the last few months. You and Dallas are just sitting talking, like you used to do…. Can you imagine that? |
| Erin: | Yeah. |
| Therapist: | So what does it feel like? |
| Erin: | A bit awkward…..but better. |
| Therapist: | How does it feel better? |
| Erin: | It's a bit like it used to be, like he gets me. |
| Therapist: | I really hope you just got a bit of a hint then about how if our relationships with people who are important to us improve, we can begin to feel a bit better? |
| Erin: | Yeah I think so. |
| Therapist: | Okay, so bringing this together, I think we both agree that all those things you've been experiencing for a while now sound pretty much like depression, and we'll talk soon about how the depression might have started. But we do know that depression and relationships are linked, and I think you're beginning to see that if we change some of the things about those relationships you might start to feel a bit better? |
| Erin: | Yeah, I guess so. |

In the above vignette, the therapist provided some new information to Erin about depression and about IPT-A, with a view to (1) increasing her understanding about her disorder and (2) beginning to understand how IPT-A may help alleviate some of the distress. As Erin learns and understands more about both her distress and the process of healing, the therapist will attempt to guide this increased understanding into the *belief* that healing will happen.

Although psychoeducation is an essential component of the Initial Phase of IPT-A, it continues throughout the entire intervention. The therapist continues to be on the lookout for opportunities to extend the young person's understanding of her distress or disorder and how the therapeutic process can impact this positively. The therapist also continually monitors the client's beliefs about the therapeutic process.

## The Interpersonal Inventory

Once the client's suitability for an interpersonal intervention has been established and psychoeducation has begun, the Interpersonal Inventory is conducted. In many ways, this inventory is where the differences between IPT-A and other interventions begin to emerge. The Interpersonal Inventory consists of five tasks, each of which has a focus on the interpersonal world of the young person. The goal of this inventory is for the therapist to begin to understand what it is like to live in the interpersonal world of her client and to attempt to understand how the network of relationships (and changes in these relationships) may have precipitated current symptomatology or may be maintaining symptoms. The role of psychoeducation in this phase is to increase the young person's understanding and insight. A key task of the therapist during this inventory is to convey a genuine interest in the client's world and in any suffering that may be a consequence.

## 1 Developing an Interpersonal Map

The first task of the Interpersonal Inventory is to conduct a detailed review of the young person's significant relationships. Additionally, the therapist takes the opportunity to explore the young person's social supports and how these supports may have changed as symptoms of distress have emerged. An effective way to begin this is by using the Closeness Circles described in Figure 5.2.

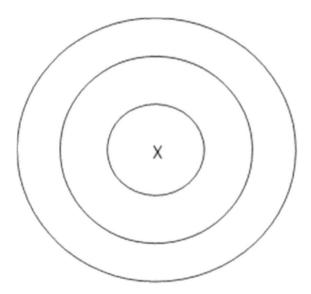

*Figure 5.2* The Closeness Circles.

The therapist explains to the young person the X in the middle represents him and the inner circle represents his closest relationships. The middle circle represents people who are close to him but not as close as those in the inner circle, and the outer circle is for people who are still in his life but not as close as those in the other two circles. There are no right or wrong places for clients to put people on their diagram. The purposes of this exercise include exploring the client's relationships, providing the young person with an opportunity to focus in a structured way on the people who are important to him, and to help the client begin to understand the connection between relationships and emotional difficulties.[1]

Therapist:   *Erin, a main part of IPT is to think about the people in your life who are important to you. To help with that, I'm going to draw some circles on this*

|            | paper, with an X in the middle. (Therapist draws circle.) The X is you. Then in this inner circle, I'm going to ask you to put the names or maybe initials of the people who are the most important to you. It might be the ones who you are closest to, the ones you think most about, maybe care most about, or at least take up a lot of your head-space. Then in this next circle, I'm going to ask you to put the names of the people who are next most important to you—they're not as important to you as these in the inner circle, but they're still pretty important in your life—still pretty close to you. Then in this outside circle, I'll get you to put other people who are not as close as those in the other two circles but they still have a role in your life. Do you get what I mean? |
|------------|---|
| Erin:      | I think so. Like family and stuff in the inner, then other people in the other circles? |
| Therapist: | Well, you can put anyone wherever you want. It's just how close they are to you that matters. Once you've finished, I'd like to spend some time talking about you and them if that's okay with you…so I can get to know how these people fit into your life, if there's been any changes lately, that sort of thing. Is that okay? |

Following Erin's construction of her Closeness Circles (see Figure 5.3), the therapist explored some of her relationship patterns. The therapist also continued psychoeducation about the link between relationships and depression.

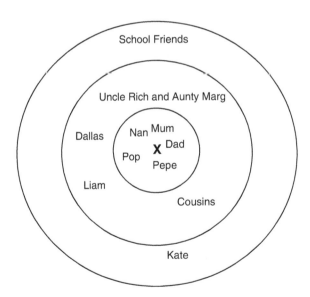

*Figure 5.3* Erin's Closeness Circles.

| Therapist: | Thanks for doing that, Erin. So I see your Mum and Dad are in your inner circle, and so is your Nan and your Pop and also your little dog Pepe. |
|---|---|

| | |
|---|---|
| Erin: | Yeah, Liam's not. He's so annoying at the moment. He used to be in the inner, but I'm just so sick of him being such a douchebag all the time. That's why he's out there. |
| Therapist: | Do you think Liam knows that? |
| Erin: | I tell him often enough. I've told him heaps of times not to come in my room, but he never listens. |
| Therapist: | Yeah that can be real annoying. How long has Liam been annoying you like that? |
| Erin: | A while. Probably since the beginning of the year—when he started high school. |
| Therapist: | And that's about when you started to get depressed. |
| Erin: | Are you saying he caused my depression? Little shit. |
| Therapist: | I'm saying when we get depressed, our relationships with people often change. Things might stress us about them that didn't stress us as much before maybe. What do you think? |
| Erin: | Dunno. Mum says I've become intolerant. |
| Therapist: | When you're depressed, it's so hard to keep a good balance. I don't know if you've become intolerant or not. I do know that when you're depressed it's so much easier to get pissed off with people, whereas when you're not depressed you're more likely to let some stuff go. |
| Erin: | I dunno. I can't stand people around me now. Before I used to spend heaps of time with Dallas and Kate. Now they just annoy me. |
| Therapist: | I notice Dallas is in your second circle and Kate in the outside circle. Have they always been there? |
| Erin: | They were both in my inner circle. Especially Dallas. I'd talk to him about everything. Anything and everything. |
| Therapist: | But now? |
| Erin: | I mainly keep to myself. As mum told you I spend ALL MY TIME in my room. That's a lie, but I don't get out much. Except to school. |
| Therapist: | Tell me about Dallas. |
| Erin: | Well he was my best mate. We did everything together—he's in most of my classes at school, we've got similar interests, especially in music. |
| Therapist: | Tell me a story about Dallas. |
| Erin: | A story?...Well, last year we went to a festival together to see some bands. He's so absentminded he forgot his ticket. So when we got there—I had my ticket—first he tried to con security to let him in and when they didn't he saw one of the small bands arriving and he told them about the ticket and said, "Can I be your roadie for five minutes?" They felt sorry for him and went "Yeah, okay", so he got in. |
| Therapist: | I notice you're smiling Erin. I don't think I've seen you smile before. Thinking of Dallas makes you smile? |
| Erin: | Yeah but I still can't bring myself to see him—except at school and we don't talk much there. Still text a bit but I just haven't got the energy. |
| Therapist: | So Erin if I had got you to do the circles, say late last year, Dallas would have been in the inner circle. What if I asked you how you hope the circles would |

|  | look like when we've finished the IPT, where would you want him to be then? |
|---|---|
| Erin: | I dunno. If I'm still feeling like this there'd be no change. But if I'm feeling better it'd be good if he was back in the inner I suppose. |
| Therapist: | Okay. Look, we'll be seeing each other each week for a while, then as you do get better, a little less often, probably once every two weeks, then even less frequently, maybe once a month. I'll keep your circles in your file and we'll get them out quite often. I'm really keen to talk about some of the other people here and to see how people move in your circles as you do begin to feel better. And maybe we can spend some time on what changes you'd like to make—if you would like people to move back to where they were—or even some people move to different places. We can talk about some strategies to help these moves take place if you like. Does that sound okay? |
| Erin: | Yeah I suppose. I just don't have the energy to think about it now though. |
| Therapist: | Sure. You've had a really tough year this year and it must seem like it's just too hard for things to change. Look, thanks again for doing this. I feel I've got a better idea of some of the important people in your life and I'm looking forward to hearing about more of them. I guess I hope that you are getting a sense of how your depression has affected your relationships with some of them, especially Dallas. So let's pick that up next session, Erin. |

The questions below provide some general examples that may facilitate exploration of the young person's Closeness Circles.

- *Tell me about your brother.*
- *How long have you known Bill?*
- *Is Georgia your girlfriend?*
- *Of all these people, who do you trust most?*
- *Who would you go to if you were in trouble of some kind?*
- *Who do you have most fun with?*
- *Who do you laugh with most?*
- *How much time to you spend with your mum?*
- *What sort of things do you and your mum do together?*
- *Tell me about some of the good things about your relationship with your boyfriend. Tell me about some of the not-so-good things.*
- *I'm just wondering about the expectations you have of your friendship with Sal. Can you tell me of a time when she lived up to your expectations? Are there times when she hasn't lived up to these expectations?*
- *When you look at all these people in your circles, is that how you want it to be?*
- *Who would you want to move if you could?*
- *If you think back to before you got depressed, say six months ago, was your Closeness Circle any different?*
- *If you had a magic wand and you could make your circles just how you wanted, how would they be different?*
- *How would you like it to be different in six months' time?*

- *Tell me about a time when you felt really close to someone in your inner circle. Who was that person? When was that? What were you doing at the time? How did you feel then?*
- *Is there anyone in the inner circle you wish was somewhere else? What's keeping them there? What would need to change for them to move? How could that change happen?*
- *Are there people in the outer circles you wish were closer to you? What's stopping them moving? Can you think of any way that would help them move?*
- *Think for a moment about the people in the inner circle. If I asked them to do this exercise, do you think you'd be in their inner circle? How do you feel about that?*
- *Are there people in your inner circle who, when they are together with you, make things uncomfortable for you?*

## 2 Linking life events to the presenting problem

The second task of the Interpersonal Inventory is to link life events to the onset of the young person's symptoms. The goals of this task are to establish the events that co-occurred with the onset of symptoms and the impact of these events on the young person. Although stressful life events will be a major focus, sometimes seemingly innocuous events may have had significant impact. The actual impact of the event can only be established by asking the young person to describe how important the life event was for him or her. In addition, adverse life events do have cumulative impact (Moffitt, 2013). A useful way to explore these events is to ask the young person to construct a timeline, beginning about six months or so before the onset of symptoms.

### Erin

In the first session, Erin and her mother described that during Erin's adolescence, she developed a keen interest in the Air Force. When she was 13 years old, she joined the Air Force Cadets. Erin took an active role in the Cadets, aspiring on graduation from high school to proceed to university studies in aeronautical engineering. The Cadets took on a pivotal role in Erin's life and occupied a substantial amount of her weekend and holiday time in training and study. Her mother observed that Erin "lived and breathed" the Cadets, and she took on leadership roles and mentored younger members. Sadly, when Erin turned 16 she undertook a battery of psychological and biometric tests where it was discovered that although she had the academic capacity and aptitude to proceed to her chosen university career, she had a particularly rare form of colour blindness that would preclude her from aeronautical engineering. According to Erin, the officer who revealed this news to her, quite unhelpfully added, "Erin you can't do engineering because of your colour blindness, but have you considered becoming a chef?"

*Therapist:* *Erin, one of the things we know about depression is that it often begins after tough things that happen in life. Especially things that stress us and*

*The Initial Phase of IPT-A* 131

*cause worry and sadness. Do you mind if we talk for a bit about your life from just before you got depressed?*

Therapist: So I'm going to draw a line here. On the right-hand end is now and on the left-hand end is, let's say, about 12 months ago.

|←————————————————————————————————————————→|
Last October                                                              Now

*Your depression kicked in about six months ago, so that was about last May. Can you think of things that were going on in your life just before then?*

Erin: Do you mean anything, or just the bad stuff?
Therapist: Let's begin with the bad stuff, and we might add other things later.
Erin: Well, the worst thing that happened was when I got my colour-blind diagnosis. That was just after Easter—April 22nd.
Therapist: Okay. So can you tell me on a scale of zero to ten, if zero was no stress at all and ten was maximum stress, what was getting that diagnosis for you?
Erin: Out of ten? ... About thirteen.
Therapist: Thirteen? Man, that's a lot of stress. Can you help me understand that?
Erin: Well, it meant I couldn't be in the Air Force.
Therapist: And that meant so much to you.
Erin: Well, I wanted to do aeronautical engineering since I started high school. And now I can't.
Therapist: I'm so sorry, Erin. I didn't realise how much that meant to you.
Erin: The psych dude said I could be a chef. He pissed me off so much. I've got nothing against chefs, but I just wanted to be an engineer. And then the next week, Pepe got hit by a car.
Therapist: Your little dog.
Erin: Yeah, and my mum and dad said they'd get me another one but I just want Pepe back.
Therapist: And Pepe's in your inner circle. He's so important to you still. Erin your tears tell me how sad you are about Pepe. And losing him just after you got your diagnosis—what a terrible, terrible time for you.
Erin: Yep, it sucks. But everyone says get over it, so I guess I'll just have to.
Therapist: But now, six months later, it still hurts you so much to think about it.... So the psych said be a chef, and your mum and dad said they'd get you another puppy, but all you wanted was for things to be back to the way they were, with your dream to be an engineer still alive and also Pepe still alive.
Erin: Yeah and even my friends said get over it. Well, they didn't say those exact words but that's what they meant.
Therapist: What did your friends say, Erin?
Erin: They were really sad about Pepe, but they all said things like you can always get another job and stuff like that.
Therapist: And you felt no one got it. The people closest to you just didn't get it. They

| | |
|---|---|
| | *didn't get how your life was changed forever. I guess that's when you started spending a lot more time in your room? Just avoiding other people?* |
| Erin: | They all started annoying me. I just wanted to be alone. |
| Therapist: | So you not only lost your dream career and your pet, but you also lost a whole lot of time with friends as well. The people who were closest to you—the people in your inner circle—you lost some of that as well. |
| Erin: | I guess so. I used to talk to Dallas about everything, now I'm just in my room. |

Erin's timeline now looks like this:

```
                        Diagnosed colour blind 13/10
                        Losing Pepe
                        Losing time with friends
─────────────────────────────────────────────────────────────▶
Last October                   April                        Now
```

Further discussion of the timeline revealed that there was collateral damage associated with these losses. Erin's schoolwork had deteriorated, which constituted the loss of her sense of self as a competent student. As part of her self-imposed isolation, Erin lost not only the social support her family and friends provided but also her capacity to contribute positively to her group of friends. She also lost the sense of being understood by friends and family as well as involvement in social events such as going to the movies and other activities she previously participated in. In addition, as a consequence of the diagnosis of colour blindness and the loss of her pet dog, Erin felt she had been forgotten by God. Prior to these events, Erin had a non-religious but nonetheless close connection with what she believed to be a universal force who rewarded good for good and bad for bad. Erin would often "check-in" with her construction of divinity to keep herself morally and spiritually balanced. Her diagnosis and loss of Pepe shattered these assumptions, and she now found it impossible to pray the way she used to and at times found herself questioning the fundamentals of her faith.

As well as identifying life events associated with the onset of symptoms and the subjective impact of these events, the timeline also provides the opportunity for the therapist to observe the interactions of process and content affect. The sadness and devastation that Erin expressed when reporting her diagnosis of colour blindness (and also when reporting her dog being hit by the car) were consistent with what the therapist expected her immediate response to these events would have been. The process and content affect were congruent. The therapist acknowledged this:

| | |
|---|---|
| Therapist: | *And Pepe's in your inner circle. He's so important to you still. Erin your tears tell me how sad you are about Pepe. And losing him just after you got your diagnosis—what a terrible, terrible time for you.* |

In another example, **Bill**, a 15-year-old boy, was reporting the death of his older brother, Geoff. Geoff, driving too fast after drinking too much alcohol, lost control of the vehicle which left the road and hit a tree. Geoff was killed instantly, leaving Bill trapped in the passenger's seat for over an hour before being discovered and then for another hour before being freed from the vehicle. When Bill was recounting the story in therapy, he told it like a news reader would have reported the accident. Bill's recount was almost devoid of any affect or emotion. His process and content affect were incongruent. Incongruence between process and content affect almost always signifies that the emotions have not been processed effectively and may need to be explored further. The interpersonal consequences of this incongruence clearly may also need to be explored. However, during this Initial Phase of therapy, when the primary aim is to establish the parameters of the young person's distress and to establish a strong therapeutic alliance, it is often best to note this incongruence in order to return to it later, during the Middle Phase when the primary focus will be alleviation of symptomatology and improvement in interpersonal functioning.

The conversations between the therapist and the young person during the construction of the timeline also affords the therapist the opportunity to consider which Problem Area is most closely associated with the young person's symptoms. Although identification of the Problem Area is addressed more formally later in the Interpersonal Inventory, the astute therapist will be looking for clues that make any one of the Problem Areas more or less likely to be linked to the development and maintenance of symptoms. For example, the Problem Area Interpersonal Gaps is usually associated with difficulties in communicating attachment needs effectively to others. The young person's descriptions of how relationships are initiated and maintained and the nature of the developing relationship with the therapist will provide data on this Problem Area. The therapist will often get a sense of how well the young person communicates by attending to the interpersonal communications that occur with the therapist during these early sessions. The dialogue above suggests that although Erin withdrew from friends and family as her depressive symptoms worsened, she displayed an age-appropriate maturity in describing the social and psychological context of this withdrawal. She withdrew from friends and family not because she lacked the capacity to initiate and maintain relationship but as a strategic social decision to minimise her distress. And Erin recognised that this strategic withdrawal came at a cost, that of loneliness. If Interpersonal Gaps was seen as less likely to be the Problem Area most closely associated with Erin's depression, only three contenders remained: Complex Grief, Interpersonal Disputes, and Role Transition. These will be explored in the next task of the Interpersonal Inventory.

In summary, the second task of the Interpersonal Inventory, linking life events to the presenting problem, can assist in exploring:

- events that co-occurred with the onset of symptoms.
- the impact of these events.

- the interpersonal consequences of these events.
- content and process affect associated with stressful life events.

### 3 Identifying the Problem Area(s)

The third task of the Interpersonal Inventory is to establish the Problem Area most closely associated with the onset and maintenance of symptoms. The psychoeducation that began at the beginning of the Interpersonal Inventory continues during this task as the therapist explains each of the Problem Areas to the young person and collaboratively decides which of the four is most closely linked to the symptoms. The identification of the Problem Area (or, sometimes, Problem Areas) will provide a focus for the remainder of treatment. None of the Problem Areas are diagnoses but rather a concise way of describing the interpersonal factors involved in the development and maintenance of psychological symptoms.

The four Problem Area identified in IPT-A are (1) Complex Grief, (2) Interpersonal Disputes, (3) Role Transitions, and (4) Interpersonal Gaps.

*Complex Grief*

Complex Grief is chosen as the Problem Area when the young person's symptoms arise within a context of significant loss. The loss may be in relation to the death of an important person, such as a family member or friend. However, the experience of loss is not limited only to loss through death. Many young people experience significant and multiple losses as they progress through their adolescent years, and for many the emotions surrounding the loss are not adequately processed because they are not given permission to grieve. Often adults and peers offer well-intentioned advice that may minimise or even negate the young person's loss experience. Erin is an example in point. As demonstrated in the dialogue above when Erin received her diagnosis of colour blindness, her losses were enormous. Not only did she lose her chosen career—her future—she also lost a large part of her past—the four years of constant and conscientious devotion to the Air Force Cadets. But she also lost a significant part of her identity. The time, effort, enthusiasm, and diligence with which she approached her time in the Cadets largely defined her sense of self. Erin believed and felt all this was taken away from her when she received her diagnosis. Adults around her compounded this sense of loss by minimising it. Erin's experience was that no one took her loss seriously; in therapeutic terms, none gave her permission to grieve. Compounding this, when her pet dog was killed on the road shortly after her diagnosis, her well-meaning parents immediately offered to buy her another puppy. Her parents' efforts to soothe her loss by replacing her pet failed to acknowledge Erin's profound sense of hurt and sadness over losing her pet and once again did not afford her the space or time to grieve for this pet that meant so much to her. As a consequence of not being heard, Erin withdrew from friends and family, thereby creating yet another loss: that of her social support network. Thus, at a time when Erin needed the support of her family and friends (and pet) most critically, they were now unavailable.

Many adolescents experience significant loss, including loss through death. Grief is a normal and healing process. Complex Grief is only identified when a disorder, in Erin's case, depression, arises directly in response to the emotions of loss not being adequately processed—when the anticipated grief response to loss transmutes into an experience characterised by lasting distress and impairment of academic or vocational functioning and ruptured interpersonal processes. (See Chapter 7.)

*Interpersonal Disputes*

In many cultures, as young people proceed from childhood to adulthood, they are faced with the joint demands of seeking personal independence through a shift in dependence on the family to inclusion in and dependence on the peer group. With this change in the nature of relationships, new skills are acquired, new types of relationships forged, and new challenges encountered. Interpersonal Disputes are not uncommon as young people enter this new territory. Disputes are often with parents but may also be encountered with peers, teachers, siblings, romantic partners, sports coaches, and others. Conflict is exacerbated for some young people who encounter abuse, parental mental illness, substance use, crime, poverty, or other stressors (Springer et al., 2007).

Conflict may be over one salient issue with one person or may be a pattern of behaviour with several significant others. Interpersonal Disputes is identified as the Problem Area when the level of dispute is no longer normative but has led to a disruption in a significant interpersonal relationship (or relationships). For many young people that creates a sense of profound debility—a feeling of "stuckness"—others have made decisions about and for them that get in the way of how they want to live their lives. This "stuckness" is often accompanied by a feeling of inevitability, often anger, and above all intransigence: the belief that there is little or nothing they can do to change the situation. And with no end in sight, depressive or other symptomatology may follow.

## Gina

Gina, for example, a 15-year-old girl, lives with her mother, father, and younger sister. Her peer group were given a fairly free reign by their parents. In contrast, Gina's mother expected certain behaviours from Gina and was reluctant to accede to what Gina believed to be reasonable requests. Gina constantly found herself having to make excuses to her friends about why she couldn't go to some of the places her friends frequented or stay out as late as they were able to. Because of this, Gina believed her mother's demands were compromising continued membership of her peer group. She felt "on the edge of being kicked out". A significant interpersonal incident occurred when Gina told her mother she was getting her tongue pierced. Gina believed this would firm up her tenuous place in the group. Her mother, however, flatly refused permission for this. A memorable argument ensued during which both Gina and her mother's positions became more entrenched. Being 15, Gina needed her mother's permission to have this procedure, and her mother refused to allow this to occur.

From a developmental perspective, at 15 Gina is in the process of disconnecting from her family on her way towards independence, via connection to her peer group. Acceptance by her peers is critical for Gina as this group offers acceptance, meets her needs for belonging and nurture, provides opportunities to model and practice age-appropriate developmental behaviours, and is central to her identity formation. Gina believes her mother's intransigence is fatally compromising her tentative membership of this group, membership that is critical to her sense of social survival. Gina believed that nothing she could do would change her mother's stance. Within this context, Gina began to develop symptoms of depression and social anxiety, including panic attacks at school and home. She ceased arguing with her mother about the tongue piercing, which her mother interpreted as now being less important to Gina, but from Gina's perspective was a reflection of giving up. Gina became surly and irritable at home, and fear and anxiety replaced the cautious friendliness that characterised her previous interpersonal style.

The therapist and Gina would consider together whether the Interpersonal Disputes with her mother were linked to her symptoms and distress. Together they would explore through the Closeness Circles how her interpersonal world had changed over recent times and how successfully her interpersonal needs were being met by those closest to her. Through the timeline, they would explore any recent interpersonal stressors, including the tongue-piercing incident and the impact of this and other recent events on her. If they identified recent disputes as central to Gina's symptoms, then Interpersonal Disputes would be identified as the Problem Area and this would become the initial focus of the therapeutic process. (See Chapter 8.)

*Role Transitions*

Role Transitions in young people occur when there is a change in life circumstances that requires them to take on a new or different role. These include, but are not limited to, the transition from primary to secondary schooling or from secondary school to university or college, beginning work or starting a new job, moving from one town (or school) to another, parental separation and divorce, a new step-parent, the onset of menarche or puberty, a change in foster home, pregnancy, a new baby entering the household, parental loss of employment, the onset of illness or disability, a new role in the family following a death, and so on. Changes such as these are normative and in most cases negotiated successfully. For some young people, however, changes that would normally be associated with a tolerable degree of distress actually precipitate the onset of disorder. The impact of changes such as these is influenced by many factors, including the age of the young person and stage of development; the psychological, social, biological, spiritual, and cultural context in which the changes occur; and, importantly, the nature of the relationships, especially supportive adult relationships, within the young person's interpersonal world.

An essential component of Role Transition is the considerable loss that usually surrounds the old role. A second consideration are the difficulties the young person may have adapting behaviourally, cognitively, and affectively to the new role. For example, in the case of parental separation, the young person loses the way things used to be—a family with two parents. Not only is the old role lost, but the young person now has to negotiate a new cognitive environment: a change in the mindset of what it means to live in a single-parent family; a new behavioural environment—adapting to spending time in different locations; and a new affective environment—working out how to distribute love and affection between two parents who now live separate lives. Often these new environments are negotiated within the context of the complex amalgam of competing emotions including anger, guilt, love, loyalty, fear, or unrealistic hope that things will change back again.

Role Transitions for some young people will be negotiated adaptively whilst for others will contribute to the experience of debilitating stress, accompanied by elevated levels of negative affect and significant impairment in their social and academic functioning.

**Chris**, a 14-year-old boy, was brought for therapy by his mother, presenting with mixed anxious and depressed mood, characterised by frequent angry outbursts at home and school. Chris was Year 9 student of average ability, living with his mother and two younger sisters. His parents had separated two years previously, and Chris had negotiated this separation quite successfully. His father lived in the next town and Chris and his sisters spent every other weekend and some school holidays with their father. Neither parents had new partners, but Chris's mother was beginning a relationship with a male friend who visited some weekends. About a year ago, Chris's father told his children that he had been diagnosed with Parkinson's disease. Not much changed for a while, but then Chris's dad began to deteriorate quite quickly, with increasingly frequent and severe tremors, outbursts of rage, tearfulness, and loss of memory. Chris talked about this as a "change in dad's personality". Chris began to worry about his father during the times when he wasn't there, particularly after his father had to leave his job, spending most of his time either at doctors or at home alone. Although Chris kept visiting as usual, his sisters often found other things to do on those weekends and Chris found himself wishing he didn't have to go. His time with his father became increasingly stressful as Chris found himself not only caring for his father but doing a lot of things around the house that his father could no longer do for himself. In addition, previously Chris would often take a friend on these visits and they would do fun things together with his father, like fishing and kayaking. Chris now found himself reluctant to ask friends as he didn't want them to see his father as he was. He described feeling embarrassed by his father and also resentful of all he had to do. Chris felt guilty about his embarrassment and about his resentment—he still loved his father a lot and couldn't understand his conflicting feelings.

Chris's primary Problem Area was Role Transition. The old role of being a son of a well father was now lost. Included in this loss were (1) the previous well-defined relationship with his father as a nurturer, guide, role model, confidante; (2) the things they used to do together—fun things like fishing and kayaking but also the relaxed time with each other; and (3) the expectations Chris had for their future together. In the new role, Chris couldn't work out how to negotiate being the son of a father who was very ill and required care and assistance. On an emotional level he was struggling with his father's "new personality": how to respond to his father's depression and rages. The stresses for Chris included unresolved grief surrounding the loss of the old role, not wanting the new role, and not understanding how to do it. He was uncertain about what the reasonable expectations were of him in supporting his father and what resources he needed to accomplish this.

If Role Transition is the Problem Area linked with the young person's symptom profile, the focus of therapy becomes first to identify the losses associated with the old role and, if necessary, assisting the young person to mourn and grieve for those losses. Second, the focus of therapy is to identify the new affective, functional, and interpersonal processes needed to successfully negotiate the new role. A strong therapeutic alliance will assist in accomplishing these tasks, which in many cases are surrounded by confusion, bewilderment, anger, and often despair. (See Chapter 9.)

*Interpersonal Gaps*

When some young people enter the therapist's office for the first time, it doesn't take long to work out that something is not right. Some young people, despite living their childhood and adolescence in the company of others, don't seem to pick up the rules of engagement. Whilst there is considerable variation amongst young people, most, without consciously trying, internalise the capacity to initiate and maintain relationships. For some though, their childhood and adolescence comprises loneliness; broken friendships; rejections; inability to communicate emotions effectively; and regularly misunderstanding others and, in turn, regularly being misunderstood by them. Most young people live in an interpersonal world in which their peer group plays a pivotal role, and this environment is central to the development of a personal identity. If, during this critical time of identity formation, the young person's behaviours, cognitions, and affects do not comply with the peer group's expectations and requirements, the adolescent may experience rejection, ridicule, and even bullying rather than the sense of belonging, nurture, and connectedness optimally provided by this group. When young people do not possess the required relationship skills to build social connections, or the skills necessary to maintain them, these normative requirements of adolescence may be jeopardised. The peer rejection that often accompanies social failure leads some young people to elevated levels of distress that may be experienced, for example, as social anxiety and depression.

It should be noted, however, that some young people with low-level interpersonal skills who do not experience social acceptance by the peer group still seem to progress successfully through adolescence. Some young people seem to be uninterested in developing connectedness with their peers and even may develop an almost compulsive self-reliance that is ego-syntonic for them. Interpersonal Gaps is only identified as the Problem Area when the young person's distress and symptom profile is linked to an inability to relate to others in a way that is meaningful for him or her.

Whilst this Problem Area relates primarily to an overarching inability to initiate and maintain relationships, more subtle expressions of these social deficits may also cause distress and symptomatology. Examples include the over- or under-expression of emotion, inappropriate and easily triggered anger towards others, being over- or under-involved in the lives of others, being overly sensitive to criticism, inappropriate sexual behaviour, and a reduced ability to recognise and understand the needs and responses of others.

## Crystal

Crystal is an 18-year-old who did not lack the ability to initiate relationships but had a history of difficulty maintaining them. Crystal's mother brought her to therapy and described her own understanding of Crystal's difficulties. She also reported accounts from Crystal's peer group, with whom Crystal's mother had a good and longstanding relationship.

Crystal was in her last year of high school and had been part of a fairly large but tightly formed group of friends since she moved to her new school five years ago. Crystal liked boys and had dated two of the boys in this group prior to forming an attachment with Ben, a reserved boy who was well liked by most of his peers and teachers. Crystal and Ben's relationship progressed steadily and before long they were dating. Crystal observed that others in the peer group thought she had treated her former partners carelessly and were concerned that she would hurt Ben. Crystal nonchalantly told them not to worry because "he is the one for me". From Crystal's perspective all was going well, but some of her peers were becoming increasingly annoyed at the cavalier way she was treating Ben. She would flirt with other boys and some of the girls; would criticise and belittle Ben in front of the others in the group; talk openly about their sexual encounters; and, from the perspective of others, generally began to control Ben's life. Others in the peer group saw this as a familiar pattern, as they had observed this behaviour with Crystal's other two boyfriends. Crystal however continued in this same manner, oblivious to the annoyance she was provoking and a gradual distancing in her relationship with Ben. For Ben, a sentinel moment occurred one day at the supermarket. He and Crystal had been shopping for groceries for an upcoming party planned by the group of friends. At the checkout Crystal noticed several packets of potato chips in the trolley. In a loud voice, seemingly unaware of the presence of many other shoppers, Crystal began to berate Ben, incessantly insisting that one of their friends was purchasing that item, that he was wasting his money, that he never listened, and that next time she'd be better off shopping by herself. Ben stood looking at the floor, but after a short while pronounced to Crystal "I'm over this" and left the shop. When Crystal had paid for the shopping and returned to the car park she found that Ben's car had gone. He wouldn't answer his phone and a short time later Crystal received a text message from Ben saying he wanted a break in the relationship. Crystal was stunned and devastated. Ben refused to take her calls and at school her peer group sided with Ben. They shunned Crystal despite her repeated attempts to tell her side of the story. Before long, Crystal ceased contact with the group of friends and she started missing school. Her mother reported she was spending a lot of time in her room, refusing to communicate with her family. Her low mood was fed by endless rumination about the end of her relationship with Ben. In these ruminations, Crystal demonised both Ben and her previous group of friends, blaming them for the breakup, convinced they were jealous of the relationship she and Ben had together.

Crystal's mother brought her to therapy after Crystal began having panic attacks when she tried to leave home. Her mother was also concerned about Crystal's low mood, unpredictable rage, and social isolation. Her therapist diagnosed major depressive disorder with anxious distress and found that this disorder was most closely linked to the Problem Area of Interpersonal Gaps. Crystal had developed a pattern of behaviour that others could see in her but she could not see in herself. This pattern alienated her from others, culminating in rejection by others. This rejection was ego-dystonic for Crystal as it challenged her identity as one who is well liked and always in control, leaving her depressed, anxious, and depleted.

In cases such as Crystal's where Interpersonal Gaps is identified as the Problem Area most closely linked to the symptom cluster, the therapist's goal is to identify the gaps in the young person's social behaviours that are precipitating and perpetuating the current distress. In Crystal's case, the gap was not in initiating but in maintaining relationships. She lacked insight about her own behaviour and how it impacted on others. A therapeutic goal in this instance would be to assist Crystal to develop an awareness of how others demonstrate their feelings and of how her behaviour impacts others and for Crystal to develop a range of alternative behaviours that, whilst still meeting her attachment needs, are consistent with the needs and requirements of others, thus maintaining social alliances. (See Chapter 10.)

**Collaboratively Identifying the Problem Area**

The process of identifying the Problem Area(s) demonstrates the collaborative nature of IPT-A. This begins with psychoeducation about the nature of each of the Problem Areas, culminating in a joint agreement between therapist and young person about which of the four is most closely linked to the young person's current life experience. The dialogue below with **Erin** illustrates this, beginning first with psychoeducation about each of the four Problem Areas and providing enough information for her to make an informed choice about which area is most closely linked to her presenting problem.

Therapist: Erin, in IPT one of the things we find really helpful is trying to link your depression with what we call Problem Areas. The Problem Areas help us understand more about where your depression came from and they also give us direction for our future sessions together. In IPT there are four Problem Areas. I want to describe them to you and then together we'll decide which one is most closely linked to your depression. Is that okay?

Erin: Yeah. Problem Areas?

Therapist: The Problem Areas help us understand more about how your depression changes things in your relationships with others and how these changes help to keep your depression going. We know you got depressed soon after your colour-blindness diagnosis. And around that time you lost Pepe and no one seemed to get how much those two things meant to you. I think that working out the Problem Area will help us understand that better and also help us work out what to do about it.

Erin: Okay.

Therapist: So I'll describe the Problem Areas to you. Now already I think that two of them probably don't apply to you, but I still want to run them by you to see if you agree. The first one is called Interpersonal Gaps, and we use that Problem Area when people have major difficulties starting relationships and then keeping them going. These people just don't seem to have what it takes to do relationships well and they get depressed because they want to be able to do relationship stuff but they just can't seem to be able to. But in our conversations and in the conversation we had with your mum, you seem to be okay in that area. You've had great relationships with friends and family in the past, and they've lasted. What do you think?

Erin: Yeah, I suppose so. But they're not going great now, though. I'm not talking to anyone.

Therapist: Yeah, I know, Erin, but I'm not sure your depression started because you had relationship problems in that way. They came after. See the difference?

Erin: Everything was okay until April. Then it all went to shit.

Therapist: So the next Problem Area is called Disputes. We use that one when the depression seems to be triggered by major conflict in people's lives. There are usually lots of fights and conflict, and for young people it's often when parents set rules that seem unfair and lead to so much disagreement that the young person feels trapped and can't do anything to solve it.

|   |   |
|---|---|
|   | Sometimes there are lots of disagreements with friends or other people like teachers, and it seems that their whole lives are just driven by conflict. People with this Problem Area often get depressed because they see there is no way out. Do you know anyone like that? |
| Erin: | Yeah maybe. I think Dallas's brother is a bit like that. He just argues with everyone all the time and then he gets depressed because he thinks no one likes him. It's not me, though. I hate conflict. I'm more a peacemaker. |
| Therapist: | So we can rule out Disputes. And are you happy to rule out Gaps as well? |
| Erin: | Yep. That doesn't seem to be me either. |
| Therapist: | Okay, then the next one is called Role Transition. A bit of a funny name, but it's like when things happen in life that lead to major changes. It's a bit like being in a play and you have a character to play and suddenly the director says that from now on you have to play a different character. But you know all the lines for the first one and don't know anything about the new one. You miss the old one and just want to go back. But you can't. In real life, for some people, it's about things like leaving home, or parents getting divorced, or maybe getting really sick. |
| Erin: | Or finding out you're colour blind. |
| Therapist: | Yeah, maybe. That changed everything for you. |
| Erin: | It was just like suddenly being a new character. And I want to be the old one again. |
| Therapist: | So Role Transition fits you? Just let me tell you about the fourth one and then we'll work out which one fits best. So the last Problem Area is called Complex Grief. It's called complex because although grief is really hard, most people work their way through it. A bit like going into a dark tunnel then coming out the other side. But when it's complex, people seem to get stuck in the tunnel. And it can be complex for lots of reasons. There are many losses in life. Sometimes people close to us die, families break up, or we might move to another country and lose friends and culture and all the things that are familiar to us. Lots of losses, but sometimes others don't realise how important the losses are for us and it's like we can't grieve. Then it might be like getting stuck in that dark tunnel and stuck there alone—because nobody else gets it. |
| Erin: | That's how I feel—stuck in a tunnel—I can't go forward and I can't go back. |
| Therapist: | Can we just think about some of your losses for a minute? When you got your diagnosis, you lost so much. It seemed like all your time over the last few years in the Air Cadets was suddenly a waste of time, but you also lost your dream of being an engineer. And then Pepe got run over and you lost your pet—but from what you've told me about Pepe, he was a great listener when things weren't going so well for you, so you lost that as well. And because people around you didn't seem to understand, you pulled back from them. You just didn't have the energy. So, in a way, you lost a lot there, too. At a time when you needed your friends and family |

|  | *probably more than ever, they weren't there. And it affected your beliefs as well. Now you're not sure what you believe anymore, and you can't seem to pray the way you used to. Your career, your pet, your family, friends, beliefs—that's so much loss, Erin.* |
|---|---|
| Erin: | It wasn't just my career—it was my life. |
| Therapist: | It was a really huge loss. I remember you said on a scale of one to ten it was thirteen. |
| Erin: | So I'm really stuck in that tunnel. And, yeah, that last one fits me. |
| Therapist: | Complex Grief? |
| Erin: | It's a bit of both really. It does feel like I'm a new character in the play, but the worse feeling is being in the tunnel. |
| Therapist: | I think I agree with you. I can see what you're saying about the new character—you don't want to leave the old one behind because you were happy and content in that role, and the new one was forced on you and you really don't want to play that role. But I can also see just how much you have lost and you're hurting so much from those losses. So are you okay to think about Complex Grief to start with? Then in our time together, we'll hopefully be able to help you find a way through that tunnel you're stuck in at the moment. |
| Erin: | Sure. |

## 4 Linking symptoms to the Problem Area

Once the Problem Area has been collaboratively identified as that most closely associated with the young person's symptoms, the fourth task of the Interpersonal Inventory is to link the Problem Area to the symptoms in such a way that the young person not only *understands* that link but also *believes* that the therapeutic process will address the Problem Area and begin to resolve her current symptoms.

At this point, a review of the current symptoms will help clarify in the young person's mind the nature of her current life experience and how these symptoms are being maintained by the relationship difficulties. The client will be reminded that these difficulties will be addressed by attention to the Problem Area. Part of the psychoeducation component of IPT is helping the young person understand in general terms how relationship difficulties and symptomatology are connected and, in specific terms, how her current experience of life is associated with the status of her relationships.

One of the central tasks of the IPT therapist is to educate the young person from the outset about the relationship between psychological symptoms and interpersonal functioning. Relationships are central to the identity of most young people, and many of them have some awareness of the role of relationships in their problems. However, many young people with psychological symptoms may be more inclined to see their problems are directly related to deficiencies in themselves. Conversely, some may lay all the blame on other people and see their current distress as being entirely the fault of others. Either of these positions, and the many in between, will influence the developing identity of the young person, shaping a sense of self-blame or worthlessness on the one hand or victimisation and powerlessness on the other. In IPT-A the therapist seeks to uncover these misunderstandings and create a more realistic appraisal of the nature of the young person's interpersonal world and his roles and responsibilities within it. The therapist will aim to create a therapeutic relationship in which the young person feels nurtured and cared for, and safe enough to tolerate appropriate feedback about his interpersonal behaviours.

Young people who are experiencing significant depression, anxiety, or other symptoms may need particular assistance in developing realistic perceptions of their relationships and may require clear and direct explanation of the link between the identified Problem Area and their symptoms. This explanation will need to be repeated at various times through the therapeutic process, using different explanatory devices until the therapist is certain the young person has an adequate grasp of this connection. The therapist's task here is not complete until the young person not only understands this link but also believes that symptoms will lessen through working on the Problem Area.

**Erin**, for example, showed some understanding of the link between her losses and her depression when she used the therapist's metaphor of being stuck in a dark tunnel to describe her current life experience. She recognised that her losses precipitated her depression and her current symptoms were a constant reminder of those losses. The therapist would work to confirm that understanding, then help Erin move from understanding to belief and the expectation that her symptoms will lessen as her grief over those losses is processed.

*Therapist:* So we've decided that Complex Grief is the Problem Area that most closely matches with how you feel at the moment. Have you got any questions about that?

*Erin:* Not really. I think it's that one, too, but I can't see how that helps. I mean it's Complex Grief or whatever, but I'm still colour blind, I still can't be an engineer or anything in the Air Force and I still haven't got Pepe. I'm still fucked.

*Therapist:* Remember how you talked about being stuck in the dark tunnel? Not being able to go forward and not being able to go back? Erin we can't make that tunnel go away, but I'm pretty confident that little by little you can move to the front end, and eventually you'll be able to see the entrance. Get what I mean?

*Erin:* Yeah, I suppose so. It's just that I'm negative at the moment. I guess I can see that. And I know what you said about Dallas is true. God, I miss him.

*Therapist:* I know you do, Erin. And I'm hoping that before long you'll want to see him again and eventually get back to where you were with him. But I guess one of the things I wanted to do today was help you see that all of the things you have lost are linked to your depression, including losing what you had with Dallas. We both know that you can't get a lot of that

|  | back, but maybe eventually being able to talk to Dallas about those things and have him understand what it all meant to you would help you feel better. And from what you've told me about Dallas, maybe he'd be pretty keen for that to happen, too. |
| --- | --- |
| Erin: | I know he would. So do you think that would help? |
| Therapist: | I think you even asking me that question means you've moved a little bit closer to the end of that tunnel. |

In the above dialogue, the therapist focussed on confirming in Erin's mind the link between her losses and her depression but also on helping her see that by reconnecting with one of the significant others in her life, Dallas, she would begin to feel better: that is, experience a reduction in symptoms. In IPT terms, she would improve interpersonal functioning by enhancing communication skills in significant relationships, which would then impact on her symptom profile. Also, in the above dialogue the therapist noted that Erin's more forthright patterns of communication may indicate an increasing degree of security with him. She demonstrated an level of affect in this session that was lacking in previous sessions, both annoyance: "I mean it's Complex Grief or whatever, but I'm still colour blind" and vulnerability: "God, I miss him".

This task of connecting Erin's depressive symptoms to Complex Grief will remain a focus for the therapist until Erin consistently demonstrates she has internalised this connection and acknowledges her need to grieve her losses by communicating the feelings associated with them to those in her life whom she cares about and who care about her. In the meantime, her therapist will act as a transitory attachment figure and will attempt to foster a relationship with Erin in which she is able to communicate these feeling of loss in a caring and safe, albeit temporary, relationship.

## 5 Exploring attachment

The fifth task of the Interpersonal Inventory is for the therapist to continue to develop an hypothesis about the young person's attachment style. Understanding the young person's attachment processes begins from the moment she walks into the office on her first visit and continues until her last visit. The Interpersonal Inventory presents a focussed opportunity to explore attachment behaviours during the Closeness Circles, construction of the timeline, identification of the primary Problem Area, and linking the symptoms to the Problem Area. The young person's attachment style is a key factor in assessment and management of mental disorders as it will not only influence the young person's responses to the therapist but will also influence the therapist's behaviours towards the young person. Chapter 3 provided a summary of attachment theory and how this theory applies to Interpersonal Psychotherapy. Chapter 3 also discusses strategies to assist the therapist in understanding the young person's attachment behaviours and style.

In the following conversation with **Erin,** the therapist asked some specific questions related to attachment, about trust and how this led to expectations of others when Erin was in need of care.

*Therapist:* In our time together so far, that first session with your mum and the other two sessions we've had together, I've been thinking about your relationships with other people and I'd like to talk about that a bit more if that's okay?
*Erin:* Yeah, okay.
*Therapist:* So just going back to your Closeness Circle; can you tell me about who you trusted when things weren't going too well for you?
*Erin:* Do you mean now or before?
*Therapist:* Well, both, really. Let's start with before.
*Erin:* Well, Mum or Dallas probably. I'd trust Mum but there were some things I wouldn't tell her. I'd tell Dallas pretty much everything.
*Therapist:* Can you tell me about a time when you did trust Dallas with something that was important to you?
*Erin:* Well, a while ago Mum and Dad were having heaps of arguments. They were fighting all the time—yelling and then not talking for hours. I thought they were going to break up or something. Dallas and I talked about that so much. He didn't say much but I knew he got it—his parents split up a few years ago. Anyway, Mum and Dad got over it and it's okay now.
*Therapist:* So Erin you were upset and worried about your parents and trusted Dallas with your worry. And he didn't let you down.
*Erin:* He didn't let me down. Heaps more than that though—sometimes I'd phone him at like two in the morning or something and he'd wake up and still be there. But we both knew I'd do the same for him if he was sad or something.
*Therapist:* You knew he'd be there for you?
*Erin:* Yeah, of course. I knew it and he knew it, too.
*Therapist:* And what about your Mum? You said she was someone else you could trust with most things. So can you tell me about a time when you were little, say five or six or something, when you were sick or scared or lost or something like that? Can you think of a time like that?
*Erin:* Yeah—I can remember one time. Once when I was little, Mum and I were shopping in a big supermarket. Mum sent me to get some stuff from another aisle. It was stuff I wanted to get like chocolate or something. I'd just found it and there was this huge crash and all the lights went out. The whole place was just so dark. People were screaming and crying— shit-scared. Is that what you mean?
*Therapist:* Sure is. So what did you do?
*Erin:* I don't know. I know I was crying. Didn't know where I was—it was really dark, I don't know what the crash was but that didn't happen again. You could hear people moving around and bumping into things—crying and some were still screaming. I think I just stayed

|            | where I was. I was still crying and scared but not as scared as when the crash happened. |
|------------|---|
| Therapist: | Where was your Mum? |
| Erin:      | Well, she was still in her aisle. But by then she would have been trying to find me. I remember just wanting to hear her voice and smell her perfume. And hug her. So I just waited. After a while, some shop people came around with torches and I found Mum. She'd actually got to my aisle in the dark and she wasn't that far away. I just couldn't hear her because of all the other noise. I remember we just left all the shopping and got out of there. |
| Therapist: | So you knew your Mum would come looking, that's why you just stayed where you were? |
| Erin:      | Course she would. Anyone's mum would've. |

In the above dialogue, first about Dallas, Erin demonstrated a clear expectation that when she needed Dallas, he would be there for her. And equally, that if Dallas needed her, she would be there for him. Bidirectional trust and reliability indicates a positive sense of self and also a positive sense of other, both pointing to a security of attachment. Likewise, in the second part of the dialogue, Erin was convinced that in her hour of need her mum would do nothing other than come looking for her—that is, provide the care and protection she needed.

Whilst a brief dialogue such as this is by no means enough to form a firm view on Erin's attachment style, the content of her narrative as well as the richness of her descriptions provide the therapist with data that support the hypothesis that Erin's attachment style is more secure than either preoccupied or avoidant. This hypothesis would be continually reviewed as the therapeutic relationship develops.

In summary, the Interpersonal Inventory consists of five steps:

1   Developing an Interpersonal Map, assisted by the Closeness Circles.
2   Linking life events to the mental disorder, assisted by use of the extended timeline.
3   Identifying the Problem Area(s) most closely linked to the young person's symptoms.
4   Linking symptoms to the Problem Area(s) in a way that the young person first begins to understand and, second, believe that as the Problem Area is addressed, his or her symptoms will begin to resolve.
5   Exploring attachment, an ongoing process.

Following completion of the Interpersonal Inventory, the therapist is in a position to build on the information derived from the holistic formulation and present this to the young person.

## The Interpersonal Formulation

The next task of the Initial Phase of IPT-A is to present an Interpersonal Formulation to the young person. It is apparent from the dialogues above that much of the formulation is drip-fed to clients during the process of the Interpersonal Inventory. For example, the diagnosis, if appropriate, has been communicated to the young person; the Problem Area has been identified by collaborative process; and the Problem Area has been linked to the young person's current distress or disorder. The Interpersonal Formulation offers the opportunity to summarise for the young person:

- how the holistic influences (biological, psychological, social, cultural and spiritual) interact to shape the young person's current experiential world.
- how recent stressors contribute to the development of symptomatology.
- the link between relationships (and relationship changes) and the presenting problem.
- how drugs and/or alcohol may be interacting with distress/disorder (if appropriate).
- how the Problem Area relates to the symptoms.
- how Interpersonal Psychotherapy provides an opportunity for these issues to be addressed, with an emphasis on a hopeful outcome.
- strengths that might assist recovery.

However, although the formulation is a summary, it is more than just a summary. We have already discussed how in the therapy room there are two experts: the young person is the expert in his own life—no one else knows what it is like to be him—but the therapist also brings expertise to the dyad. The formulation is an opportunity for the therapist to demonstrate this expertise by providing information, links, interpretations, understanding—in short, by helping the young person to make more sense of his current experience of life.

One young person, after the therapist had discussed the formulation with her, provided the following observation:

**Jane,** aged 23

> *Before therapy, my life was like walking around in a room full of rubbish. I could smell it all the time, it was under my feet, it was everywhere. When you told me that what was going on for me was depression I was so relieved. It was like putting all the rubbish in a big box. I could still see it, still smell it, but at least I could walk around the box without the rubbish under my feet. Then when we worked out my depression was about Role Transition, is was like putting all the rubbish in a much smaller box. And this was a box I could reach into and throw the rubbish out the window.*

## The Treatment Agreement

The final task of the Initial Phase of IPT-A is to discuss the responsibilities of the young person and his or her family during the therapeutic process and to prepare the young person for the next phase of therapy: the Middle Phase.

The Treatment Agreement should include the following:

- the approximate number of sessions.
- the frequency and duration of sessions.
- the Problem Area to be addressed.
- the expectations of both therapist and young person.
- treatment boundaries and telephone contact.
- the role of the parents in therapy.
- the role of the school.

These components are discussed below.

### The approximate number of sessions

IPT-A is a time-limited intervention. However, the time limitations are not dictated by a rigid formula but by the evolving nature of symptom reduction, within the context of the developing therapeutic alliance. Clinical experience suggests an approximate guide of eight to fifteen sessions will usually be on the therapist's mind when contemplating the Treatment Agreement. The precise number of sessions will be influenced by factors such as the severity of the young person's distress and functional impairment; attachment behaviours and style; the level of insight the young person displays; the quality of social and interpersonal support provided by the family and friends; age and stage of development; connectedness to school or employment; the young person's commitment to being involved in therapy; and, of course, the young person's progress during therapy.

### The frequency and duration of sessions

Once the number of sessions has been negotiated, the therapist and young person will discuss the frequency and duration of sessions. In IPT-A it is usually best to attempt weekly sessions where possible during the Initial and Middle Phases and then make a collaborative decision about titrating sessions at the beginning of the Consolidation Phase to bi-weekly, then spaced even further apart as the therapy reaches its conclusion. The duration of sessions will usually be 50 minutes (the therapeutic hour), but this may vary, for example in school situations where standard lesson times may be 40–45 minutes.

### The Problem Area to be addressed

As the Problem Area has already been discussed at length and agreed upon, including this discussion in the Treatment Agreement serves primarily as a reminder of this key element of therapy. It also provides an opportunity for the therapist to highlight two things. First, discussion of the Problem Area will occupy a central role in future sessions, emphasising yet again the importance that the identified Problem Area has in interpersonal relationships generally and, specifically, in the young person's current distress. Second, that during sessions if another Problem Area emerges as significant, the flexibility is there to transfer to that Problem Area if this is collaboratively decided as the best option.

### The expectations of both therapist and young person

IPT-A is not a passive therapy. Young people are expected to take an active role in the process, including completing homework. IPT-A homework is likely to include tasks such as practising new interpersonal skills and communication patterns, reflecting on associated affect, and observing how these may be related to the current experience of symptoms. Young people need to know that the focus of therapy is for the most part on the present, not the past, and during sessions they will be expected to discuss events that have occurred between sessions, including communications with significant others that have gone well and examples of interactions that have not. The role of the young person will shift during the course of therapy. The therapist has a relatively active role during the Initial Phase as much of this phase consists of data gathering and psychoeducation, but as therapy progresses, the therapist will become less directive and more focussed on the interpersonal incidents brought to session by the young person. During the course of therapy, the therapist will expect the young person to bring to therapy the subject matter for discussion, and the therapist's role will be to ensure that the therapeutic processes remain aligned with the Problem Area and associated communication patterns identified as salient in the Initial Phase.

### Treatment boundaries and telephone contact

During discussion of the Treatment Agreement, the therapist will inform the young person about confidentiality and its limits, emphasising that all sessions will remain confidential unless the therapist comes to the conclusion that the young person is at risk of serious harm to themselves or to others. Should that circumstance arise, the therapist will discuss with the young person what steps could be taken to offer protection. Parents will also be informed of the confidential nature of the sessions and reminded that the therapist is not at liberty to discuss session content unless the young person gives explicit permission to do so. This conversation with the parents should be conducted in the presence of the young person so the young person and parents get precisely the same message.

Mufson et al. (2004) recommends weekly telephone contact between sessions for the first weeks of treatment and offers the young person the opportunity to call the therapist should the need arise. These discussions continue to afford the therapist the chance to demonstrate respect for the young person and provide further occasions to strengthen the therapeutic alliance by emphasising the mutuality of the client's and therapist's roles. For example,

*Therapist:* *For the first few sessions, I'd like to phone you between sessions just to see how you're going. It's not like a therapy session, just a few minutes to see that things are going okay with you. Probably about midway between sessions, so if we meet every Tuesday, maybe I could phone on Fridays. Would that be okay? So what would be the best time and the best number to get you on? And if you need to call me for any reason, please feel free to. I won't always be able to answer, but if you leave a message I'll get back to you.*

More recently, therapists have used text or email messages instead of phone calls for this communication. The decision of which modality to use is up to the therapist and the young person. The key message for the young person is that the therapist is thinking of her even when she is not in the room.

### The role of the parents in therapy

In most IPT-A interventions, particularly for younger clients, parents will be involved in the Initial Phase of treatment. They may bring their young person to the first session of therapy; provide valuable information about the young person's presentation at home; and also provide information about relevant family history, including the young person's younger years. Once the diagnosis has been established and the therapeutic modality selected, the therapist will provide some psychoeducation to the parents about the nature of the young person's presenting problems and how therapy will proceed. This, of course, hinges on the young person's acceptance of parents' involvement. Whilst most clients are agreeable to their parents' involvement, some will oppose it. For example, if the identified Problem Area is Interpersonal Disputes and the primary dispute is with the parents, the young person may initially be reluctant to include the parents in any manner. Likewise, if there is a history of abuse involving the parents, the young person may refuse parental involvement. Additionally, there may be many reasons why some parents are unavailable to be involved in therapy, such as work commitments, the young person living apart from parents, the parents' own mental disorder, substance use, physical health issues, imprisonment, geographic isolation, or unwillingness to be involved.

Parents can be educated to be collaborative therapists in the home environment—to reinforce some of the new interpersonal skills learnt in therapy and to act as safe others with whom the young person can practice new interpersonal skills. More generally, parents can be educated to develop a set of behavioural expectations, particularly social expectations, appropriate to the young person's level of distress and functional impairment and to adjust these expectations as the young person progresses in therapy. Where there is an unwillingness for either the young person to assent to parental involvement or the parents to be involved, it remains the task of the therapist to continue to encourage parental involvement, with the caveat that some young people's relationships with parents are so toxic that any involvement would likely compromise the therapeutic process.

152  *The Initial Phase of IPT-A*

**Erin** (with Erin's mother, Julie, present)

Therapist: *Thanks for joining us again, Julie. Erin and I have had three sessions together now and we'd like to fill you in on how things are going. And Erin please feel free to add anything you'd like to as we go. Erin has already let me know that she has told you a bit about what we've been talking about and she said she's okay about me adding some things now. I just want to say that Erin's depression has been pretty serious. You've noticed at home some of the changes in Erin over the past six months or so—she's been sad and irritable, spending a lot of time alone, not wanting to talk much, not doing as well at school, not seeing much of her friends at all—that sort of thing—and she just can't seem to snap out of it. Anything else, Erin?*

Erin: *And pissed off with Liam and Dad.*

Julie: *Erin!*

Therapist: *You said you haven't been sleeping too well either, Erin, and you seem to be tired all the time, even when you do sleep. So overall, those kind of things happen when you're depressed. Julie, I think Erin has recently told you about how devastated she was when she got her colour-blindness diagnosis and all that meant for her. It took me a while to understand how serious that was, too. She had some other pretty major losses about then as well—Pepe got run over—and something else that happened is that Erin was feeling so bad about things that she started spending much more time in her room, just thinking, and she lost nearly all contact with her friends. The longer she was away from them, the harder it became for her to contact them again. So she sort of lost her friends as well. And you told me, Julie, that Erin also pulled back from her family.*

Julie: *I kept telling her to call Dallas or Kate. She's such good friends with them—but she wouldn't.*

Therapist: *I know—it was so hard for her. Depression does that to you. The things you know you need to do, you just can't seem to bring yourself to doing.*

Erin: *I just don't have the energy. I kinda want to see Dallas but at the same time I don't.*

Therapist: *So, Julie, Erin's depression started after she lost all these things, and now we have to help her find a way to start living her life again. But to begin with, it's so important for us all to understand how much all those losses meant to her.*

Therapist: *Julie, those tears?*

Julie: *I just want her to be happy again—her old self.*

Therapist: *Erin?*

Erin: *I want to be my old self again. I just don't know how. And I can't.*

Therapist: *Julie, understanding how hard this is for Erin is an important first step. I really do believe Erin will begin to feel better before too long, and when that starts to happen maybe we'll get together again and review things, if*

|  | *that's okay with Erin. But in the meantime, you could encourage Erin to have meals with you but don't stress too much if she's not up to it. Encourage her to see her friends a bit more but again only if Erin's good with that. As far as jobs around the house goes, what do you think, Erin?* |
|---|---|
| Erin: | *No, I'm not allowed to do anything. (Erin smiles.) That's been okay—my room's spotless, but that's because I compulsively clean 'cos I've got nothing else to do. Plus I've been doing my washing.* |
| Julie: | *She's been pretty good with that sort of thing. Too good, really—I just want her to get out more.* |
| Therapist: | *Julie, one thing you could do. I'm concerned about Erin's constant tiredness. Most likely it's all part of her depression, but just to make sure, could you get her along to your doctor just to check it out? I'll write to him today but if you could do that pretty soon, it would be good. Okay Erin?* |
| Erin: | *S'pose.* |
| Therapist: | *Well, thanks you two. Julie, I just want to spend a bit more time with Erin before we finish. I'll see her again next Friday. Do you have any questions?* |

## *The role of the school*

The American Academy of Child and Adolescent Psychiatry in their Practice Parameters for Depressive Disorders (Birmaher et al., 2007) and Anxiety Disorders (Connolly and Bernstein, 2007) recommend that in addition to family involvement, the young person's school should also be included in any treatment approach. These parameters identify four areas to be addressed:

1   School personnel could benefit from psychoeducation to help understand mental disorder and its effects on students (NICE, 2017). Part of this educational process is acknowledging that their primary roles are teaching and learning but that mental disorder presents a substantial barrier to the fulfilment of these roles. This was illustrated in the Australian report *The Mental Health of Children and Adolescents* (Lawrence et al., 2015). Lawrence notes that both school attendance and school performance are significantly impacted by mental disorder and that young people with a depressive disorder missed an average of 23 days per year because of their disorder and those with an anxiety disorder missed an average of 20 days. This was in addition to days missed due to other reasons. This report also found that students with any disorder were much more likely to perform at below-average level across a range of subjects than were students with no disorder.
2   Issues related to confidentiality should be discussed with school personnel as teachers often operate under a different level of confidence than that of therapists.

3 The therapist, along with the young person's family, should advocate for variations in, for example class schedules, workload, and assessment tasks consistent with the level of the student's functional impairment until symptoms have resolved.
4 Some students may qualify for a disability assistance under local or state legislation that may require the therapist's endorsement.

School psychologists, guidance officers, counsellors, social workers, and school nurses, as well as teachers and administrators, can create an environment where students with mental disorder are nurtured and cared for. Likewise, providing a point of contact such as a year supervisor or equivalent, can assist vulnerable students to negotiate often daunting requirements of the school setting.

Reluctance on the part of the family or student to establish contact with the school should be respected and explored. In these cases, the therapist would outline the contribution the school could make towards recovery and perhaps negotiate specific levels of contact, such as with the school psychologist, who could retain a similar level of confidentiality to that of the therapist.

## Orientation to the Middle Phase of treatment

By about session 3 or 4, all of the above tasks of the Initial Phase and, prior to this, the holistic assessment, will have been completed. Gunlicks-Stoessel et al. (2019) suggest that by week four, a response to IPT-A should be observed. They suggest that if this is not the case, augmentation of therapy, for example a change to twice-a-week sessions or, in some cases, antidepressant medication, may be warranted. Following this consideration, all that remains is to prepare the young person for the next part of the treatment process, the Middle Phase.

Orientation to the Middle Phase consists primarily of revisiting the symptoms, distress, and impairment the young person is experiencing and relating these again to the identified Problem Area. The young person is reminded that as the Problem Area is addressed in therapy and as relationships begin to change, she will start to feel better. Case summaries from other clients with similar Problem Areas or stories such as the story of Jane, related earlier in this chapter, who saw her life prior to therapy as a room full of rubbish, can often help reinforce the effectiveness of the Problem Area focus for symptom resolution.

Metaphors such as the tunnel metaphor that **Erin** related to well can equally be used effectively:

*Therapist:* *Erin when we begin our next session on Friday, we'll start to focus on the Problem Area of Complex Grief that you saw as the one most closely linked to your depression. Do you remember that?*

Erin: *That one was the closest. I remember there was another one about changing actors that was pretty close too.*

Therapist: *That's right, changing actors—Role Transition. So we decided to go with the grief one because of all the things you lost—particularly losing your life's dream when you got the colour-blindness diagnosis. And there were the other things as well, like Pepe, and you also lost your relationship with Dallas and your other friends because you just didn't have the energy to deal with people. I remember you told me it was like being stuck in a long black tunnel—you couldn't go forwards and you couldn't go back. You were stuck.*

Erin: *I still can't see how I'm going to get out, though.*

Therapist: *I do remember, Erin, that as you thought about what it might be like to talk to Dallas again, and to tell him what it is really like for you, and for him to be listening and being there for you, that you felt yourself move a little bit in that tunnel. Do I remember right?*

Erin: *Maybe. I dunno. Yeah, maybe. I think Mum finally got it at last. I couldn't believe it when she cried. She hardly ever cries—maybe she's beginning to get it. I know Dallas would get it if we talked.*

Therapist: *And the tunnel?*

Erin: *Yeah, maybe if Dallas and Mum finally got it I wouldn't feel so lonely. The tunnel? It'll be a long time before I see any light.*

Therapist: *Well, next session we'll try to work out how you can take some steps forward in that tunnel. I think that as we work out how to talk to some of the people in your circles so that they actually begin to understand what all of those losses really mean for you and how your life changed, you'll feel less alone. That's like taking some steps towards the light. What do you think?*

Erin: *I hope so.*

Therapist: *Okay, Erin, that's about it for today. So between now and next session I just want you to think a bit about that tunnel and see if you can think of anything else that might help you move towards the light. We'll talk about that next week. I'll call you on Tuesday, about 4:30, when you get home from school. And don't forget, if you want to check anything out before our session next Friday, give me a call or message me.*

## Summary

The Interpersonal Inventory, comprising the five tasks described above, is central to the Initial Phase of IPT-A. Following the holistic assessment, the Initial Phase provides the therapist the opportunity to explore the interpersonal world of the young person and, in so doing, to assist the young person gain a better understanding of how his or her interpersonal relationships relate to their distress or symptoms. Through the Closeness Circles, the timeline, the identification of the Problem Area, connecting this Problem Area with the distress or symptoms, and developing an hypothesis about the young person's attachment style, the therapist will be shaping the therapeutic alliance such that it becomes for the young person a safe place in which she can freely learn, question, emote, and heal.

## Note

1 Therapists may find it helpful to complete their own Closeness Circles prior to using this technique with clients. Although this technique is deceptively simple, unexpected questions and feelings often arise during its completion. For example, a dichotomy between who I *should* put in the inner circle versus who I *want* to be that close may arise. In addition, putting names on paper with closeness being the criterion often elicits surprising responses. If the therapist has already completed his or her own Closeness Circle, he or she may be in a more empathic position to deal with responses that may arise in clients.

## References

Birmaher, B., Brent, D., et al. (2007). Practice parameter for the assessment and treatment of children and adolescents with depressive disorders. *Journal of the American Academy of Child and Adolescent Psychiatry*, 46(11), 1503–1526.

Connolly, S., & Bernstein, G. (2007). Practice parameter for the assessment and treatment of children and adolescents with anxiety disorders. *Journal of the American Academy of Child and Adolescent Psychiatry*, 46(2), 267–283.

Deitz, L., Mufson, L. Irvine, H., & Brent, D. (2008). Family-based interpersonal psychotherapy for depressed pre-adolescents: An open-treatment trial. *Early Intervention in Psychiatry*, 2(3), 154–161.

Gunlicks-Stoessel, M., Mufson, L., et al. (2019). Critical decision points for augmenting interpersonal psychotherapy for depressed adolescents: A pilot sequential multiple assignment randomized trial. *Journal of the American Academy of Child and Adolescent Psychiatry*, 58(1), 80–91.

Hlastala, S., Kotler, J., McClellan, J., & McCauley, E. (2010). Interpersonal and social rhythm therapy for adolescents with bipolar disorder: Treatment development and results from an open trial. *Depression and Anxiety*, 27(5), 457–464.

Jacobson, C., & Mufson, L. (2012). Interpersonal psychotherapy for depressed adolescents adapted for self-injury: Rationale, overview and case summary. *Americal Journal of Psychotherapy*, 66(4), 349–375.

Lawrence, D., Johnson, S., Hafekost, J., Boterhoven De Haan, K., Sawyer, M., Ainley, J., & Zubrick, S. (2015). *The mental health of children and adolescents: Report on the second Australian Child and Adolescent Survey of Mental Health and Wellbeing.* Department of Health, Canberra.

Moffitt, T. (2013). Childhood exposure to violence and lifelong health: Clinical intervention science and stress-biology research join forces. *Development and Psychopathology*, 25, 1619–1634.

Mufson, L., Dorta, K., Moreau, D., & Weissman, M. (2004). *Interpersonal psychotherapy for depressed aadolescents* (2nd ed.). New York: Guilford Press.

Mufson, L., Moreau, D., Weissman, M., & Klerman, G. (1993). *Interpersonal psychotherapy for depressed adolescents.* New York: Guilford Press.

Mychailyszyn, M. P., & Elson, D. M. (2018). Working through the blues: A meta-analysis on interpersonal psychotherapy for depressed adolescents (IPT-A). *Children and Youth Services Review*, 87, 123–129.

National Institute for Health and Care Excellence (NICE). (2017). *Depression in children and young people: identification and management. Clinical Guideline.* Published September 2005, updated 2017. nice.org.uk/guidance/cg28

O'Shea, G., Spence, S., & Donovan, C. (2015). Group versus individual interpersonal psychotherapy for depressed adolescents. *Behavioural and Cognitive Psychotherapy*, *43*(1), 1–19.

Springer, K., Sheridan, J., Kuo, D., & Carnes, M. (2007). Long-term physical and mental health consequences of childhood physical abuse: Results from a large population-based sample of men and women. *Child Abuse and Neglect*, *5*, 517–530.

Tang, T-C., Jou, S-H., Ko, C-H., Huang, S-Y., & Yen, C-F. (2009). Randomised study of school-based intensive interpersonal psychotherapy for depressed adolescents with suicidal risks and parasuicide behaviours. *Psychiatry and Clinical Neuroscience*, *63*, 463–470.

Tanofsky-Kraff, M., Wilfley, D., et al. (2010). A pilot study of interpersonal psychotherapy for preventing excess weight gain in adolescent girls at-risk for obesity. *International Journal of Eating Disorders*, *43*(8), 701–706.

Young, J., Mufson, L., & Davies, M. (2006). Impact of comorbid anxiety in an effectiveness study of interpersonal psychotherapy for depressed adolescents. *Journal of the American Academy of Child and Adolescent Psychiatry*, *45*(8), 904–912.

# Part III
# The Middle Phase of IPT-A

# 6 The Middle Phase of IPT-A

**Contents**

| | |
|---|---|
| Introduction | 161 |
| Assessment is an ongoing process | 162 |
| Explaining client and therapist roles in the Middle Phase | 162 |
| Staying on track | 162 |
| Techniques for working on the Problem Area | 163 |
| Plan and rehearse changes | 164 |
| Markers of improvement | 165 |
| Involving parents and others in the Middle Phase | 165 |
| *Parents* | 166 |
| *Referring parents for mental health and other interventions* | 167 |
| *School staff* | 167 |
| Summary | 167 |
| References | 168 |

**Introduction**

The Middle Phase of IPT-A focusses on addressing the issues raised in the Interpersonal Formulation. The aims of the Middle Phase reflect the general aims of IPT-A:

- to reduce the symptoms of depression or other disorder
- to assist the young person to communicate more effectively about his or her needs for closeness and support, especially in relation to the major Problem Area
- to enhance the young person's social support system

During the Middle Phase, the young person increases his or her range of interpersonal skills to deal with their current distress or symptoms. In learning how to cope with present challenges, clients acquire lifelong coping skills that provide resilience to future adversity.

## Assessment is an ongoing process

Assessment continues through the Middle Phase. Specific aspects of the Problem Area will be explored in order to develop approaches that effectively deal with the major factors contributing to distress. As new information comes to light, the Interpersonal Formulation may be revised, treatment agreements may be adjusted, and the hypothesis about the young person's attachment style refined.

## Explaining client and therapist roles in the Middle Phase

The collaborative partnership established in the Initial Phase continues in the Middle Phase, but with the young person's role in therapy shifting significantly. In the Initial Phase the client and therapist provide a lot of information. In the Middle Phase, the focus changes to building interpersonal competencies in the young person and developing the necessary skills and confidence to implement these. This includes discussing her relationships and associated affect in some detail. Disclosure is facilitated by increasing trust in the therapeutic relationship.

The therapist's role remains an active one in the Middle Phase and is guided by an awareness of being a transitory attachment figure. The therapist explicitly cultivates the collaborative nature of therapy, individualises treatment, and monitors symptoms. As the Middle Phase progresses, the therapist deliberately modifies the nature of the therapeutic relationship so that the young person takes on more responsibility for identifying interpersonal patterns that are helpful and those that are contributing to symptomatology.

This change in the therapeutic relationship will in most cases be discussed transparently with the young person. The therapist, for example, might explain that she may not ask as many questions in order to create space for the young person to raise issues and feelings he is experiencing in relation to the Problem Area. If this change in the therapist's behaviour is not explained, the young person may attribute his own rationale to account for it, such as that he has done something wrong or has disappointed the therapist in some way.

The therapist may suggest that the transparency around roles provides examples of how the young person's experience in therapy might inform the ways he negotiates other relationships. This will be elaborated in later sessions, especially during the Consolidation Phase.

As work on the Problem Area progresses, the young person is continually consulted so that decisions are made jointly with the therapist and draw on the young person's expertise and knowledge of his situation. The therapist models an expectation that the client can understand key aspects of his experience and make wise choices about the best ways to reach his goals.

## Staying on track

Although there is considerable flexibility in the Middle Phase in terms of how Problem Areas are addressed, it is essential that they remain the focus or therapy.

The therapist will continually be on guard for distractors from the task of working on the Problem Area. For example, Crystal, who was introduced in Chapter 5, developed depression and social anxiety associated with Interpersonal Gaps. Crystal often wanted to discuss peer group issues that the therapist believed were distractions that assisted Crystal to avoid facing the Interpersonal Gaps that were central to her symptoms. In this case, the therapist acknowledged Crystal's interest in peer group activities and reminded her that in order to reduce her distress, her Interpersonal Gaps needed to be addressed.

Staying on task also involves anticipating and managing crises. Crises may include suicidal ideation or behaviour, self-harm, or dangerous and damaging behaviour. In managing these issues, the therapist should look for ways to help the young person understand how they connect to the Problem Area. If peripheral issues are raised by the young person or her significant others, the therapist should first explore their relevance to the Problem Area as this may not be immediately clear. While acknowledging the young person's concern, the therapist needs to generally steer away from issues that depart from the Problem Area or relate issues of concern to the Problem Area. It is often helpful to refer to the treatment agreement.

The Problem Areas can be thought of as a focus that targets the work of the Middle and Consolidation Phases. They are shorthand conceptualisations that facilitate a strategic approach to maximising therapy outcomes, which is essential, given the time-limited nature of IPT-A. What is most important is that the young person finds the conceptualisation of the Problem Area acceptable and meaningful for her circumstances.

It is not uncommon for more than one Problem Area to contribute to the client's distress. When this is the case, it may be possible to address these, even within a time limited intervention. For example, Interpersonal Gaps and Interpersonal Disputes sometimes coexist. Assisting young people to develop skills to manage conflict may reduce the distress associated with Disputes and also reduce some of the behaviours related to Interpersonal Gaps, such as those that are impeding initiating and maintaining relationships. Generalising learning is a major focus of the Consolidation Phase.

## Techniques for working on the Problem Area

Although the aims of working on the Problem Area remain consistent for all clients, the strategies and techniques vary according to the young person's circumstances and needs. The techniques included in this book do not form an exhaustive list. If the therapist is familiar with other approaches and feels these techniques may be more effective in engaging particular clients and addressing their issues, the therapist should certainly consider using alternative approaches, whilst always ensuring that the work is directly focussed on the Problem Area.

For some young people, the clinical techniques discussed in Chapter 4 will be sufficient for resolving or partially addressing the Problem Area, and this may be all that is required to bring about significant improvement in symptoms.

Additional techniques are included in the Problem Area chapters (Chapters 7–10) to help make accessible the concepts or responses that might otherwise be difficult for the young person to understand or express. With some young people it will not be necessary to use any of the techniques as described. For example, in the case of Admir, discussed in Chapter 8, although he might well have benefited from approaches outlined in that chapter, such as Mapping, these techniques were not essential to his progress. Time that may have been spent on them to further develop his insight, which had already improved to adequate levels through discussion with the therapist, was instead devoted to developing the social skills and confidence necessary to implement effective conflict solving strategies.

## Plan and rehearse changes

A key aspect of operationalising the insights gained in exploring Problem Areas is to assist the young person to communicate his needs, especially in relation to care and support. The therapist creates a safe space within which the young person can identify and express his needs. Next, a bridge must be constructed from the young person discussing his needs with the therapist to an ability to communicate these needs effectively to significant people in his life. Social skills development and confidence building are key components of the bridge.

The therapist determines where to focus for maximum gain. Even among young people experiencing Interpersonal Gaps, many clients do not need global social skill development. The existing competencies need to be uncovered and reinforced so that the young person can consciously draw on them. Social skill development can then selectively focus on the aspects which most challenge the young person and which are most salient to his symptoms.

A common theme across the Problem Areas is that the young person has not been able to find ways to meet his needs, including his attachment needs. IPT-A provides some catch-up time. It is an opportunity for accelerated growth in the hothouse atmosphere of therapy. Even a few sessions, providing they precisely target the key issues and vital communication skills, can produce profound improvements in the effectiveness of the young person's communication with his significant others. This can elicit the care and support he needs to help him deal with the Problem Area. If this support is not forthcoming in his current relationships, then new avenues of support can be developed. For young people with few social competencies, or who are burdened with additional adversity, the improvements may not be as profound but may nevertheless be sufficient to bring some improvement in their needs being met. The concept of good enough improvement is central to time-limited therapy. Even small improvements can change the young person's life trajectory. As a client starts experiencing some successes, feelings of hopelessness will be challenged, making other small changes possible, and thus positive momentum builds.

Continuing the horticultural metaphor, just as a hothouse plant often needs to experience a gradual transition to the environment outside, or hardened off, in order to avoid shock due to sudden changes in temperature, humidity, or sunlight intensity, so, too, the young person's new growth may be soft and vulnerable to shocks outside the protected environment of therapy. In IPT-A, many young people will need preparation in order to apply the growth and learning gained in therapy to the real world. The components of this preparation in IPT-A are identifying and rehearsing effective communication strategies, building confidence, and developing the young person's ability to keep herself safe—psychologically, emotionally and, where appropriate, physically—when communicating their needs to others. These competencies include identifying safe people and choosing a time, place, and methods most likely to produce the desired outcomes.

## Markers of improvement

The understanding that the young person develops during the Initial Phase about the connection between her symptoms and the Problem Area is reinforced during the Middle Phase. Identifying and monitoring markers of improvement is a key part of this process and also helps to promote hope of positive outcome. This might include symptom reduction, solutions to problems, communicating more effectively, and having more of her attachment needs met.

Therapist questions that may assist the young person to identify signs of improvement include the following:

- *What are your goals for the Problem Area? How will we know when you are making progress in achieving them?*
- *As your depression improves, what signs might you notice? What might I notice? What might your parents or friends notice?*
- *As you become less depressed, what will be different?*
- *When we work out ways to reduce the conflict with your parents, what might change for you? For example, how do you imagine it would affect how you're feeling? And how might it affect the way you relate to others?*

## Involving parents and others in the Middle Phase

Therapy may be enhanced when it embraces the influence of parents and a range of other people who are important for the young person. They can be a valuable source of information in understanding the client and in improving her interpersonal support. However, caution must be exercised, as no matter how well the significant others know the young person, their opinions and suggestions will be subjective and influenced by their own needs and concerns.

Parents and others may not be aware of the full extent of the young person's circumstances, especially her internal world. Parents and teachers tend to underestimate the level of distress that young people are experiencing, especially when internalising disorders, such as depression and anxiety, are present

(Beaver, 2008; De Los Reyes et al., 2015). Additionally, as part of the individuation process, adolescents often keep some information private from their parents. Also, in order to fit in with peers, they may not share some aspects of their experience with their friends and associates.

It may be helpful to explain to parents, teachers, or other significant people that distress in adolescents can be expressed by behaviours such as acting out, asserting independence, and feigning indifference. These behaviours can easily be misinterpreted as a lack of care and respect or deliberate disobedience. Adults may respond punitively, which is likely to be counterproductive and compound the young person's difficulties. They may also miss opportunities to respond in ways that help to open communication and convey support.

In determining the appropriateness of inviting the young person's significant others to attend therapy, the potential pros and cons need to be weighed. The first issue to consider is the young person's wishes. His preference should be respected. However, this does not preclude exploring the reasons for reticence on the part of the young person regarding inviting others to participate in a therapy session. It might be that the young person's concerns can be readily addressed so that he is comfortable with the prospect of involving others in this way. For example, in the case of Pippa, discussed in Chapter 9, she declined the option of having her divorced parents attend therapy. Pippa's reticence was based on a fear that her parents would argue with each other. On discovering this, the therapist offered separate sessions for each parent. This arrangement was acceptable to Pippa and allowed the therapist to facilitate Pippa communicating her needs to her parents more effectively.

Before involving others in a therapy session with the young person, the capacity of the other to be attuned to the young person's needs should be considered.

Parents, school staff, or other significant people might also be invited to contact the therapist regarding any developments that may be relevant to therapy. Additional issues specific to each Problem Area regarding involving significant others are identified in the four Problem Area chapters.

It is always the young person's final decision about who if any of his or her significant others attend therapy sessions or are contacted by the therapist.

### Parents

Parents' goals regarding therapy will have been explored during the Initial Phase. In the Middle Phase, these aims, which may be quite broad, are revisited and refined in relation to the Problem Area. The nature of the work during the Middle Phase can be discussed so that the parents can support it. This should include a reminder that IPT-A is present focussed rather than being oriented to the past as they may be keen to talk about historical issues, including wanting to return to settle old scores or justify their position.

In addition to providing psychoeducation to assist parents to understand and support the needs of the young person, the role of parents or others may include active participation in therapy sessions and being involved in assisting the young person with skills practice activities outside therapy.

## Referring parents for mental health and other interventions

When the young person's parents are experiencing mental health, drug and alcohol or other issues impeding their parenting capacity, a key way to support the young person's recovery may be to assist the parents to access assessment, treatment, and social support for themselves. Some parents may be resistant to acknowledging or addressing their own issues; however, many will welcome the therapist's observations and suggestions. Some will not only be grateful that the therapist has reflected on their circumstances and needs, they may be reassured that this capacity for care and attention would in turn benefit their young person. This is discussed in the case of Admir in Chapter 8.

## School staff

School staff can be a source of valuable information for the therapist and are also well placed to monitor the young person's functioning and support her in practising skills she is learning in therapy. With consent, the therapist could contact the school directly and also support the parent's role in discussing the young person's needs with the school. School staff might be requested to make adjustments to reduce the demands and stress that may be contributing to the young person's symptoms.

School staff will usually welcome information relevant to academic performance, and it can be helpful if the therapist frames their communication in those terms with specific examples. Suggestions from the therapist for school adjustments may be more readily received after eliciting the school's concerns and goals.

If the young person is willing, it can be helpful to share safety plans with trusted school staff. This might include examples of strategies the young person can use to manage difficult affect. With this information, school staff may be able to more effectively manage crisis presentations and do so in ways that reinforce the work of therapy. For example, a teacher's response to a young person experiencing acute distress might include this:

> I can see that you are distressed. This seems like a good opportunity to practice some of the things you've been working on with your therapist. Let's get the safety plan out that you developed with her to remind us of the strategies you might use.

## Summary

The Middle Phase assists the young person to describe his or her experience of the Problem Area. A major component is developing clients' social skills so that they can more effectively elicit the care and support that they need. The therapist keeps therapy on track by ensuring it is focussed on the Problem Area. The roles of the young person and the therapist evolve during the Middle Phase so that the young person takes more responsibility for identifying and addressing interpersonal behaviour that is related to his or her symptoms. Finally, in the Consolidation Phase, the aim is to generalise the young person's enhanced social competencies to other challenges he or she may be dealing with currently or may face in the future.

## References

Beaver, B. (2008). A positive approach to children's internalising problems. *Professional Psychology: Research and Practice, 39*(2), 129–136.

De Los Reyes, A., Augenstein, T., Wang, M., Thomas, S., Drabick, D., Burgers, D. & Rabinowitz, J. (2015). The validity of the multi-informant approach to assessing child and adolescent mental health. *Psychological Bulletin, 141*(4), 858–900.

# 7 Complex Grief

**Contents**

| | |
|---|---|
| Introduction | 169 |
| Defining and assessing the Problem Area of Complex Grief | 170 |
| Working on Complex Grief in the Middle Phase | 172 |
|    *Essential Processes in IPT-A for Complex Grief* | 174 |
|    *Potential barriers* | 181 |
|    *Indicated Processes in IPT-A for Complex Grief* | 186 |
| Summary | 202 |
| References | 203 |

## Introduction

Loss in life is guaranteed, and grief is the process of adjusting to loss. It is the inescapable cost of forming attachments, and grief is sometimes referred to as the interest paid on love. Grief is a normal, natural, healthy response hardwired into us as a species. Grief is a process whereby we adjust emotionally, cognitively, physically, socially, and spiritually when our attachments to people, things, or aspects of self are severed. When the healing mechanism of grieving becomes blocked or impaired, Complex Grief reactions occur, with serious consequences for our functioning as well as our physical and mental health.

The aim of using psychotherapy for Complex Grief is to restore the grieving process so that individuals can adjust to their new circumstances following loss. IPT-A is distinguished from other therapies by achieving this through a particular focus on the improvement of interpersonal functioning. Psychological equilibrium is threatened when attachment bonds are broken. Assisting clients to meet their attachment needs constitutes a central part of an IPT-A intervention. This involves individuals more effectively communicating their experience and needs to others, which in turn increases the likelihood that they will receive the support and care they need. Improving communication also has the benefit of activating adjustment. While some of the essential work of grief can be carried out alone, through internal reflection and solitary activities, some of it is necessarily an interpersonal process (Attig, 2011; Klass et al., 1996). Communicating with others helps us to clarify and work through our responses to loss. It supports us to gain perspective and to create meaning about our loss (Neimeyer, 2001). These processes are played out in relationships and they are key in healthy adjustment to loss. IPT-A is indicated for moderate to severe depression (e.g., NICE, 2017); however, therapy will not be necessary for most young people experiencing adaptive grief reactions (e.g., if they do not have a mental disorder; see Stepped Care, Chapter 1).

Because loss cuts to the quick of our humanity, working on this Problem Area can be a double-edged sword for the therapist. The therapist often witnesses important growth in the young person. As rewarding as this might be, it can be a challenging place to work. The client's distress may elicit significant reactions in the therapist. For example, it might trigger aspects of the therapist's own history of loss, which can provide fertile ground for the therapist's personal and professional growth. Self-reflection, supervision, professional development, and sometimes personal therapy are particularly pertinent professional responsibilities when working on this Problem Area. The attention to self by the therapist may be necessary to maintain clinical poise in the face of the client's raw pain.

The aims of working with this Problem Area are to assist clients to

- understand the connection between Complex Grief and their symptoms
- explore their reactions to the loss and gain insight into their responses and those of their significant others
- deepen their existing support network by assisting them to communicate about the loss and their related needs
- extend their support network, if necessary, to include new supportive relationships

This chapter outlines the *Essential Processes* for addressing Complex Grief in IPT-A. A number of *Indicated Processes* that may be necessary for some adolescents and young adults are also described, including psychoeducation about loss and activities drawn from the creative arts.

## Defining and assessing the Problem Area of Complex Grief

The Problem Area of Complex Grief is defined as responses to loss that are generally maladaptive. These responses hinder the person's ability to adjust to loss in ways that enable him or her to function well following the loss. Complex grief is distinguished from an adaptive grief reaction by its timeframe, level of distress, and impact on functioning. In adaptive grief reactions, distress and a degree of impairment may be present, but the symptoms are self-correcting and constitute a healthy process by which people adjust to loss. Distinguishing adaptive grief from depression can be a complex task involving consideration of the impact of symptoms on functioning (intensity, frequency, and duration) and the presence of specific symptoms as markers of depression rather than adaptive grief, e.g., erosion of self-esteem, guilt, psychomotor changes, and suicidality (American Psychiatric Association, 2013).

A broad definition of Complex Grief works well for most young people. This encompasses loss resulting from bereavement and other forms of loss. In the IPT literature, there is some variation in the definition of this Problem Area. For example, Mufson et al. (2004) refers to this Problem Area as Grief and restricts it to loss resulting from bereavement. Mufson addresses non-bereavement losses within the Problem Area of Role Transition. Stuart and Robertson (2012) include both bereavement and non-bereavement losses in the Problem Area they refer to as Grief and Loss. The inclusion of non-bereavement loss within this Problem Area helps to communicate to the young person that the therapist recognises that the impact of these forms of loss can be significant. When loss is unacknowledged or unrecognised by others, which is sometimes referred to as disenfranchised grief, it can increase the risk of a Complex Grief reaction (Rando, 1993).

A sense of disenfranchisement was a major factor in Erin's Complex Grief, as discussed in Chapter 5. Erin's grief was complicated by a perception that her family and friends did not understand the importance of her loss and were dismissive of her feelings. IPT-A assisted her to understand her responses to loss and to help other people to understand the impact of the loss on her.

As young people lack the greater life experience of adults, they may be more susceptible to doubting the validity of their experience and therefore dismiss their responses to loss as out of proportion or unacceptable, particularly if they sense that people who are important to them do not endorse their responses. Additionally, the developmental imperative for adolescents to conform to peer expectations may increase their sensitivity to feeling excluded.

When loss comes thick and fast, its multiplicity may contribute to grief becoming complex. Adaptive grief takes time, and if an additional loss or other adversity occurs before the young person has adjusted to an initial loss, then their coping mechanisms may be overwhelmed.

Some groups of young people experience elevated rates of loss and their experience of loss may have particular characteristics. Forewarned with this demographic information, the therapist can be alert to exploring issues that may be particularly relevant to different populations of young people. For example, multiple loss is common in Indigenous and First Nations people due to the impact of dispossession and trauma, often spanning centuries. The range of resulting loss impacting these young people and their families, include premature death and disability, substance use, mental disorder, incarceration, loss of culture, out-of-home care, neglect, and abuse (e.g., Wynne-Jones et al., 2016). The case of Michelle, discussed below, encompasses some of these issues.

For some young people experiencing transitions, their distress and impairment are related directly to the loss associated with the transition, rather than the transition itself. When this is the case, Complex Grief may be chosen as the primary Problem Area rather than Role Transition. For example, this may apply to some young people experiencing migration or same-sex attraction. There is multiple loss in any migration experience, whether it is an international move or relocation within a country. Additionally, asylum seekers and refugees have usually experienced not only numerous losses but often also trauma in their country of origin, during their journey to safety, which may include many years in transit, and sometimes in their new host country (e.g., Mares, 2016).

Same-sex attracted young people, especially those growing up in families or religious and cultural communities in which same-sex attraction is unacceptable, may experience loss in the form of rejection by family, friends, community, and religion (for example, the case of Grant in Chapter 9). Complex Grief rather than Role Transition is chosen as the primary Problem Area when the young person's distress and impairment are related directly to loss.

A stepped care approach (discussed in Chapter 1) is perhaps nowhere more pertinent than in relation to loss. Most young people experiencing grief and loss do not need psychotherapy. They will recover from the loss without mental health intervention. The therapist assesses the appropriate level of intervention required. Some young people will benefit significantly from psychoeducation, self-help, and supportive counselling. For those at elevated risk of Complex Grief reactions, watchful waiting (to identify emerging symptoms of disorder) or IPT-A as a preventative intervention may be warranted. Elevated risk may be related to a range of factors including pre-existing anxiety or depression; history of trauma; lack of perceived support; or the circumstances of the loss, e.g., violent, sudden, or unexpected. In the case of Michelle, below, her presentation clearly warranted mental health intervention due to the severity of her symptoms, including suicidality, the nature and number of the losses she experienced, and the transgenerational trauma and abuse experienced by her family and relatives.

In order to individualise IPT-A, the therapist assesses the young person's needs, including the nature and circumstances of her grief, her competencies, risk factors, and the adequacy of her support. This will help the therapist to determine whether the *Essential Processes* outlined below are likely to be sufficient for the young person to adjust to her loss or whether some additional *Indicated Processes* may be required.

## Working on Complex Grief in the Middle Phase

The goal of IPT-A for Complex Grief is to reduce symptoms by assisting clients to adjust to the loss, so that they can function well in the new situation, including accessing the support they need. This may be facilitated by creating the

Complex Grief 173

safety, confidence, and skills necessary for clients to explore and communicate their experience of loss to the therapist and to significant others or to adjust to the loss in other ways.

The arc of therapy in the Middle Phase of IPT-A for Complex Grief is summarised in Figure 7.1. *Essential and Indicated Processes* are identified.

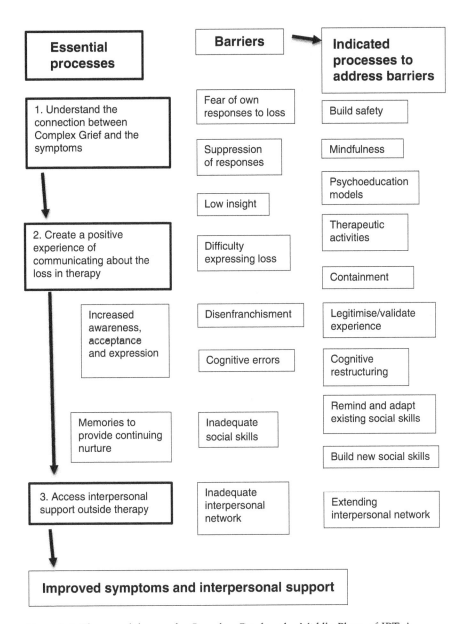

Figure 7.1 The arc of therapy for Complex Grief in the Middle Phase of IPT-A.

Although *Indicated Processes* may be potentially beneficial for many young people experiencing Complex Grief, because IPT-A is time limited, they are only used if required and to the extent necessary for the young person to progress through the *Essential Processes*.

The *Essential Processes* in the Middle Phase are the following:

1. Understand the connection between Complex Grief and the symptoms
2. Create a positive experience of communicating about the loss in therapy
3. Access interpersonal support outside therapy

### Essential Processes in IPT-A for Complex Grief

*Understand the connection between Complex Grief and the symptoms*

As we have already mentioned, it is essential that the young person understands the connection between the Problem Area and their symptoms. This provides the rationale for the work in the Middle Phase and encourages belief in a positive outcome. This understanding is established in the Initial Phase, as seen in the dialogue with Erin in Chapter 5 about the timeline. The connection is reinforced in the Middle Phase, for example, in the case of **Vijay,** aged 17, who experienced multiple and anticipatory loss.

*Therapist:* We decided a couple of sessions ago that your depression was related to grief, and today the connection has become even clearer. You've really helped me understand how the losses have affected you. You coped well with all those moves your family made as you were growing up. As you have described them to me, I've understood more about how stressful they were for you and your family. You found it really hard to make new friends, but you worked at it, only to have your family move again after a year or two. You didn't tell your parents how much you minded because you knew there was no option for your dad and it was happening for the other military families as well. But it sounds like you really hated it. You said it was like leaving part of yourself behind. Have I understood this correctly?

*Vijay:* Yeah.

*Therapist:* Last year your dad was seriously injured, and you've been really worried, not knowing if he might get worse. Earlier this year your big sister left home and you really miss her. Then your mum had to work long hours so you don't see her much. Recently your dad has deteriorated and you've heard he might not live much longer. This is a huge list and it's been going on for years. Most people would struggle to cope with injury and possible death of a parent and you've had all these additional losses as well. You haven't had time to grieve. Things have been happening too thick and fast, so a backlog of sadness has built up.

|  |  |
|---|---|
|  | *And now you're worried your dad might be dying. Am I right, or do you think I'm exaggerating it?* |
| Vijay: | *I hadn't put it together like that. Thinking of it all as loss—but you're right. It has gotten harder and harder.* |
| Therapist: | *You mentioned earlier that you didn't want to be sad or angry around your mum and dad. Our sessions will give you time and space to talk about what it's been like for you. As you do that, you'll lessen the load you've been carrying around and I think you'll find the improvement in your depression that you are beginning to notice will continue.* |

*Create a positive experience of communicating about the loss in therapy*

The distress caused by significant loss can be maintained and magnified by social isolation. In Complex Grief, many young people have formed a view that no one understands their experience of loss. This belief can become self-fulfilling as they give up attempting to communicate their feelings about the loss and their need for closeness and support. In IPT-A, the therapist unambiguously steps into this space and actively creates an experience where the young person feels well listened to and understood by the therapist. This demonstrates to the young person that it is possible for others to be genuinely interested in understanding them. This positive experience in therapy challenges the young person's negative assumption about the prospects of others being interested in him or about his own capacity to communicate effectively.

The therapist creates this encouraging experience by explicitly inviting the young person to tell his story about the loss and by demonstrating that she wants to hear the details. The invitation to the young person to tell his story should be explained and contextualised so that the young person understands the rationale. This is another opportunity for the therapist to demonstrate transparency. For example,

|  |  |
|---|---|
| Therapist: | *Part of the way we, as humans, cope with loss is to talk about it. It might be to go over what actually happened, or to talk about feelings, questions, doubts, worries, confusion, needs, anything at all. It is a key part of grieving, and many people need to go over it again and again. It can help us take in that the loss has happened and understand what it means for us. I'll be inviting you to tell me about how this loss has affected you. I'm really keen to understand the details and different aspects of what it has been like for you. We'll take some time for this. Then we can think about who else in your life you'd like to discuss this with, how you'd like them to respond, and how we might help that happen. How does that sound?* |

The therapist can anticipate and acknowledge potential barriers to the young person relating his experience:

Therapist:   It sounds like you're concerned this could be like opening a can of worms, in terms of you getting upset. As far as I'm concerned, it's fine if you become upset here. In fact, this is a great place for that to happen. I can help you deal with it, and we will probably both learn from it. Remember, I mentioned before that emotions can be like steam in a pressure cooker? When you express your emotions, you release the pressure inside, and it's less likely the emotions will burst out when you don't want them to.

Some young people will need more psychoeducation than this in order to accept their responses and express their grief in therapy. Several models and tools to help young people understand and accept their responses to loss are included in the *Indicated Processes* section later in this chapter.

The therapist can use questions to help clients describe their experience. For example,

- Tell me about ...
- What did you love most about?
- What do you miss most?
- Are there things about the loss or the way it happened that you feel angry or guilty about?
- Are there things you said or didn't say that you think about?
- Can you help me understand what that was like for you?

The therapist's body language and responses provide evidence of his interest and understanding. Comments that accurately summarise or refer to the client's experience also show the therapist has been listening carefully and understanding:

- It sounds like a particularly difficult aspect for you of your father's death is...
- I can see that this would be really hard on you and her. Am I right in thinking this is one of the most difficult things for you?
- So you really minded that you weren't allowed to visit him in hospital?
- Am I right in thinking you felt left out and angry that you didn't get to attend the funeral?

The therapist can amplify the learning for the client from telling his story, by inviting him to reflect on the process and the qualities present in the therapeutic relationship. Continuing the case of **Vijay,**

Therapist:   What has it been like, you telling me about how you feel about your dad and the uncertainty around his health?
Vijay:   It's been hard. But kind of good.
Therapist:   Can you tell me some more about what was hard and good?
Vijay:   Well, it's hard to talk about, but it's good the way you listen.

| | |
|---|---|
| Therapist: | I'm curious, what gave you the sense I was listening? |
| Vijay: | You look like it. And you didn't interrupt. |
| Therapist: | Anything else? |
| Vijay: | Not sure. |
| Therapist: | I was mainly listening, but I did say a few things. How do you feel about what I said? |
| Vijay: | Good. Like it showed you understood. |
| Therapist: | So in addition to telling your story in a way I could understand, you also noticed a few things I was doing. Did the way I responded to what you were saying help you tell your story? |
| Vijay: | Yeah. |
| Therapist: | Let's get your Closeness Circles out. I'd like to hear who you'd most like to talk with about the things we've discussed and how you'd like them to respond. I know it's been hard talking to me about this and it probably will feel hard talking to other people, partly because you're worried about upsetting them. But just as you found it helpful to talk about it with me, I think a really important part of you feeling better will be finding ways to help other people understand what's going on for you. You'll feel reconnected with your family and you'll all be in a better place to support each other. |

The therapist hypothesised that Vijay had some characteristics of anxious avoidant attachment and made a point of acknowledging that it wasn't easy for him to relate this experience. Time was spent helping Vijay understand his conflicting need to access support and his doubts about trusting and relying on others.

In this way, the therapist prepared Vijay for the third *Essential Process* in this Problem Area, accessing interpersonal support outside therapy. This included asking him who else might respond in ways that he found helpful in the therapy session, such as listening well, without interruptions and with understanding. The dialogue also demonstrates how the second and third *Essential Processes* can provide opportunities to reinforce the first, understanding the connection between Complex Grief and the symptoms.

In the case of **Michelle**, aged 14, these processes occurred in a different order. Michelle came to therapy after a suicide attempt. She presented as mature beyond her years, which seemed to be related to her experience of multiple losses. Michelle and her family identified as Aboriginal. Their losses included premature death and disability in their extended family and a keenly felt erosion of their traditional culture. Michelle was greatly distressed by her grandmother's recent stroke, which left her speech impaired and with memory loss. Michelle had suddenly lost the "normal" grandmother she had known, including the reliable support she had always found in her. Michelle's brother had died six months previously by suicide. Michelle's parents were struggling to cope with caring for her grandmother and with the grief of their son's death. Michelle had withdrawn from her family and friends. Not knowing how to respond to her parents' grief isolated her from them. This was compounded by feelings of shame about her reaction, which left her feeling unable to access her usual sources of support that she turned to when in need. Consequently, Michelle felt alone in her grief.

Michelle appeared to be securely attached, and this is reflected in the way she subsequently engaged in therapy; acted on the therapist suggestions, including completing tasks outside therapy; and in the straightforward ways she ultimately accessed support. These characteristics become apparent as her case unfolds in stages through this chapter.

In order to promptly address Michelle's safety, the first two therapy sessions occurred in the week following her suicide attempt. Therapy focussed on developing a safety plan and assisting Michelle to communicate her experience to her parents (thus beginning the third *Essential Process*, accessing interpersonal support outside therapy). Michelle's parents demonstrated that, despite their own grief, they had the desire and capacity to support her. Following this, as often occurs when young peoples' attachment needs are addressed, Michelle's suicidality rapidly decreased. The IPT-A intervention continued, including frequent review of her suicidality and safety plan.

In addition to assisting the young person to communicate her experience to the therapist and her significant others, another way to meet attachment needs following loss is through memories. We can continue to be nourished by a person or thing following a loss, even though the circumstances may have changed, or the person or thing is no longer physically present in our lives (e.g., Klass et al., 1996). Keeping positive memories alive is central, and the therapist can facilitate this through discussion and encouraging the young person to create concrete symbolic representations of the loss, including using activities such as those described below.

Attig (2000, 2011) states in relation to loss through death, that building an enduring love for the person can sooth the pain of our loss. Memories are the vehicle for this, and they need to be nurtured so that the lost person can carry on shaping our lives in positive ways and their love continue to nourish us.

The therapist fostered Michelle's continuing bond with her grandmother:

*Therapist:* *It sounds like a particularly difficult aspect for you regarding your Nan's stroke is missing the way you used to talk with her and the reassuring things she would say to you. She still tries to talk to you, and it upsets you when you don't understand her. You feel embarrassed and don't know what to say. I can see that this would be really hard on you and her. Am I right in thinking this is one of the most difficult things for you?*
*Michelle:* Yeah.
*Therapist:* *Could you tell me about a time when you felt well supported by your Nan?*
*Michelle:* Back in year 5 when the kids were giving me a hard time for being black.
*Therapist:* *And your Nan?*

| | |
|---|---|
| Michelle: | She told me not to worry about it. That they were young and didn't know any better. |
| Therapist: | Do you remember anything else about how she was then? |
| Michelle: | She told me how smart I was and kind. How everyone who knew me loved me. |
| Therapist: | Your Nan does sound lovely. Do you remember anything else? |
| Michelle: | Nan even offered to go up to school. |
| Therapist: | And that was important? |
| Michelle: | Yeah. She hated going to school. Said it reminded her when she was little. You know they used to get punished for speaking (traditional) language at her school. |
| Therapist: | Yes, I know and think it was really wrong. So even though it would have been very difficult for her, she was willing to go to your school to try and stop you being bullied. |
| Michelle: | And she felt embarrassed up there because her reading isn't very good. |
| Therapist: | The more I hear about your Nan, the more I like her. Do you think she still loves you and would say those things to you if she could speak now? |
| Michelle: | Yeah. |
| Therapist: | From what you've told me, it's very clear she loves you a lot! Because she can't speak to you the way she used to, you're going to have to fill in the dots with your memories so that her support can continue to benefit you. To help you do this, you'll need to keep your memories of her fresh. Writing them down will help, or drawing. I'd like you, even when you're an old woman like your Nan, to be able to remember the details of her love and support for you. Would you be interested in writing or drawing some of your memories? (Michelle nods.) |
| Therapist: | Great. It could be big things or small ways she showed that she loved you, compliments she paid you, things she taught you, anything at all. See what you can come up with over the next week and I'll be interested to hear about it. You could also ask your parents if they remember things about the way she was with you when you were little. |

At the following session, Michelle described how not only had she made a list of positive memories, she had read her list aloud to her grandmother. She stated that her grandmother had clearly been moved and that they had cried together but they were "good tears", in the sense that she felt closer to her grandmother and her grandmother was smiling and laughing among her tears as Michelle related her memories.

During the next session, discussion about Michelle's continuing connection to her brother proceeded in a similar way.

| | |
|---|---|
| Therapist: | I was wondering if we could talk about your brother. He's not here for you to talk to the way you can with your Nan. But is it okay to think about him in a similar way? |
| Michelle: | I guess so. But how, when he's not here? |

*Therapist:* You've been feeling less sad recently and it seems to be related to remembering all those good memories of your Nan and realising they are still true, even though she can't speak to you. I was thinking you might be able to use the memories of your brother in the same way.

The therapist facilitated a discussion to help Michelle remember the ways her brother had shown his care for her. Between sessions Michelle assembled mementos of her brother, including gifts and cards he had given her. She decorated a box in which she intended to keep these reminders of him. These processes provided effective ways for Michelle to continue to feel nurtured by the love her brother had shown her during his life. Other creative activities discussed later in this chapter could have provided additional means for Michelle to achieve this. Michelle's therapy then focussed on the third *Essential Process* of IPT-A for Complex Grief, accessing interpersonal support outside therapy.

Sometimes the simple question "What do you find most difficult about your loss?" can quickly assist the young person to relate their loss to the therapist. For example, **Mark**, aged 17, became depressed after he was diagnosed with cancer. He had become socially withdrawn and avoided most of his friends as well as avoided contact with teachers and family gatherings. When asked what was most difficult about his diagnosis, he commented:

*"I hate the way people keep asking me how I am, like they're expecting me to spill my guts all the time. Or they say I'm sorry about your illness. What am I supposed to say to that?"*

Further discussion revealed that Mark feared that he wouldn't know how to respond to questions or might get upset in public. Mark was trying hard to be positive rather than sad all the time and felt the condolences of others and enquiries about how he was coping undermined his efforts. When the therapist explored this, it became clear that Mark feared crying in front of others. He worried about feeling humiliated and judged as weak, partly related to perceptions of how he should behave as a male but also related to a dread of people pitying him. Additionally, Mark was no different from many adolescents in feeling that fitting in and being "normal" was crucial in order to be acceptable or attractive to his peers. This meant not being different. He was particularly sensitive to perceived difference based on his illness and felt that sharing feelings, especially sad emotions, would accentuate his difference.

Mark felt the common adolescent urge to assert his independence and at the same time experienced a vulnerability and need for support and guidance characteristic of earlier developmental stages. He attempted to exercise autonomy through noncompliance with medication, neglecting academic assignments (which he normally enjoyed), and increased substance use. This caused conflict with his parents, which was distressing for all concerned.

Mark struggled to make sense of his diagnosis and grappled with "why me?" He rejected his religious beliefs, and this added to his isolation from friends and family who were part of a religious community.

As Mark discussed his responses to his diagnosis, he expressed sadness, confusion, and anger. For Mark, this led to greater insight into his support needs, which in turn led to a reduction in conflict. He was then able to negotiate other ways to express autonomy.

When a loss is significant, attachment needs are likely to be accentuated. The losses experienced by both Michelle and Mark were compounded by their sense that they could not discuss their loss with people who were important to them. The therapist assisted Michelle and Mark to tell their story of loss in therapy. By creating a positive experience, where they felt listened to and understood, the therapist met some of their attachment needs and prepared the way for these needs to be met by their significant others.

Potential barriers

For some young people, discussing their loss using verbal methods, such as those outlined above, is all that is required of them to effectively communicate their experience of loss, including expression of the associated affect. This will be sufficient for them to move on to the next *Essential Process* in Complex Grief, that of communicating their experience of the loss to people outside therapy. Other clients will struggle with the invitation to tell their story in therapy. When this is the case, the therapist identifies the barriers and provides indicated therapy processes (Figure 7.1) to address whatever is preventing the young person from relating her experience.

In summary, assisting the young person to communicate her experience of loss in therapy has several benefits. It

- helps the therapist understand how best to support the young person's adjustment to the loss
- increases the young person's awareness and acceptance of her responses and needs in relation to the loss, which will assist her to help other people understand her experience and ultimately respond in ways that meet the young person's needs
- gives the young person the experience of being listened to well, with respect, interest, and understanding
- gives the young person opportunities to practice ways to communicate her experience, which ultimately assists her to communicate with her significant others

*Access interpersonal support outside therapy*

In the third *Essential Process*, the therapist facilitates communication between the young person and their significant others. The young person's attachment bonds may have been broken or threatened by loss and by their failure to access supportive connections with others following the loss. In the second *Essential Process* above, the therapist consciously steps into the role of a transitory attachment figure by demonstrating his interest, care, and capacity to understand the young person's experience of loss. This is followed by helping the young person, through discussion and, if indicated, role rehearsal, to make the transition to accessing attachment supports outside therapy. When the young person does this successfully, there is often significant improvement in symptoms. The young person's sense of isolation may dissolve as he experiences care, concern, and understanding from the therapist and particularly when these are provided by his significant others. As we saw in the case of Michelle, her suicidality rapidly diminished when she was able to relate her experience to her parents and grandmother and feel their support.

Continuing with **Vijay**, the therapist explained this process:

*Therapist:* When you described to me how your dad's injury has affected you, it helped me understand you much better. You gave me details about what you have been experiencing, and that made it easier for me to appreciate more precisely how and why you've been feeling so miserable. I was really interested to hear what you said, and I felt closer to you as a result of the examples you shared with me. I suspect if you can describe your experience to some of the important people in your Closeness Circles the way you have to me, they will have a much better understanding of what's been going on for you. I imagine many of them will feel moved in the way I have. They will feel more connected to you and you will feel closer to them. What do you think about what I'm saying?

*Vijay:* Maybe. I hadn't thought about it like that.

*Therapist:* I know this matters a lot to you, so it's important that we prepare in a way that is most likely to lead to the kind of responses you want. We can do some planning, for example, figure out who might be the best people to start with, how to check if they are receptive, and what's the best time for this kind of conversation to go well. We can practice the ways you could communicate with them to build up your confidence. You could then talk with them by yourself or, if you prefer, you could invite them into a session here, where I could support you to say the things you want to say and possibly help them understand what you need. How does that sound?

Anticipatory grief poses challenges and also provides opportunities to complete unfinished business that might otherwise further complicate the young person's grief. The following dialogue with Vijay about his boyfriend, Chris, and father provides an example of this.

*Therapist:* We've been talking about how difficult you're finding the uncertainty around your dad's health and not knowing if he might die sooner rather than later. As hard as this is, it also gives you the opportunity to think ahead and use the

## Complex Grief    183

| | |
|---|---|
| | remaining time you have with him well, to say things you want to say, or ask him things, and minimise the chances of regrets after he's gone, like feeling you wish you'd said or done something. Is it okay if we talk about this? |
| Vijay: | I've been wondering about that. |
| Therapist: | And? |
| Vijay: | Chris thinks I should call him out for being a homophobe. |
| Therapist: | And you? |
| Vijay: | He's right. Dad is a homophobe. But he's still my dad. Chris thinks I'll always wonder how much Dad really loves me if I don't talk with him about this before he dies. |
| Therapist: | And what do you think? |
| Vijay: | I go round in circles. Like he was really upset when I came out. Now he is so sick, part of me feels bad about upsetting him. He always used to say homophobic stuff. He doesn't do that so much anymore, and he did make an effort to make Chris welcome. But sometimes he says stuff which is really off, and he treats Chris differently to the way he treats my sister's boyfriend. |
| Therapist: | How do you mean? |
| Vijay: | Well, he doesn't ask about Chris in the same way. |
| Therapist: | I'm guessing you haven't spelt out to your dad how you feel about this because you're not sure if you should or what you would say? |
| Vijay: | Yeah, like it might all go wrong and I'd really regret it. |
| Therapist: | You probably know many LGBTQI people are unsure how to talk with their parents or others about things like this. I can understand it feels even more complex for you because you don't know how much longer your dad will be alive. How about we experiment with different things you might say and how your dad might respond? It might help you figure out if, how, and what you might say. |
| Vijay: | That'd be good. |
| Therapist: | Imagine your dad sitting in this chair. Just for now put your concern about upsetting him to one side—we will think about that, but not just yet. What might you say to him about this, or anything else that's on your mind? |

Through role rehearsal, chair work, and discussion, Vijay clarified that he wanted to tell his father about his sadness at the prospect of him dying and how much he would miss him. He decided to also mention how difficult it had been for him to come out and how important it was to him that his father had welcomed Chris. He opted to wait until he'd seen how his father responded before deciding whether to approach the behaviour he found difficult in his father.

In order to focus the third *Essential Process* effectively, the therapist and the young person need to share a good understanding of their current interpersonal functioning and support needs. For example,

- How well does the young person feel understood and supported by others?
- What does the young person need, or would ideally want, by way of support from others?

- How has the loss impacted other important people in the young person's life?
- How much does the young person understand about the impact of the loss on others?
- Has the young person asked the other person about this?
- Has the other person shared information with the young person about his or her reactions to the loss?

As mentioned, many clients believe that no one can understand their experience of loss. The questions below may help with assessment in the Initial Phase of treatment and will also assist the young person in exploring strategies for communication with others about the loss.

- *How well do you think other people understand how the loss has affected you?*
- *What have they done or said that suggests they do or don't understand?*
- *What have you told them about how the loss has affected you?*
- *Of the things you haven't told them,*
  1. *what has held you back?*
  2. *how do you imagine they would respond if you did tell them?*
- *Do you think the loss has affected them? If so, in what ways?*
- *Who else would you like to share this with (e.g., the things we have discussed, the picture you've drawn, your writing, etc.)?*
- *What are some examples of what you might tell them?*
- *What might be a good time to talk with them about this—perhaps when you are both less likely to be disturbed and when you aren't tired or distracted?*
- *Of the people you know, who do you think would be better at understanding your situation and responding in the ways you need?*
- *What could you tell them about what you need or want from them by way of response? Do you want them to just listen, to comment, to tell you what they think, to give you a hug, to encourage you to cry or express your emotions, to try to distract you or cheer you up? Or do you want them to help you in some practical way?*

Some young people are fortunate in having robust support networks. For them it may be sufficient to help them adjust their communication in a few significant relationships so that other people have a better understanding of their attachment needs following the loss. This may be all that is required for the young person's attachment needs to be met.

For example, after Michelle's parents made clear to her that they wanted to understand and support her through her grief, she found it easier to reach out to her extended family and friends. She told them how sad and angry she was feeling. Michelle was disappointed when some people responded in ways that she experienced as being dismissive. With the therapist's encouragement, she then selected a few people who, based on past experience, she felt had the greatest capacity to understand her needs. She gave them information about how she would like them to support her and what she didn't find helpful.

Michelle's apparent confidence that her family and friends would respond to her needs positively and her relative ease in communicating with them was consistent with the therapist's hypothesis of her secure attachment style. It is telling that, even though she experienced some peoples' initial responses as unhelpful, she understood that they were trying to help and was able to give them feedback about how they could best assist her. In addition, she demonstrated a capacity to recognise her needs and the differing potential between her significant others to provide the type of interpersonal support she wanted. A less securely attached young person would be unlikely to show such confidence regarding the availability of help. A young person with a preoccupied attachment style would be focussed on gauging and testing the availability of care. Their behaviour may be counterproductive and alienate the very people they are seeking assistance from. Young people who are avoidant in their attachment would be likely to assume that effective support would not be available for them and so not attempt to communicate their needs to others, or if they did attempt this, it would be done less directly than Michelle was able to communicate. Further information about attachment is available in Chapter 3.

**Erin** (see Chapters 4 and 5) was also able to access much of the support she needed from her existing network with the therapist's encouragement.

*Therapist:* Erin, I know you've been disappointed about the way your parents have behaved around you discovering you are colour blind and regarding Pepe being killed. You feel they've neither supported nor understood you. Help me understand what you would like from them. If they were being supportive, what would it look like or sound like?

*Erin:* They'd be interested more in how sad I feel. Like they'd be asking me about it. They haven't even bothered to ask. They just offered to buy me a new dog and said I could study other types of engineering.

*Therapist:* You mentioned you tried to talk to them about it early on but you quickly got the impression they didn't understand and then you gave up.

*Erin:* Yep.

*Therapist:* Have you thought about trying to help them understand?

*Erin:* Why should I? If they really cared, they'd figure it out.

*Therapist:* You know, some people aren't good at figuring this stuff out unless it's spelt out to them and it doesn't mean they don't care. I don't know if that's true for your parents, but I did get the impression that they cared a lot about you. For example, some parents think they shouldn't ask too many questions because that would be prying and might push the young person away or that the young person will open up to them if and when they are ready. If you were to make it a bit easier for them, knowing they can't read your mind, could you toss them a few hints about what you've been finding most difficult and how they could be more supportive? What might you say to them?

For other young people, their existing support network will be inadequate, even with improved communication from the young person. These clients may require assistance to expand their sources of support by developing skills and confidence to initiate new relationships or to deepen connections with people who are currently in the outer bands of their Closeness Circles.

For example, continuing the case of **Mark**, the therapist reiterated the possibility of eventual rapprochement with his parents and friends who he felt alienated from because of disagreements about religion. In the meantime, the therapist assisted Mark to develop new sources of support. Revisiting his Closeness Circles, Mark identified people with whom he'd like to deepen his connections, including his grandparents and uncle, who lived overseas, and several acquaintances at school.

After discussing with the therapist how best to proceed, Mark asked his grandparents and uncle for more frequent Skype chats. He explained to them how he was feeling and they responded by scheduling visits to see him. Following some role play with the therapist, Mark invited two fellow patients he had met at clinic appointments to hang out with him. He was delighted when they and their parents not only accepted but offered to provide transport. The therapist also informed Mark of a support group for young people with similar health conditions, as a possible additional source of support.

For Mark, Vijay, and Erin, it was sufficient for them to identify options and rehearse their communication approaches with the therapist in order for them to effectively communicate with others outside therapy. For other young people, this may be best achieved by inviting their significant others to a therapy session so that the therapist can support and coach both parties to communicate effectively. As mentioned, this occurred early in Michelle's therapy in order to promptly address her suicidality.

Further information about role play and the empty chair approach is included in Chapter 4. The approaches for developing communication skills included in Chapter 10 may also be relevant for assisting young people to communicate about loss.

### *Indicated Processes in IPT-A for Complex Grief*

For some young people, the *Essential Processes* described above will not be sufficient to bring about adequate improvement in their symptoms. They will need additional *Indicated Processes*. Barriers may include the young person fearing their responses to loss, low insight, or difficulty finding words to express their experience. Further discussion with the therapist may eventually lead them to develop insight, acceptance, and an ability to express their experience, but sometimes additional *Indicated Processes* will produce more rapid progress. Further attention to psychological safety is often required when addressing this Problem Area. This may be in relation to the young person trusting the therapist, the process of therapy, or their emotions.

In the case of Erin, her sense of disenfranchisement and associated cognitive errors were key factors preventing her from communicating with her parents and her best friend regarding how she felt about her losses (see Chapter 4). She withdrew from these important people because she believed that they felt she was overreacting and weren't interested in understanding her. Erin came to doubt the validity of her reactions. She benefited from psychoeducation about responses to loss and brief cognitive restructuring, which helped her to identify and dispute the thoughts that were leading her to withdraw in her significant relationships. These *Indicated Processes* enabled Erin to make progress with the third *Essential Process*, accessing interpersonal support outside therapy.

Examples of *Indicated Processes* in IPT-A for Complex Grief are included in Figure 7.1. The application in Complex Grief of three *Indicated Processes* is discussed below: the involvement of others in therapy, psychoeducation, and therapeutic activities that rely less on verbal exploration and more on creative expression. The other *Indicated Processes* in Figure 7.1 are discussed in Chapter 4 and elsewhere in this book.

The therapist only spends sufficient time on these *Indicated Processes* for the young person to be ready to more effectively communicate his or her support needs. It should be noted that, as the young person discusses the loss, barriers may resolve themselves. When young people feel listened to and respected, their ease in communicating their experience of the loss is likely to increase. The therapist can ensure this positive experience occurs in the therapy room and also guide the young person to positive experiences of communicating outside therapy. Where gaps in social skills are identified, new skills can be taught. If the young person's social support network is lacking in quantity or quality, it can be extended through developing new connections or deepening existing ones as, for example, in the case of Mark above.

*Involving the young person's significant others in therapy*

Although adolescents often want to assert their independence, following a significant loss, they may look to adults for guidance. Their significant others can play an important role in supporting the young person through grief and may be able to do so more effectively with information and encouragement from the therapist. This may take the form of psychoeducation, discussion, or coaching. Examples of therapist dialogue inviting parents to a session are included in Chapter 8.

Parents, teachers, and others may appreciate advice about how best to support the young person. For example, knowing that the young person is going through a challenging time, they may feel that the best way to assist them is to give the young person as easy a time as possible by lowering expectations. This can, however, have the opposite effect, where the young person feels further destabilised when suddenly there are changes in multiple areas of life. If home, school and extracurricular routines and rules are maintained, this can provide much-needed refuge from grief. Familiar rhythms can provide reassurance that some things haven't changed, together with momentum and support for life moving forward. This advice is relatively straightforward when a young person is experiencing an adaptive grief reaction and does not have a mental disorder. In IPT-A, however, when the young person is depressed or experiencing other disorders, this advice is aligned with an understanding that the young person's current level of functioning may not be at his or her premorbid level.

When the people that the client relies on for support are also grieving, as may be the case for family, friends, or a school community following a bereavement, injury, or disaster event, the care available to the young person may be reduced while these people attend to their own grieving. It may not be the role of the therapist to assist these additional people directly, but the therapist may be able to make a referral or facilitate the young person's significant others accessing care. Aiding key people in the young person's support network can dramatically increase the capacity of those people to care for the young person.

**Michelle's** therapist recognised that the level of grief in Michelle's extended family and community was profound. Although Michelle's parents increased their care and attention for Michelle when they became aware of the level of her distress, they struggled with their own grief. During the first two therapy sessions, with Michelle's consent, the therapist provided psychoeducation to her family, including how best to care for Michelle and strategies to help keep her safe. The therapist also liaised with other agencies including Michelle's school and community health service to establish a local grief and loss peer support group.

Psychoeducation for parents may be necessary to address the common misunderstanding that they can protect young people from grief by not displaying or discussing their own feelings. This attempt at protection denies young people opportunities to learn how people grieve. The aim is to strike a balance between protecting young people from feeling overwhelmed by parental grief reactions while allowing them opportunities to learn and to be reassured that it is possible to cope with painful experiences.

Cultural norms regarding grief and expectations of adolescents can vary significantly between cultures and between different generations within a culture. The therapist must ensure that their practice is culturally appropriate (e.g., Wynne-Jones, 2016) when working cross-culturally.

*Psychoeducation to assist understanding and acceptance of loss*

Some young people are confused, overwhelmed, or frightened by their responses to loss. This can be a powerful hindrance to accepting, communicating, or sometimes even recognising their responses. They may be greatly aided by education about reactions to loss: their own reactions and those of others. Learning that their reactions sit within a broad range of responses that people commonly experience in relation to loss can be a huge relief. This can break the

Complex Grief    189

logjam of what has been unexpressed, which has been contributing to their grief being complex.

A central aspect of assessing this Problem Area is to gauge the young person's emotional literacy in relation to loss. Some young people will need a thorough and broad education about the emotions of loss and what to do with them. Other young people will have good emotional literacy already and require no education or only brief information focussed on gaps in their understanding.

**Nathan**, aged 15, for example, was alarmed and confused about his responses to his father's death. He had difficulty accepting his emotional reactions to his loss. Following some psychoeducation, his processing of the loss proceeded with its own momentum as he found it easier to talk about his experience, first with the therapist and then with some of his significant others. In contrast, **Nile**, also aged 15, needed psychoeducation in order to accept his responses to his bereavement. But this wasn't sufficient for him to express his grief to others. Several further sessions were spent on psychoeducation activities (described below) to help explore his experience of loss before he was ready to communicate his feelings and needs to others.

Sharing theory and models about grief and loss with young people can do the following:

- Provide maps of the territory of loss. There will be many individual pathways across this territory. Thus, models should not be offered in a prescriptive way or imposed as an ideal illustration of what is normative.
- Provide reassurance about the process of grieving and adjusting to loss.
- Help young people frame, understand, and legitimise their own and other people's experience of loss.
- Suggest possible next steps or options in adjusting to the loss.
- Help young people process their emotions and ultimately communicate with their significant others about the loss and their needs in the changed circumstances resulting from the loss.
- Help the young person's significant others to understand the young person's needs.

Four psychoeducation activities are included below followed by two activities for working on loss. The diversity in young people's preferred learning styles can be addressed by choosing from a range of formats and mediums when introducing these models. This might include verbal description; visual representation like a handout, website, whiteboard or screen image; and, in some cases, tactile or ambulatory experience (see below).

*Activity number 7.1: Stages of grief and loss*

Models of stages in the adjustment process following significant loss can help young people understand and accept their own and other people's responses to loss. Kübler-Ross's (1969) model—denial, anger, bargaining, depression, and acceptance—can be a useful starting point and other models are available (e.g., Bowlby and Parkes 1970, Konigsberg 2011, Kübler-Ross and Kessler 2014)).

These models are used to convey that there are recognised stages that people may go through following significant loss. They are not intended to imply that healthy grieving involves progressing through all the stages in a linear way. Some of these models are bereavement-specific. If the young person's loss is not a bereavement, then using more generic language for loss will be beneficial. Invite the young person to apply the model to her own experience, including which aspects are more or less relevant or true for her. The young person could be invited to develop her own individualised model, representing her unique experience of the loss. Where part of the young person's difficulty around the loss concerns a lack of understanding or acceptance of how other people are responding to the loss, it may be useful if she considers how the models might help her to understand the other person. For example,

*Therapist:* I've explained a bit about these stages people might go through. Have you had any thoughts about examples you've noticed in your family or other people?

*Fernando:* Yeah, lots. Since mum got her diagnosis, it's like everyone changed. Like you said in the stages. My sister just pretends nothing's changed. It's like she doesn't care. My little brother has been really angry and getting in fights. Dad started going to church all the time, much more than he used to. And he keeps on at Mum to stop smoking and to eat healthy stuff. I told him he was being weird and it wouldn't make any difference, and we argue. But you talked about bargaining. Maybe that's what's going on with him?

*Therapist:* You may be right. I guess what is pretty clear is that everyone in your family is finding it hard to adjust to this news about your mum, which is to be expected. You are each dealing with it differently. That's created misunderstandings and arguments and pushed you apart. How might understanding this help?

An option for introducing these models is for the therapist to physically move to different parts of the room as she describes each stage, giving examples and possible applications that the young person might relate to. The young person can then be invited to physically move with the therapist through the stages, giving feedback about which stages he recognises or relates to in himself or others (see the dialogue with Nazim in Activity number 7.3 below).

*Activity number 7.2: Different experiences of grief*

Some people expect that there should be a diminution of the intensity of the loss and the associated pain over time. However, this may not be what they actually experience. The loss may not diminish even after many years. It can still feel just as big, significant, or painful. When this mismatch of expectation

Complex Grief 191

and experience occurs, some people are inclined to judge their own or other's grief, concluding that it is abnormal or pathological.

Many people who experience this non-diminishing trajectory of loss continue to function well and their responses are clearly not pathological. They change as a result of the loss in adaptive ways. They grow through dynamic interaction with the loss. They are stretched and expanded by their endeavours to incorporate the loss into their identity, their relationships, and their sense of meaning. Tonkin's (1996) model of growing around grief helps validate this experience of loss. It is adapted in Figure 7.2 and is readily grasped by adolescents. The trajectory of loss lessening over time is represented with a series of two circles, one inside the other. The external circle represents the person, and the internal circle depicts the pain or significance of the loss. Initially, the circle inside is nearly as large as the outside circle. With the passing of time, the internal circle gets smaller, representing the diminution of the loss, and the external circle or the person stays the same size. Another trajectory, that of growing through loss, is initially represented in the same way with the internal circle nearly as large as the external circle. Over time, the internal circle remains the same size, representing the loss not diminishing, while the external circle gets larger as the person grows through the loss.

A third trajectory provides a helpful addition for some young people. It combines elements of the previous two trajectories. In this pathway people grow through their grief, and perhaps, as a consequence of that growth, the pain of their loss eventually decreases.

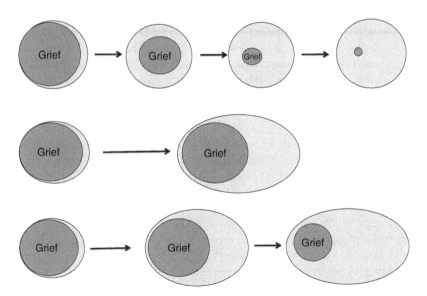

*Figure 7.2* Different experiences of grief.

After explaining the model, it can be useful to invite the young person to comment on aspects which are similar to, or different from, her own experience or that of others.

This model suggests that the loss doesn't necessarily disappear from our life. It can become incorporated into it. Our experience of the loss may change as our life changes and it may affect reactions to future situations. This latter point can be re-examined in the Consolidation Phase. Revisiting the model there can be part of a conversation about how to generalize learning from the current loss to cope with future challenges.

*Activity number 7.3: Body oriented approaches to grief and loss*

Some young people find it easier to identify and talk about their body sensations than their emotions. For these young people, discussing their physical responses to the loss can be a more productive place to start. Noticing what's happening in their bodies often in turn assists the young person to identify and discuss associated thoughts and feelings. This is one way that mindfulness can be integrated into therapy. Mindfulness is discussed in Chapter 4 and in the case of Kylie later in this chapter.

Even for young people who are relatively more emotionally literate, it may be helpful to include some discussion of body sensations to complement and expand their understanding of reactions to loss. A number of models and metaphors can be used to facilitate discussion of the body's response to loss. Noticing ebbs and flows of energy is one approach.

> Therapist: *There will be times when we feel tired and want to rest and times when we want to be active. There may be periods when we want to focus on the loss, to think about it, to remember and to mourn, and there may be other times when this doesn't feel right, when we need to think about other things, the future, and moving forward with our lives. Have you noticed anything like this in yourself or others?*

These changes and shifts may be more rapid in children and adolescents than in adults. The fluctuations can be distressing and confusing for some young people. Models that suggest that changing responses are normal can provide reassurance and permission for the young person to accept and allow these natural oscillations to occur.

The concept of yin and yang in Chinese medicine is somewhat akin to this and may be helpful particularly for those young people familiar with martial arts such as tai chi, chi gong, karate, or judo. Yang can be thought of as action and yin as yielding. Western culture tends to emphasize the value of action (yang) to the detriment of appreciating the power of yielding, letting go, or resting (yin). Yin and yang are understood as interrelated parts of the whole. Balance between the two creates health, just as bright day and dark night form a single day. Yang becomes yin and yin becomes yang as action becomes rest and returns to action, in a continual cycle. Yielding or rest produces restoration and creates space or energy for action.

Similarly, for young people interested in physics, Isaac Newton's notion that "for every action there is an equal and opposite reaction" could be used to introduce the idea of a natural ebb and flow in our reactions to loss.

Other young people may find naturally occurring cycles in nature, such as seasons, helpful in reflecting changing responses to loss. For example, the bursting forth of energy in spring follows the diminishing energy of autumn and the fallow and restorative time of winter.

Stroebe and Schut (1999) describe a natural process of oscillation between periods of being focussed on the loss and periods of avoidance or attention on moving forward with life. Times of respite can be an important part of adaptive grief.

The above metaphors can help young people understand body or energetic perspectives in loss and lend themselves to movement, as illustrated in this dialogue with **Nazim**, aged 16:

*Therapist:* Nazim, over here (therapist moves to the relevant side of the continuum) represents those times when we feel we have no energy and we just want to flop. We may want to sleep a lot and things may feel overwhelming and too much. We may want to pull the bedclothes over our head and not face the world. We may be thinking about the loss, or maybe we aren't aware of thinking about anything at all. Then at other times (therapist moves to the other end of the continuum) we will experience the opposite. We might have a lot of energy and feel a need to do things, to sort things out, or to move forward with our lives. It might be difficult to be still or reflect. It may feel like we have an energy that we need to release or express. There may be other times (therapist moves to a point along the continuum) where we experience a mix of both. We might be starting to think about doing things, and energy is building but not quite sufficient yet to act on our thoughts. Do you think any of this relates to your experience?

*Nazim:* Well, I feel low energy a lot of the time.

*Therapist:* What have you noticed?

*Nazim:* I don't know, just like I don't want to do anything.

*Therapist:* That's certainly what can go on for people when they are at this end of the continuum. There may be more. Can I invite you to come and stand with me up here? This might seem a bit strange, but moving while we explore an idea can sometimes help our understanding. It can activate different parts of our brain. I can give you some examples of things people might experience, and you could let me know about parts of your experience that come to mind. Is that okay?

*Nazim:* I guess so.

Most people have a default mode and may be more comfortable with one side of the continuum and avoid the opposite. However, this can inhibit their grieving and adjustment to a loss. It is often necessary to allow ourselves to move back and forth between different states in order to progress through grief. The dialogue below with **Kylie**, aged 21, illustrates one way of approaching this.

Therapist: Kylie, one of the things we've learned about your grief is that it has been important for you to be active. You've been telling me how you really needed to sort some things out and you've been successful with getting a lot of that done. This is a real strength you have. In other parts of your life, you are good at solving problems. You think things through logically, and you believe in your ability to make a difference for the better. You notice how other people do things, and you're good at adapting their skills and applying them to your own situation. This ability you have has helped you deal with some aspects of your mum dying and it will be helpful in dealing with other challenges you may have in life. I think you can feel proud of it. Have I understood this aspect of you correctly?

Kylie: I hadn't thought about it as something to be proud of but the way you say it, I guess it is a good thing.

Therapist: You have also been telling me that you don't feel comfortable letting yourself just stop and do nothing. Could you help me understand that a bit more?

Kylie: Well, it doesn't achieve anything, does it? I just feel low, and nothing changes.

Therapist: Does part of you sometimes feel like doing nothing or just feeling your feelings, whatever they might be—sadness or anger?

Kylie: Well, yes, but what's the point? What does it achieve?

Therapist: What do you imagine would happen if you let yourself do that?

Kylie: I'll just feel bad.

Therapist: And what might happen then?

Kylie: I don't know, I might feel worse?

Therapist: And what do you think would happen then?

Kylie: (Looking alarmed/distressed) I'll be a waste of space, a loser. No one will want to be with me.

Therapist: Could you explain that to me?

Kylie expressed a belief that she would be boring and people would avoid her if she became too sad. The therapist acknowledged this as an important point to return to after completing the explanation of the oscillation concept.

Therapist: You might be right, Kylie. If you stop being active for a while, then you may notice painful emotions because you aren't distracting yourself with activity. But that might be exactly what you need to do to help move

> through your grief. You've discovered that you can avoid painful feelings by keeping busy, but you have also noticed that the emotions can sneak up on you at times when you don't want them to, like when you're in public. I am suggesting that if you give some attention to your feelings it can make it less likely they will come bursting out at other times. What do you think?

Kylie: It's kind of the opposite of what I do.

Therapist: *There are times when we need to be active in dealing with issues like loss and times when we need to stop the activity to allow ourselves to rest and reflect. You're great at this side of the continuum. (Therapist points to the activity side of the continuum.) Highly skilled, in fact. You've been avoiding this side. (Therapist indicates the other side of the continuum.) You haven't really allowed yourself to stay with the sadness for very long. You feared that if you did it would get worse. One option would be to experiment, to see if this is what actually happens. You can try the experiment in therapy where, if you do "fall apart" in your terms, you would be safe. Outside therapy, you could try short breaks from being active, and you can always switch back to being active if you feel you can't cope with what happens.*

Kylie's lack of comfort with the emotions of loss meant she avoided talking with others about how she and they were feeling. The activity helped identify this obstacle to Kylie accessing interpersonal support. A combination of psychoeducation about emotions, cognitive approaches to challenge negative beliefs about emotions, and mindfulness increased Kylie's ability to tolerate emotional distress, which in turn enabled her to communicate with others about her loss.

*Activity number 7.4: Defining steps to healing*

The young person's role in therapy is explained in the Initial Phase of IPT-A, and this is revisited and adjusted in the Middle Phase. In Complex Grief, this can be extended to provide specific education about what they can do to help themselves adjust to the loss.

The psychoeducation models discussed above help young people identify and understand their own and other people's experience of loss. Models can also suggest ways through grief, albeit with the above-mentioned proviso that they are not used prescriptively (e.g., Worden's 2002 "tasks of mourning").

Clinical tool 7.1 My tasks following loss and Clinical tool 7.2 Helpful things I can do after loss aim to make transparent for young people what they can do to assist themselves to adjust to all forms of loss, not only bereavement, and incorporate the interpersonal focus of IPT-A. Clinical tool 7.1 is suitable for an older or more astute young person. Clinical tool 7.2 is designed for a younger adolescent or for adolescents with less insight.

> **Clinical tool 7.1   My tasks following loss**
>
> N.B. *This clinical tool template should be individualised for each client.*
> Following a significant loss I can assist my adjustment by
>
> - accepting that the loss has happened
> - acknowledging my pain, or other reactions, to the loss
> - adapt to a life where what I have lost is no longer present
> - finding ways to continue to be nurtured by what I have lost, including remembering
> - sharing these things with people who are important to me so that they can understand
>   - what the loss means to me
>   - how best to support me
>   - how they can help me with these five tasks
>
> (Adapted from Worden, 2009)

> **Clinical tool 7.2   Helpful things I can do after loss**
>
> N.B. *This clinical tool template should be individualised for each client*
> Following my loss I can help myself feel better by
>
> - accepting that the loss has happened
> - allowing myself to be upset if that's what I feel
> - keeping my good memories
> - talking about how I feel and what I need with people who are important to me so that they can understand
> - asking for help when I need it
>
> (Adapted from Worden, 2009)

The above examples are provided as generic clinical tools that can be used as client handouts. They should be individualised for each client as in examples Figure 7.3 for Mei, aged 16, and Figure 7.4 for Jake, aged 12.

Handouts and discussion such as this can help to demystify therapy for the young person, clarifying his role in therapy, and outlining what he can do outside therapy to help himself.

The concept of repressive coping style is an important consideration in relation to the second points in Figures 7.3 and 7.4. People with this coping style tend to deny their emotional distress and direct their attention away from threatening information (e.g., Derakshan and Eysenck, 1997). Repressive coping can promote resilience in some individuals by preserving cognitive

Following Mum's death, I can help myself by:
- accepting that Mum has died
- acknowledging my pain, or other reactions, to Mum dying
- adjusting to a life where Mum is no longer present
- finding ways to continue to be nurtured by Mum, including remembering her
- sharing these things with people who are important to me so that they can understand:
    - what Mum's death means to me
    - how best to support me
    - how they can help me with these five tasks.

*Figure 7.3* Mei's handout: My tasks now mum has died.

Now that I have moved so far away from my friends, I can help myself feel better by:
- accepting that this move has happened
- allowing myself to be upset if that's what I feel
- keeping my good memories, staying in touch with my old friends and also making new friends
- talking about how I feel and what I need with people who are important to me so that they can understand
- asking for help when I need it.

*Figure 7.4* Jake's handout: Helpful things I can do after moving.

ability under stress and protecting from adverse emotional consequences of bereavement or trauma but can be maladaptive in other situations (e.g., Bonanno and Mancini, 2008; Parker and McNally, 2008). Recognising this coping style challenges the assumption that catharsis is a necessary component in the healing of a significant loss. While catharsis is an important aspect of clinical work for many young people, it may not be required for all to adjust to loss. Attempting to encourage the young person, regardless of coping style, to focus on difficult emotions may not only be counterproductive but could be seen as potentially abusive for those with a repressive coping style. A more respectful approach would be to assist the young person to evaluate his or her coping style. This would include considering the potential advantages and disadvantages both in coping in the immediate aftermath of loss and also its effectiveness in dealing with the loss during the subsequent months and years. Some young people may conclude that the benefits of repressive coping clearly outweigh alternatives. Others may see the greatest benefits early on in the loss, when they might otherwise feel overwhelmed. However, they may recognise that with the passage of time, exploring their emotions could be beneficial, not least so that they can communicate with others about their experience.

For young people experiencing significant ambivalence about their loss, sensitivity will be required in explaining and exploring suggestions about the role of memories (e.g., in Clinical tools 7.1 and 7.2 and Figures 7.3 and 7.4). For example, if the relationship or situation was abusive or negative in other ways, some memories may not be positive or nurturing. Ambivalence is a risk factor for complicated grief reactions, and young people with these experiences will usually need opportunities to identify and process their ambivalence. Freud (1917) in his paper Mourning and Melancholia, identified elevated risk for grief progressing into depression when the grief was related to repressed hostility towards an ambivalently regarded lost object.

The therapist can provide concrete examples of how these tasks of grieving can be worked on in session and outside therapy and involve the young person in collaboratively selecting activities to progress these tasks.

*Creative activities to explore, process, and communicate about loss*

Creative activities can facilitate expression and make therapy accessible and engaging for young people who find it difficult to express their experience with words. They may include drawing, writing, collage, quilting, weaving, basket-making, memory boxes, website design, music, dance, theatre, other performance, rituals, and commemorations.

These activities invite the client to create something concrete to represent her loss. This requires the young person to reflect on her experience and may involve her in processing the loss on mental, emotional, and somatic levels. The activities externalise the young person's internal experience and, in doing so, can render it more accessible and easier to communicate to others. These activities can prepare the young person and give her something concrete to talk about, as opposed to trying to express an internal world that she may otherwise experience as nebulous and unclear. The process of externalising can bring insight and new perspectives. Emotional content that has not been expressed previously may emerge.

These activities can bring a sense of containment or comfort as they express and organise things that may have felt confused and jumbled. Some young people report that they feel less overwhelmed following the activity.

It will not be necessary to use any of these activities with some young people. They may be capable of exploring the themes addressed in the activities using other therapeutic processes, such as discussion, as with Michelle and Mark above. The therapist can offer choice and ask the young person about her preferences. For example:

> I've noticed you don't find it easy to talk about your boyfriend's death. Some people find it easier to write or draw as a way of expressing how they feel about their loss. I remember you said you enjoyed art at school. We have some choices here. We could continue talking as we have been, and it doesn't matter if it takes a while, it often does, or I'm wondering if you would prefer to do something like art or collage?

In summary, creative activities can assist young people to

- create a concrete symbolic representation of their loss
- identify and express their feelings and thoughts about their loss
- develop perspective and insight
- communicate with others about the loss
- develop a sense of meaning in relation to the loss
- gain a sense of containment and agency

Principles for using experiential and creative activities in therapy

Key principles for using experiential and creative activities in therapy are summarised below. Some of these principles are further elaborated in the discussion that follows.

- **Explain the rationale** for the activity. Examples of therapist dialogue are included below. For most young people brief explanations will be sufficient. Anxious clients may need some reassurance—for example, "There is no right or wrong with this activity, just experiment. You could start by touching the pencil or crayon to the page and see what emerges".
- **Emphasize choice.** Make clear that the activities are optional and that the young person has choices—for example, "You can choose what you focus on and how much you tell me about what you produce. You can keep some of it private if you wish. If you prefer, you could do the activity on your phone".
- **Reduce awkwardness and foster self-direction.** For example, "Some people prefer to do this not being watched. I'll do some things at my desk while you're drawing. It's just so you don't feel too much in the spotlight. I'll check in with you after about ten minutes, but let me know any time you're ready to discuss".
- **Exercise caution in offering interpretations**, not least because you will usually be guessing—for example, "Please tell me about what this means for you or what it was like producing it".
- **Build communication with significant others.** For example, "Who else would you like to share this with?"
- **Foster safety,** including with regard to the young person talking with others about the activity—for example, "It's great that you are keen to discuss this with your boyfriend. Let's have a think about how you'd like him to respond and how you could increase the chances of that happening".
- **Experience the activities for yourself** before inviting clients to do them. This will give you a greater insight into the potential power, impact, and nuances of the activity.

*Activity number 7.5: Drawing about loss*

Drawing activities can be broad and general, such as a simple invitation to represent the loss. Alternatively, an activity might focus on specific aspects of the loss, for example, representing a particular memory about the person or thing that has been lost. The former may be especially helpful early on in the Middle Phase, while the latter can help to explore aspects of the loss that have emerged as particularly important or problematic. An invitation to produce a drawing about loss could be something like this:

Therapist: Joe, we talked about how drawing might be helpful and you mentioned that you were willing to give it a go. I'd like to invite you to do that now. Would you draw something to represent moving so far away from your friends? It could be anything at all. It might be a specific memory or something more general. Sometimes people feel nervous or self-conscious about drawing. Maybe they feel they are not good at art or are concerned about getting it wrong. There is no right or wrong with this. Whatever emerges is likely to be helpful. It could be a realistic representation, it could be abstract, symbolic. It might be random lines or a blur of colour. Whatever emerges is fine.

Inviting the client to think of wishes in relation to the loss and to represent these wishes on the page can be a potent way of accessing aspects of the loss that may have gone unexpressed. This might include regrets and feelings of guilt. It may also elicit beliefs about fairness and the meaning of the loss. For example,

Therapist: I'd like to invite you to draw three wishes in relation to the loss of your grandma. One of the things about wishes is that they can include things that might not be possible in everyday reality. As I mentioned there's no right or wrong with these activities. Whatever you come up with will be fine. Do you have any questions about what I'm suggesting?

For some young people, a simple request such as this is all that is necessary for them to undertake the activity. If the therapist is aware of information about the young person that is relevant to the activity, it can be used to individualise the introduction. Other young people, such as **Kylie**, aged 21 (mentioned above), will prefer to understand the rationale for the activity before engaging in it. Kylie is highly intelligent, and the therapist chose language that might not be suitable for a young person who is less interested or astute:

Therapist: You are good at logical thinking and that has served you well in many situations. However, our rational mind can dominate and crowd out other ways of being, blocking our emotions, imagination, or creativity. Giving some space to these aspects can help us to understand ourselves. For example, there may be parts of our experiences that our rational mind tells us are unacceptable, silly, embarrassing, childish, or selfish. However, these aspects may be important in understanding what we need and in adapting to loss. Thinking about wishes in relation to loss *can help us tap into feelings and other responses. I'd like to invite you to draw some wishes in relation to your mum. Remember, wishes don't have to be rational or even possible.*

*Activity number 7.6: Writing about loss*

Writing is another way to externalise the experience of loss, to facilitate exploration and expression, and to gain perspective and insight. The young person could be invited to write about the loss in session or as a journal activity outside therapy.

As with other creative activities, some young people may be hesitant and concerned about not understanding what is required of them in the activity or getting it wrong. Reassurance can be given and trigger questions may help the young person begin.

*Therapist:* There is no right or wrong, and the aim isn't to produce perfect literature. You can just experiment by putting words on the page and seeing what emerges. It could be a letter, e-mail, text, a story, fairy tale, simple bullet points, or random words on the page. You don't need to be concerned about spelling or punctuation. Some people find it helps to think of a particular memory and what was happening at the time.

Writing on a page is a different tactile and kinaesthetic experience compared to typing on a screen. Both might be beneficial therapeutically. As with artwork, writing can be scanned or photographs taken to enable digital storage.

After an appropriate period of writing, the client may be invited to talk about what the experience was like for him. Inviting the young person to read his work aloud can add a powerful dimension. Giving the words voice may be a qualitatively different experience from expressing them on the page or screen. Writing may be the first time the young person has expressed his experience in words. Reading aloud may be the first time he gives voice to his feelings and thoughts. This additional dimension of expression, speaking his experience rather than just putting silent words on a page, may amplify the young person's affect, both in intensity and variety, and move him along significantly in understanding and processing his responses to the loss. If the young person seems daunted by this, he may find it easier to read out just part of his writing.

Guidance can be given for how the young person approaches the task of reading aloud.

*Therapist:* As you are reading, I'd like you to look up from time to time and notice that I'm here and I'm listening to you. You could make eye contact, if you feel comfortable doing that, and then continue reading.

A key part of activity-based therapy is to invite the client to reflect on her experience of the activity. In IPT-A, the therapist is particularly alert to factors that might influence the young person's ability to communicate her experience to others. Reflection can be informed by a mindfulness approach, as in the case of **Adela**. When Adela read aloud, the therapist noted that she was uncomfortable making eye contact and whenever she did, then her voice and facial expression suggested she was fighting back tears. The therapist checked what Adela was experiencing and sought to assist her to understand how this dynamic might be affecting her symptoms and her ability to talk to others. It is important to note that the therapist had introduced some mindfulness approaches to assist Adela to identify emotions in previous sessions, so she was already familiar with this approach:

*Therapist:* What did you notice about what you experienced as you read aloud?
*Adela:* It was really hard.
*Therapist:* What was the hardest?
*Adela:* Looking at you.
*Therapist:* What did you notice happened when you did look at me?
*Adela:* It was hard to say the words.
*Therapist:* What did you actually experience? Did you notice any thoughts, feelings or sensations in your body?
*Adela:* My voice got trembly. I felt a bit sick.

Through further exploration of her experience, Adela was able to identify that reading aloud and looking at the therapist intensified feelings of sadness and fear. The therapist asked what she thought the fear was about, and this enabled her to identify several sources of discomfort regarding crying, including a concern she previously had not articulated that if she started crying she would be overwhelmed and might not stop and that she would be judged negatively by others. This provided a useful prompt for the therapist to provide further psychoeducation about the role of emotions in loss, to address containment and affect regulation, and to explore Adela's fear of negative evaluation by others.

After discussing the young person's experience of the activity, as illustrated above, the therapist explores who else the young person has discussed these issues with and who she would like to communicate with about these things.

## Summary

Attachment needs will be challenged by significant loss. Our task as therapists is to assist our clients to find ways to meet their need for closeness and support in the changed circumstances brought by the loss. This may involve reconnecting or deepening connections within existing relationships or developing new relationships. Many young people will need some psychoeducation in order to be able to identify and express their responses to loss and to effectively communicate their experience to others. Additionally, young people can continue to be nurtured through their memories of the person, thing, or aspects of self that have been lost. They may need encouragement to do so, and some young people will need to actively shore up their memories. Fortunately, there are many ways to do this, including discussion with the therapist; communication with their significant others; and using creative activities, including those discussed in this chapter.

## References

American Psychiatric Association. (2013). *Diagnostic and statistical manual of mental disorders* (5th edition). Arlington, VA: American Psychiatric Publishing.

Attig, T. (2011). *How we grieve: Relearning the world* (Revised edition). New York: Oxford University Press.

Attig, T. (2000). *The heart of grief: Death and the search for lasting love.* New York: Oxford University Press.

Bonanno, G., & Mancini, A. (2008). The human capacity to thrive in the face of potential trauma. *Pediatrics, 121*, 369–375.

Bowlby, J., & Parkes, C. (1970) Separation and loss within the family. In E. J. Anthony & C. Koupernik (Eds.). *The child and his family.* New York: Wiley, 167–216.

Derakshan, N., & Eysenck, M. (1997) Repression and repressors: Theoretical and experimental approaches. *European Psychologist, 2*, 235–246.

Freud, S. (1917). Mourning and melancholia. *The Standard Edition of the Complete Psychological Works of Sigmund Freud, Volume XIV (1914–1916): On the History of the Psycho-Analytic Movement, Papers on Metapsychology and Other Works,* 237–258.

Hillin, A. (2012). *Grief, loss, transition and change: creative ways of working with children, adolescents and adults workshop handbook.* Sydney, Australia: Anthony Hillin.

Klass, D., Silverman, P., & Nickman, S. (1996). *Continuing bonds: New understandings of grief.* Philadelphia, PA: Taylor & Francis.

Konigsberg, R. (2011). *The truth about grief: The myth of its five stages and the new science of loss.* New York: Simon & Schuster.

Kübler-Ross, E. (1969). *On death and dying.* New York: Macmillan.

Kübler-Ross, E., & Kessler, D. (2014). *On grief and grieving: finding the meaning of grief through the five stages of loss.* New York: Scribner.

Mares, S. (2016). The mental health of children and parents detained on Christmas Island: Secondary analysis of an Australian human rights commission data set. *Health and Human Rights Journal, 18*, 219–232.

Mufson, L., Dorta, K., Moreau, D., & Weissman, M. (2004). *Interpersonal psychotherapy for depressed adolescents* (2nd ed.). New York: The Guilford Press.

Neimeyer, R. (2001). *Meaning, reconstruction and the experience of loss.* Washington, DC: American Psychological Association.

National Institute of Clinical Excellence (NICE). (2017). *Depression in children and young people: identification and management.* London: National Institute for Health and Care Excellence.

Parker, H., & McNally, R. (2008). Repressive coping, emotional adjustment, and cognition in people who have lost loved ones to suicide. *Suicide and Life-Threatening Behaviour, 38*, 676–687.

Rando, T. (1993). *Treatment of complicated mourning*. Champaign, Illinois: Research Press.

Stroebe, M., & Schut, H. (1999). The dual process model of coping with bereavement: rationale and description, *Death Studies, 23*, 197–224.

Stuart, S., & Robertson, M. (2012). *Interpersonal psychotherapy: A clinician's guide* (2nd ed.). London: Arnold.

Tonkin, L. (1996). Growing around grief—another way of looking at grief and recovery, *Bereavement Care, 15*(1), 10.

Worden, J. (2009). *Grief counselling and grief therapy: A handbook for the mental health practitioner* (4th Ed.). New York: Springer Publishing Company.

Wynne-Jones, M., Hillin, A., Byers, D., Stanley, D., Edwige, V., & Brideson, T. (2016). *Aboriginal grief and loss: A review of the literature*. Australian Indigenous HealthInfoNet. Available at http://healthbulletin.org.au/articles/aboriginal-grief-and-loss-a-review-of-the-literature/

# 8 Interpersonal Disputes

**Contents**

| | |
|---|---|
| Introduction | 206 |
| Defining the Problem Area of Interpersonal Disputes | 207 |
| The nature of Interpersonal Disputes in young people | 208 |
| "Normal" disputes between adolescents and parents | 208 |
| Damaging disputes | 209 |
|    *Seven steps* | 210 |
| Assessing Interpersonal Disputes | 210 |
|    *Confirm Interpersonal Disputes as the major Problem Area* | 210 |
|    *Explore and clarify the dispute(s)* | 211 |
| Identifying the issues in dispute and the relationships concerned | 213 |
| Determining if the dispute is resulting more from the client or from the other person | 215 |
| Exploring expectations of others | 215 |
| Are disputes a recurring theme? | 216 |
| When the dispute can't be resolved | 217 |
| Addressing Interpersonal Disputes | 223 |
|    *Identify current strategies for dealing with disputes* | 223 |
|    *Identify alternative options for dealing with disputes* | 224 |
|    *Choose an approach to deal with the current dispute(s)* | 226 |
|    *Rehearse the social skills necessary to implement the approach* | 226 |
|    *Integrate the approach in life* | 227 |
| Find a nonjudgmental description of the problem | 232 |
| List the major needs and concerns of all parties | 232 |
| Generating solutions | 233 |
| Involving parents or others in working on Interpersonal Disputes | 236 |
|    *When a parent has mental health issues or other impediments* | 236 |
| When the parent is amenable to addressing their impediments | 236 |
| When a parent is not amenable to addressing their impediments | 238 |

| | |
|---|---|
| Concluding the Middle Phase | 239 |
| Summary | 239 |
| Notes | 239 |
| References | 240 |

## Introduction

If young people perceive a dispute is preventing them from meeting needs that they see as essential to their wellbeing, the negative impact on mental health may be profound. This is particularly true when the dispute occurs in important relationships (e.g., Allen et al., 2006). Furthermore, if the young person believes that there is little possibility of resolving the conflict[1] in a way that her needs will be met, profound feelings of helplessness and hopelessness may result. This negative belief about the possibility of change on issues that the young person sees as integral to her well-being may become entrenched and can come to dominate the young person's perception of herself and her life more generally. Distress and depression can be triggered or reinforced.

The therapist challenges this feeling of hopelessness so that the client believes in the possibility of change. This may be achieved through better understanding the current patterns of communication in the relationship, identifying alternative options for dealing with conflict, and developing the social skills and confidence necessary to utilise these skills in real-life situations.

During Interpersonal Disputes, the client's attachment needs will be in play. The therapist addresses these needs by stepping into the role of transitory attachment figure. The young person's attachment style is likely to have a significant impact both on the way she behaves in disputes and the way she responds to therapy.

Interpersonal Disputes can be challenging to work on for both the client and therapist, but they can also provide unique opportunities for change. The crisis produced by significant conflict may make the young person and her significant others available for therapy in ways they wouldn't be otherwise. In learning how to cope with the present conflict, the client can acquire lifelong skills that provide resilience to future adversity.

This chapter describes the Problem Area of Interpersonal Disputes and outlines the aims and objectives of working on disputes. Three techniques that are particularly helpful for this Problem Area are discussed: the Conflict Curve, Conflict-Solving Styles, and Mapping.

The case of Admir is described in some detail to demonstrate many of the stages and strategies for addressing disputes. Other brief case examples illustrate the scope of the Problem Area and the range of techniques that can be utilised.

## Defining the Problem Area of Interpersonal Disputes

The disputes that contribute to depression and other mental disorders in young people are often with authority figures. For adolescents and young adults, this is commonly parents, caregivers, or other family members and may also include people such as teachers, sports coaches, employers, or managers. Often young people's disputes are directly about normative conflict with their parents. Jan, for example, aged 13 and with preoccupied attachment, developed anxious symptoms about her parent's requirement to be home by 9:00 pm. Jan's friends were allowed to stay out later than this. Jan believed that the curfew was not only unfair, but, crucially, it threatened her membership of her friendship group. She felt it excluded her from conversations about activities she had not been part of and she feared that the group would leave her behind. She perceived her parents as being intractable and lacking interest in understanding how important this issue was for her. We will consider the conflict between Jan and her parents in more detail later in this chapter.

Disputes where the power difference implicit between adults and young people is not present, such as friends or romantic partners, may also lead to depression or other disorders. For example, Tracy, aged 20, also appeared to be preoccupied in her attachment style. She has been going out with her boyfriend for four years. Over recent months, she has felt increasingly upset by what she perceives as her boyfriend's flirting with other women, including when she and he are out with friends together. Tracy reported that her attempts to discuss her feelings with her boyfriend always lead to arguments. Consequently, she has become pessimistic about change. She feels angry, sad, and also embarrassed and humiliated by her boyfriend's behaviour. She is frightened to leave the relationship, believing that their mutual friends would side with her boyfriend and she would be left socially isolated. Tracy's increasing sense of being trapped in a no-win situation with little hope of change has coincided with the onset of her depression.

Sometimes the other person in a dispute does not understand how important the issue is for the young person and does not comprehend the full impact of the dispute for him. This may be because the young person has not effectively explained his needs and feelings. Where this is the case, increasing the young person's capacity to effectively communicate his needs regarding the issue in dispute may bring about significant change in relation to the current dispute and also in the young person's symptoms. Developing the young person's communication abilities also has the potential to improve the way both parties feel about their relationship and may open up possibilities for more effective communication in other relationships.

Normalising issues of difference and disagreement in relationships and teaching conflict resolution skills can go a long way to countering feelings of helplessness and hopelessness that are so integral to depression. Central to IPT-A is the promotion of young peoples' sense of agency and confidence that they can create change in their relationships. As mentioned in Chapter 3: Attachment, building a sense of agency through increased personal competence is particularly important for clients such as Jan and Tracey, whose attachment style is preoccupied. Learning new ways to approach the dispute helped both of them to recognise that they could influence the outcomes of important relationships. Tracey learnt that communicating her needs to her boyfriend and learning about his needs in the relationship enabled them to work out an arrangement that they were both happy with. Even if the other party to the dispute will not change, the young person can change herself, including her behaviour and perspective, and this in turn can transform the conflict. An increased sense of her own ability to change her situation can be important for any young person as it challenges the sense of hopelessness and personal inadequacy common in depression.

The other party to the dispute may not respond to the young person's attempts to change the dispute, in ways that meet all of the young person's needs. However, some of the client's needs may be met, and this could be sufficient to transform his or her mood and outlook. The possibility that the other person may respond in negative ways should be anticipated and discussed proactively in session so that the client is prepared for this eventuality.

## The nature of Interpersonal Disputes in young people

"The young are heated by nature as drunk men by wine" Aristotle

The variation between different cultures' understanding of adolescence and their expectations of adolescents is perhaps nowhere more pronounced than in relation to conflict between young people and adults, especially parents.

Hall (1904) introduced the concept of adolescence into psychological literature. He and others characterised it as a period of "storm and stress", and this view has been widely held in some Western cultures. Many people in these cultures see some level of disputes between adolescents and adults as normal and, although often upsetting for those involved, something that generally passes and therefore not a cause for major concern. Disputes with parents and other authority figures may be viewed as a sign of individuation and movement towards independence which, in this cultural perspective, is generally welcomed as a sign of a healthy developmental trajectory for young people (Arnett, 1999).

Other cultures may want quite different outcomes for adolescent development. Increasing independence and separation from the family would be viewed with alarm (Lam, 1997). Rather, a sense of respect or even veneration for adults may be expected together with increasing family commitments and responsibilities as young people move through adolescence. In this cultural context, conflict between young people and adults may be viewed differently.

### "Normal" disputes between adolescents and parents

Despite perceptions that adolescence can be a period of conflict with authority figures, especially parents, the majority of adolescents only experience minor conflict with their parents and others (e.g., Hadiwijaya, 2017). For those who do experience significant conflict, this conflict can be adaptive for the adolescent–parent relationship (Branje, 2018).

When conflict does occur between young people and parents, it often reflects an underlying disparity in motivations. On the one hand, parents are often concerned about safety and risk taking. However, the adolescent developmental imperative of individuation will often lead young people to seek independence and push boundaries.

The family can be a safe context for young people to engage in their separation and individuation processes. Conflict can provide an opportunity for the young person to learn important social skills and gain insight about himself and others. However, conflict can cause distress for those directly involved and for the whole family. In order to minimise and manage stress, parents and young people have the challenge of achieving a balance between maintaining appropriate boundaries and limits while loosening restrictions in timely ways.

## Damaging disputes

By definition, as a Problem Area in IPT-A, Interpersonal Disputes constitute damaging conflict. These are distinguished from what we might consider to be normal levels of dispute by the intensity of distress they cause as well as the frequency, duration, and the impact on functioning for the young person and for those involved in the conflict. They may be unpleasant, reoccurring, involve angry exchanges, and involve more than one issue. Additionally, conflict can be characterised by suppression and withdrawal, and this may also be damaging. The damage tends to be compounded when workable solutions cannot be found, and the people involved in the dispute become increasingly dissatisfied with the relationship. They may then start to question the motives of the other person and come to believe that the person is not interested in understanding or respecting their concerns.

IPT-A focuses on conflict when it is associated with the onset and maintenance of the young person's depression or other disorder. When a dispute is

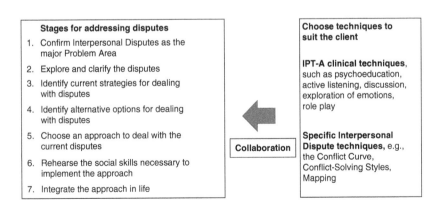

*Figure 8.1* Seven stages for working on Interpersonal Disputes.

present but not related to the young person's symptoms, this will not become a focus of therapy due to the time-limited nature of IPT-A.

These characteristics of destructive disputes (pervasive, acrimonious, and unresolved) provide useful areas of enquiry in assessing this Problem Area.

### Seven steps

Seven stages for working with Interpersonal Disputes in IPT-A are outlined in Figure 8.1 and discussed below.

## Assessing Interpersonal Disputes

### Confirm Interpersonal Disputes as the major Problem Area

The therapist will check for recurring conflict during the holistic assessment and Initial Phase of IPT-A. As noted above, the mere presence of disputes is not sufficient to confirm this as the major Problem Area.

In assessing conflict, it can be particularly useful to observe interactions between the young person and others, including how conflict arises and whether and how it escalates or resolves. When the other parties to the conflict are not present in therapy, then the therapist must rely on gathering information from the client and other informants. These accounts, of course, may not be impartial. Nevertheless, the information may still be helpful in piecing together an understanding of the dispute.

The Interpersonal Inventory provides an ideal opportunity to identify disputes. For example, during the Closeness Circles activity, the therapist invites the client to talk about conflict in any of his or her relationships. If disputes are identified, the therapist explores the level of distress caused by the dispute and ways the client and others have attempted to communicate or deal with their differences. This would usually include asking for specific examples and recent Interpersonal Incidents (see Chapter 4: Clinical techniques). Exploring an example of a dispute in some detail may yield information about the client's level of insight and understanding about his or her own and the other person's needs and their existing communication skills.

This information, in combination with the use of timelines (see Chapter 5: The Initial Phase) will help to identify if Interpersonal Disputes is the major Problem Area associated with the onset of the depression or other disorder. Additional pointers for this Problem Area are the following:

- the presence of conflict prior to the onset of the depression or other disorder
- client perception that the conflict has major negative consequences for important needs
- a recurring pattern of Interpersonal Disputes in multiple relationships
- client feelings of hopelessness or helplessness about resolving the conflict and meeting his or her needs

The benefits of arriving at this decision about the Problem Area collaboratively with the client, together with what to do when more than one Problem Area is associated with the disorder, are discussed in Chapter 6: The Middle Phase of IPT-A.

At the beginning of the Middle Phase, the therapist ascertains how much insight the young person has developed or retained from the Initial Phase about the Problem Area and why it is central to the work that they are about to embark on in therapy. Here is an example of therapist dialogue with **Admir**, aged 16, who appeared to be secure in his attachment style. Admir's case is discussed in segments through this chapter to illustrate many of the stages and strategies for addressing disputes. Information gained from Admir's holistic assessment is summarised in Figure 8.2. Admir's timeline revealed a clear escalation in conflict with his mother prior to the onset of his depression.

*Therapist:*    *It's good to see you again, Admir. As you know, this is our fifth session, so we would normally have another seven sessions after today. I'll ask you how your week has been in a moment, but first of all, let's recap from last week. Would you mind telling me what you remember from our last session? This isn't a test. It's helpful for me to know what seemed relevant or significant from your perspective.*

*Admir:*    *We talked about the arguments with Mum and you also asked me about other stuff like if I'd had any big changes or losses.*

*Therapist:*    *Yes, and do you remember what I said about why that was important?*

*Admir:*    *Well, when we did the timeline it showed how the arguing with Mum got worse before I got really low.*

*Therapist:*    *And how does knowing that help us move forward?*

*Admir:*    *You were saying if we can sort out the arguments with Mum, my depression would improve.*

*Therapist:*    *You seemed to agree with that logic last session. Now you've had a week, are you still thinking that makes sense?*

*Admir:*    *I guess so.*

Admir demonstrated that he had grasped the concept that his conflict with his mother was central to his depression and had retained this understanding. He understood the rationale for therapy focusing on this Problem Area. Given Admir's grasp of these key concepts of IPT-A, Admir's therapist could proceed straight to addressing disputes. However, if it appeared that Admir had not understood these things, further psychoeducation would be needed before proceeding to work on the Problem Area.

### *Explore and clarify the dispute(s)*

Clearly, the therapist requires a good understanding of the dispute in order to assist the young person to address it. Additionally, the process of clarifying the dispute can increase the young person's insight and understanding of his own needs and

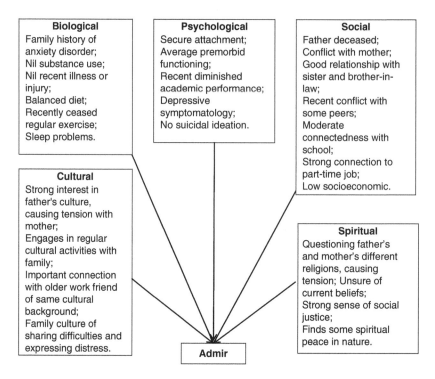

*Figure 8.2* Admir—holistic assessment summary.

those of the other party regarding it. This may go a considerable way to helping the young person to generate solutions or strategies for managing the dispute.

Eliciting the following information is helpful in confirming this Problem Area and can help inform how best to address the dispute:

- *What issues are in dispute?*
- *Who is involved?*
- *Is the dispute resulting more from the client or from the other person?*
- *What are the expectations of the relationship for each person involved? (Are the expectations realistic and compatible?)*
- *Is conflict a recurring theme in more than one relationship?*
- *What are the responses to the conflict, including cognitions, affect, and interpersonal behaviour for the client and the other party(ies)? (Is the conflict causing major distress? Is there a sense of hopelessness about change?)*
- *What are the most distressing aspects of the dispute?*
- *What is the trajectory of the dispute? (Is it getting worse, remaining static, or improving?)*

- *What helps and what makes the conflict worse, including things internal to the client or the other party and external factors such as stressors?*
- *What specific changes would the young person and the other people in the dispute like to see?*
- *How much insight does each person have about the other people in the dispute?*
- *What existing strategies and skills do the parties use for dealing with conflict?*

The therapist invites the young person to tell his or her story about the dispute and may explain that it's only when we have a good understanding of the dispute and the needs of those involved that we will be best placed to find effective solutions.

Identifying specific ways in which the young person's communication may be contributing to the dispute is key. Common patterns in misunderstandings include an expectation that the other person should understand their needs without explicitly stating them. Other examples might be that the young person uses a hostile manner that triggers arguments, or his communications are unintentionally ambiguous so that he is easily misunderstood, with the result that the young person feels frustrated and angry when the other person doesn't understand or respond in the way he thought he had clearly requested.

Some young people will have little awareness of their emotional responses to the dispute or lack the ability to communicate their feelings. When these dynamics are in play, the therapist assists the young person to recognise and express her responses, which might include feelings of sadness, anger, disappointment, resignation, and hopelessness, especially where the dispute has been chronic and when she sees no prospect of change.

The techniques outlined in Chapter 4 can be used to explore and clarify the dispute. Additionally, specific conflict resolution techniques can assist some young people, as described below.

## Identifying the issues in dispute and the relationships concerned

When conflict is a recurring theme for the young person, rather than isolated to one relationship, the conflict is probably, at least partly, due to the young person. Either his expectations of the relationship may be unrealistic, or he may lack conflict-solving skills.

If Admir was only experiencing conflict in relation to his mother, the conflict may say more about his mother than about Admir. However, further assessment identified that he was also experiencing conflict with some of his male peers at school, suggesting that the problem may, at least in part, lie with him.

After identifying that it was the conflict with his mother that is causing Admir the most distress (compared to disputes with his peers), the therapist explored the issues that are in dispute with his mother. Admir had previously mentioned that his mother "nagged" him about cleanliness and homework.

He disclosed an additional dispute with his mother. He felt his mother was denying his father's cultural and religious background and wanted him to identify solely with her heritage. Admir's parents had been refugees from a war zone. They were from communities on opposite sides in the conflict—from different religious and cultural backgrounds. Admir was born after his parents' journey to safety. When he was aged 12, his father died in a road traffic accident.

The therapist explores which aspect of the dispute is most distressing for the young person. This not only provides an opportunity for the therapist to increase her understanding and check assumptions, it encourages the young person to reflect on his inner world and can pave the way for identifying needs and emotions that the young person may not be fully aware of. For some young people, this will be a key aspect for assisting them to manage or resolve the dispute, as unconscious emotions and needs can inhibit conflict resolution.

Initially, Admir identified the chronic nature of the disputes and the fact that his mother often cried when they argued as the most distressing parts of the experience for him. It was only after further enquiry by the therapist that Admir stated that his mother's apparent lack of interest in understanding his needs or feelings upset him. He described his mother as refusing to discuss or acknowledge that he had more than just her heritage.

*Therapist:* What upsets you most about the arguments with your mother?
*Admir:* When I try and talk about it, she just ignores me or becomes hysterical.
*Therapist:* Could you give me an example of what you mean by hysterical?
*Admir:* She cries and carries on, telling me I don't understand. But she won't tell me what I don't understand.
*Therapist:* And what's that like for you?
*Admir:* I hate it.
*Therapist:* Could you tell me more about that?
*Admir:* I don't know. All of it. I hate the arguing and that she won't talk when I ask about Dad. She knows he's important to me, but it's like she just doesn't care.

At this point the therapist provided a summary and some brief psychoeducation for Admir to encourage hope and a sense of the way forward. This included:

*Therapist:* Admir, I'd like to revisit some things we touched on in our last session. I think they're relevant to where we go next.

- Some degree of conflict is probably inevitable in relationships.
- Many people find conflict difficult, or uncomfortable. They feel unsure how to deal with it and don't feel they deal with it well.
- When conflict goes on for a long time and is about important issues and with important people, and when it feels stuck, as it does for you, this can lead people to feel hopeless about it ever changing and that can be enough to create depression. As I've mentioned, that's what I suspect is going on for you.

|  |  |
|---|---|
|  | *Do you think it is accurate for your situation?* |
| Admir: | I guess so. I don't think she's going to change. |
| Therapist: | The good news is there are ways of dealing with conflict to minimise the difficulties and these skills can be learnt. If you're willing, that's what I suggest we focus on over the next few weeks. So that you have some ways to deal with conflict and so that it doesn't have such a negative effect on you and your mum. It doesn't necessarily mean you'll get your way completely, or it might be that your mother doesn't change at all. But hopefully you'll start to see that you have some options about how you deal with conflict. It might be that as you change the way you deal with your mother, she starts to change the way she responds to you. How does that sound? |
| Admir: | Well, I'd like to hear what else you think I could do, but I don't think she'll change. |

## Determining if the dispute is resulting more from the client or from the other person

Determining what and who is contributing to the conflict is crucial to focusing therapy for maximum benefit. For example, if the young person's behaviour, communication, or expectations appear at least in part to be contributing to the conflict, these things can be addressed. If, however, the dispute seems to be largely due to the other party, a different approach will be required. The readiness of the other person to engage in change will be explored. If that person is unwilling or unable to change, the work with the young person may need to focus on helping him manage the conflict to minimise his distress and meet his unfulfilled needs through other relationships. Determining if the dispute is resulting more from the young person or the other person is not about allocating responsibility or blame but rather identifying the factors contributing to the conflict and understanding how best to address these.

## Exploring expectations of others

A mismatch of expectations is a common cause of disputes. If the young person's or the other person's expectations in the relationship seem unrealistic, this suggests a direction for treatment. Modification of expectations may be sufficient to change the conflict.

In the case of Admir, as mentioned above, three issues were in dispute with his mother: his personal cleanliness, schoolwork, and cultural and religious heritage. In relation to cleanliness, there was significant divergence between the expectations of Admir and his mother. Admir felt that one shower a day was sufficient. His mother often wanted him to have three or even four showers a day, which he felt was unreasonable. Regarding homework, Admir and his mother did not have different expectations about the importance of homework. However, Admir had difficulty concentrating at home and at school. He was concerned that he was falling behind in his assignments. He resented that his mother only seemed to want to criticise him, or in his words "nag" him. Admir's expectation of his mother in relation to his heritage was that she acknowledge his father's background and allow him to discuss and explore this heritage and to identify with aspects of it.

*Therapist:* Admir, you would like your mum to show more understanding in the difficulties you're having concentrating on your schoolwork. You also want her to acknowledge your father's background and to discuss this part of your heritage because you feel it's part of who you are. Can you help me understand more of the detail of this? For example, if your mother was doing these things, what would change? What would she be doing or saying differently? How might she show you that she was trying to understand what it's like for you?

On the surface, at least, Admir's expectations seem reasonable and appropriate for a 16-year-old boy towards his mother. Whether they are realistic, in the sense of being achievable, is another matter. The likelihood of his expectations being met is obviously dependent on his mother, and this is discussed later in the chapter.

### Are disputes a recurring theme?

If the young person is only in conflict with one person, it might say more about that person than the client. However, if the young person is in dispute with numerous people, it may be more likely that the client has unrealistic expectations and/or lacks insight and conflict resolution skills. Again, this can provide a useful direction for treatment: modify expectations, increase insight, and/or develop conflict resolution skills.

Work on conflict requires the therapist to consider multiple perspectives on the issue. The young person's perspective, while central to therapy, must be understood in a wider context. Indeed, part of the therapist's role is to assist the client to consider the other party's perspective. This can be achieved through discussion (as in the case of Jan, discussed below), role play, and chair work. Young people and adults are usually more receptive to considering the other person's point of view when they have had adequate time to discuss their own perspective and when the therapist has demonstrated an understanding and empathy for their views. The therapist steps into the role of an understanding adult (a transitory attachment figure) through summarising, paraphrasing, nonjudgment, and focussed attention. In this way, Admir felt understood by the therapist, if not his mother. The sense of feeling understood was a significant part of his recovery.

## When the dispute can't be resolved

Sometimes the other party to the dispute may be unwilling or unable to modify his or her behaviour. Despite the best efforts of the young person and the therapist, the dispute may be unsolvable. The relationship may need to continue if the conflict is with people on whom the young person is dependent, or who has authority over them, such as parents, caregivers, or teachers. However, the relationship the young person hoped for is lost and is replaced by a new relationship, which is often a hollow shell of what it once was or of what the young person wanted in the relationship. The relationship may become characterised by superficiality, where the young person doesn't disclose information that is important to him and he simply goes through the motions of interacting to get through the day. When this is the case, the therapist may need to assist the young person with mourning the loss of the relationship he hoped for and finding other relationships that are rewarding. In Admir's case, this might involve deepening his connections with his sister and brother-in-law. Addressing the role of parents and others in disputes is discussed later in this chapter.

By the end of exploring and clarifying this Problem Area, the therapist should have identified the following:

- the issues in dispute
- who is involved in the conflict
- the impact of the conflict on those involved, including levels of distress and impairment
- recurring problematic communication patterns
- unrealistic and non-reciprocal expectations in relationships.

As with many things in IPT-A, the actual decision regarding which dispute to focus on initially is often less important than the process of involving the client in reaching this decision collaboratively. The competencies that are developed will be generalised to other disputes and possibly to other Problem Areas so that the client becomes more confident and competent in dealing with social problems. Generalising learning is a key focus for the Consolidation Phase (see Chapters 11 and 12).

The Conflict Curve and Mapping are concrete techniques that many young people find helpful for exploring and clarifying disputes. The Conflict Curve is discussed here and Mapping is included in Step 7 later in this chapter as it is particularly helpful in generating solutions.

### *Interpersonal Disputes technique number 1—The Conflict Curve*

Interpersonal Disputes can be of different levels of intensity and the intensity of the conflict can be an important factor governing the choice of strategy for dealing with the conflict.

When young people are depressed, they may be particularly prone to polarised thinking and viewing their world and themselves negatively. They may experience conflict as always intense and always present. Scaling can be a helpful method for exploring and challenging this biased perspective.

Scales such as the Conflict Curve (Cornelius and Faire, 1989) are particularly useful in relation to Interpersonal Disputes. Not only does the curve differentiate different levels of intensity of conflict, it also provides an opportunity to engage the young person in considering how the nature of conflict may vary with its intensity. The technique prepares the way for introducing the notion that different ways of responding to conflict may be more or less appropriate at different levels of dispute intensity.

As the name suggests, the Conflict Curve places different levels of conflict on a curve (Conflict Curves for Admir and a younger client, Jan, are included as Figures 8.3 and 8.4 below). This visual dimension is particularly useful for some young people. It can be noted that as the steepness of the curve increases, it becomes more difficult to resolve the conflict without assistance. The angle of the incline becomes increasingly slippery, making it difficult to move back to a more level or balanced state unless someone or something gives you a hand up or throws you a lifeline.

The Conflict Curve, as described by Cornelius and Faire (1989), identifies five levels of conflict. The Discomfort stage describes low-level conflict, so low that it may not be recognised as a dispute. It is the beginning of the experience of difficulty or difference in a relationship. There is often a feeling that something is not quite right in the relationship, but the exact nature of the difficulty may not yet be identified. Because it is relatively minor, it may not be acknowledged. If it is addressed, it can be managed without help from outside the relationship.

The Incidents stage includes more serious disputes, involving some distress. Incidents may take the form of short, sharp, irritable exchanges; however, the issues can also be dealt with using the existing resources and coping skills of the people in the relationship.

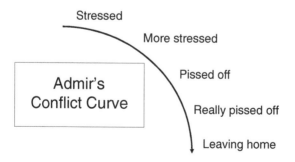

*Figure 8.3* Admir's Conflict Curve.
Adapted from (Cornelius and Faire, 1989) and http://www.crnhq.org/

When disputes reach the Misunderstandings stage, something qualitatively different is happening. The parties to the dispute are misunderstanding each other. This often involves attributing meaning or motivations to the other person's behaviour. This might include attributions such as "they don't care about me", "they're doing this deliberately", "they're trying to take advantage of me", or "they are punishing me". When people misconstrue the motives of the other, the distress and irritation may increase. They often start behaving in ways which undermine trust in the other person and the relationship. This is amplified in the Tension stage. When we believe that the other person in a dispute does not have our best interests at heart and is deliberately mistreating us, we may respond by behaving defensively or treat the other person as we perceive they are treating us. In the Crisis stage, mistrust and distance have increased to the point where the relationship is disintegrating. In the Tension and Crisis stages, it is difficult for the people in the relationship to resolve the conflict without assistance from outside the relationship.

The Conflict Curve can:

- provide the young person with psychoeducation regarding different levels of intensity of dispute
- introduce the notion that different approaches to managing conflict may be appropriate according to the intensity of the dispute
- assist the young person to develop insight into his or her own responses to conflict and that of others
- assist the therapist to understand the young person's experience of, and responses to, disputes.

Admir showed obvious interest as the therapist explained the Conflict Curve. The therapist led him in a process of individualising the model by inviting Admir to use his own language and examples.

*Therapist:* *Now let's develop your own version of the curve. Give me an example of the worst argument you have experienced with your mother?*
*Admir:* *Well a lot of it is pretty bad. I guess one of the worst was a few weeks ago when I had already had a shower and she started on at me again to have another one.*
*Therapist:* *What happened?*
*Admir:* *I told her no, I'd already had one.*
*Therapist:* *And then what happened?*
*Admir:* *She kept on at me. In the end I yelled at her and told her she was crazy. She started crying and telling me what a bad son I was for speaking to her like that. Then I yelled at her to F off.*
*Therapist:* *What happened then?*
*Admir:* *Not much. I went out.*

| | |
|---|---|
| Therapist: | What was it about that argument that makes you rank it as one of the worst? For instance, was it something about how you were feeling, or was it more about how your mother responded, or about what happened between you both afterwards, or maybe a mix of these? |
| Admir: | Well, I felt bad that I'd sworn at her, and when I came back she ignored me, and she didn't give me any dinner. She'd been crying. She didn't speak to me for a few days. She went and told my sister and her husband that I told her to F off, and they started going off at me as well. I hate it when she does that. |
| Therapist: | What was the worst thing for you about that argument? |
| Admir: | I don't know. I just felt bad. |
| Therapist: | Can you imagine an even more extreme level of conflict between you and your mother? |
| Admir: | What, like if I left home? |

Admir had difficulty identifying his feelings about his mother's behaviour. Rather than interrupt the focus of individualising the Conflict Curve, the therapist made a mental note to return later to assist Admir to identify his feelings. The therapist did this by acknowledging that both Admir and his mother had been distressed and then specifically explored his emotions in relation to his mother crying, ignoring him, not giving him dinner, and involving his sister. This enabled Admir to connect these emotional responses to his feelings about other issues of dispute with his mother. Ultimately Admir concluded that what bothered him most about the arguments was a sense that his mother didn't care about his feelings and needs.

The therapist continued to facilitate Admir to develop an individualised version of the Conflict Curve.

| | |
|---|---|
| Therapist: | If you put your words on the curve, what would you call "crisis", that worst level of conflict? |
| Admir: | Maybe F off. No, I can't say that can I? What about totally pissed off? |
| Therapist: | You can call it whatever you like, and you can change it as we go along if you want. Why don't you write on this blank version of the curve what you want to call the worst sort of argument? |

Admir wrote "Leaving home".

| | |
|---|---|
| Therapist: | Now, let's think about the opposite end of the curve, really low-level conflict, so low it's barely noticeable and may not bother you or your mother too much. Can you think of an example and what term you'd use to describe such low-level conflict? |

Admir chose the term *Stressed*.

*Therapist:* Now what about some points in between? Can you give me some examples of arguments between those two extremes and what you might call them?

When Admir had identified the stages on his individualised Conflict Curve (Figure 8.3), the therapist invited him to review the diagram and consider any implications.

*Therapist:* As we look at how this all fits together on your version of the curve, are there any changes you would like to make to fine tune it?
*Admir:* Maybe I could change really pissed off to unforgivable.
*Therapist:* Go ahead, you can make it what you want. Can you help me understand the difference?
*Admir:* Well, it's not just that I was really pissed off. I think she thought it was unforgivable because I told her to F off and that's why she was so mad and told my sister and brother-in-law. She thought I had gone too far.
*Therapist:* So part of what makes this serious conflict is that you think she felt you'd crossed a line and couldn't forgive you?
*Admir:* Yeah.
*Therapist:* And what about how you felt towards your mum?
*Admir:* Well she'd crossed my line by telling my sister and brother-in-law.
*Therapist:* Can you help me understand what that meant to you?

Admir stated that his mother knows that he hates it when she involves other family members in their conflict. However, through enquiry the therapist discovered Admir has never actually stated this clearly to his mother or requested that she not do this. The therapist made a mental note to return to this after completing the discussion of the Conflict Curve.

*Therapist:* When you look at the curve, do you see anything it might tell us about your conflict with your mother?
*Admir:* Maybe. It's not all of the really bad stuff all the time, but that's what I remember most.

The therapist complimented Admir on this observation and briefly related it back to information shared with Admir in the Initial Phase of IPT-A about how depression can affect perception by amplifying negative aspects and filtering out positive information. This is a classic example of how opportunities often emerge during the Middle Phase to reinforce key psychoeducation messages shared earlier in therapy.

The scaling implicit in this process helped Admir recognise that he tended to remember the worst interactions with his mother and lose sight of the fact that it wasn't always that bad. This technique prepared the way for an exploration of how he is currently attempting to deal with conflict and introduced the idea that the level of conflict might help in choosing the most effective approach for managing the dispute.

The case of **Jan**, aged 13, illustrates another common cause of disputes between young people and their parents. Her dispute revolved around the time Jan's parents wanted her home after being out with friends. When the therapist introduced the Conflict Curve, Jan found some of the language was not meaningful for her. However, as the therapist helped her identify some concrete examples from her life, she quickly comprehended that the level of the conflict may help in choosing the strategy most likely to be effective. Jan was excited about the prospect of learning new ways to deal with the dispute.

The therapist encouraged Jan to produce her own scale that reflected her experience of the conflict with her parents. She produced a four-point scale—low, medium, high, extreme. She volunteered "It's like the bushfire sign with the different colours when you drive into the National Park". Jan provides an illustration of the suggestion given earlier about using practical and concrete approaches when clients are at earlier developmental stages. The therapist encouraged Jan to draw the scale using the metaphor of the fire danger sign. Jan worked with crayons, choosing green, yellow, orange, and red to indicate increasing intensity of conflict. Jan enjoyed the activity, and as she focused on this concrete task she seemed happy to talk about the dispute. The therapist's judgment was that, although the activity might take more time than using didactic instruction to teach Jan about the Conflict Curve, it would be a more effective route for Jan to understand the concept of scaling different levels of dispute and also to integrate this concept into her relationships.

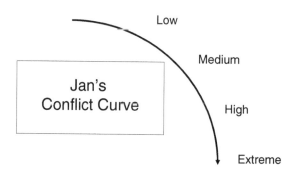

*Figure 8.4* Jan's Conflict Curve.
Adapted from (Cornelius and Faire, 1989) and http://www.crnhq.org/

The activity took about 20 minutes and led into a discussion about the way Jan currently attempts to cope with arguments of different levels of intensity and the outcomes for her of these patterns of conflict. Jan reported feeling angry with her parents, feeling hopeless about the possibility of change, and experiencing guilt about the way she spoke to her parents, which often involved yelling and slamming doors. When asked what she thought the arguments were like for her parents, her initial response was that they weren't interested in her. (In the Initial Phase of treatment, Jan demonstrated limited capacity for insight about other people's motivations in relationships.) The therapist enquired further.

*Therapist:* Jan, you've told me quite a bit about how you feel about the conflict: that you don't like it, that you feel angry, and you're not very hopeful about your parents changing. Can you help me understand what you think it's like for your parents when these arguments happen?
*Jan:* I don't know. Well, they seem angry too.
*Therapist:* What do you think they're angry about?
*Jan:* They say "no" like they really mean it. Well, they're probably worried that something bad might happen to me, but it really pisses me off because they don't understand what it's like for me. They just tell me to do what I'm told, not argue. Like they don't care.

Given time and encouragement Jan displayed some insight that her parents were probably motivated by trying to keep her safe, but at the same time she felt they weren't interested in hearing how important the issue was for her.

The therapist continued to include Jan's metaphor of the bushfire sign in the work that followed, including during some of the techniques outlined below. For example, after Jan and the therapist jointly brainstormed additional options for dealing with disputes, Jan was invited to think about what colour (or level) of dispute these strategies might work best with and mark that approach with the corresponding colour.

At a joint session with Jan and her parents, with Jan's permission, the therapist encouraged Jan to share the metaphor for levels of conflict with her parents. The therapist provided some modelling and coaching for Jan and her parents in using Jan's colour-coded language when they talk about conflict.

## Addressing Interpersonal Disputes

### Identify current strategies for dealing with disputes

Once the young person has some awareness of the ways he is responding to the dispute, therapy moves on to identifying alternative options, choosing an option to focus on initially then, through skills rehearsal, preparing to implement this option. For **Admir**, the discussion around the Conflict Curve proved sufficient for him to not only identify his current ways of dealing with conflict but also to identify alternative strategies for managing conflict with his mother.

*Therapist:* You mentioned before that you are interested in learning some new ways of dealing with conflict, and that's where we're heading. We will be assisted in this if we understand how you currently deal with conflict with your mother. You've said: you told her she was mad, you swore at her,

|  |  |
|---|---|
|  | and eventually you removed yourself from the situation. How else have you tried to deal with the conflict? |
| Admir: | Sometimes I hide from her. I used to try and reason with her and tell her that she was being over the top, but that just seemed to make her angry. |
| Therapist: | It's great that you have been trying to adjust your approach depending on your mother's responses. I'm interested in talking more about that, but first can I check if you've tried any other ways of dealing with the conflict? |
| Admir: | That's about it. |
| Therapist: | This is encouraging. It shows that you have been able to try different approaches, so you can be flexible rather than stick to one way all the time. Tell me some more about how your mother has responded to these different approaches. |

Admir gave some examples of his mother's responses, in all of which they ended up arguing.

After a thorough exploration of the way the young person is currently attempting to deal with the dispute, the therapist will be well placed to assist him to identify alternative options.

### Identify alternative options for dealing with disputes

Discussion, questions, and brainstorming can all be helpful in generating ideas about alternative ways to deal with the dispute. The therapist may need to reassure the young person that while the point is to eventually find some effective strategies, sometimes the best way to identify novel ideas and promote creative problem solving is to avoid censoring early on in the process, as this may cramp the creative flow of generating options. In this vein, there is no such thing as a silly idea.

|  |  |
|---|---|
| Therapist: | Admir, although you've tried a number of approaches, you always seem to end up arguing with your mother and you really don't want that to continue. You want her to get off your back. I'm wondering if some of those approaches might have led to a different outcome if you hadn't got angry and swore at her. It must be really hard not to get angry when she goes on at you so much, but you've mentioned that when you swear it really sets her off. Let's look at some alternative things you can do to avoid this pattern, which you both easily slip into. Imagine your mother is telling you to take a shower. What are your options? Let's try and think creatively here, don't worry if you come up with ideas that sound a bit weird. It's just about identifying as many different options as we can at this stage; then we'll think about which ones might actually work. Is that okay? |
| Admir: | I guess so, but I can't think of any. |

If the young person could readily identify alternative options, he probably would have already attempted to use these. However, with encouragement from the therapist, the young person may be able to think of additional strategies. Many young people respond well to a suggestion of imagining what other people might do in this situation. This might include real people, such as friends and family; people they look up to or admire; or fictional characters in books, films, or TV programs.

*Therapist:* Let's come at it a bit differently. What might someone else do, maybe a friend, or your sister, or someone from work, or someone from your favourite TV show or YouTube.
*Admir:* My sister sometimes changes the subject with mum. She'll start talking about the baby or ask mum to hold the baby.
*Therapist:* And does it seem to work?
*Admir:* It works for a while.
*Therapist:* Can you give me an example of how your sister does this—what she might actually say?
*Admir:* She'll say yes. I just want to feed the baby first, or I want to get the baby down to sleep, and that shuts Mum up. She doesn't seem to give my sister such a hard time as me.
*Therapist:* Would I be right in thinking that your mother thinks the baby's feeding and sleep are important?
*Admir:* Yeah.
*Therapist:* What things does she think are important for you that you could maybe use in negotiating with her about showering?
*Admir:* What, like studying?
*Therapist:* Yes, you've mentioned that she always wants you to do more study.
*Admir:* You mean tell her I'm going to do some study and I'll shower after that?
*Therapist:* Maybe. At the moment, we are just identifying options. Then I'm going to ask you to think about which ones you might like to try and how you might set them up, and we could even have a bit of a practice here together about what you might say to your mother.

Admir identified a number of alternative options. He thought about trying to negotiate a compromise with his mother by asking if he agreed to have two showers a day would she agree not to try and make him have more. He warmed to the idea of humorous responses and came up with the idea of highlighting that other people were limiting their water use due to drought-time restrictions and he wanted to do his bit to help prevent the city running run out of water. After reflection, he fine-tuned this option to suggest it as a temporary drought measure, which he thought might be more acceptable to his mother.

Admir was particularly amused when he came up with the option of pretending to take a shower by wetting his hair then going on Snapchat while the shower ran for a while.

*Therapist:* Even though initially you felt blank about what else you could try, by staying with it you've figured out quite a few options, including a couple of strategies that you've noticed your sister using. There might be other things you could try. Let's see what else we can come up with.

The process of generating numerous options, especially if some are realistic and potentially workable, often has significant therapeutic value. It directly challenges the young person's sense of being stuck and their pessimism about the prospect of positive change in the dispute. This positive impact will be further enhanced by the next stages of choosing an option and developing confidence in implementing strategies to deal with the dispute.

### Choose an approach to deal with the current dispute(s)

The young person chooses which option he would like to focus on initially and then develops social skills and confidence to operationalise this strategy.

The therapist invited Admir to consider which of the options he had identified might be more effective in different levels of conflict intensity and select one he might like to try out initially.

*Therapist:* Looking back at your Conflict Curve, which of these ways of responding to your mum do you think might work best at the high conflict end, you called it Really pissed off or Leaving home?

Admir stated that he would find it difficult to remember what he could do differently once he was involved in an argument with his mother because he would be too angry. The therapist suggested a circuit breaker so that he and his mother could calm down and try a different approach rather than continuing to argue. Admir liked this idea and wanted to try calling timeout when he and his mother started to argue so that they couldn't speak for ten minutes to give them some cooling down time.

The therapist noted that it wasn't the first time Admir had mentioned his anger in relation to conflict. The Interpersonal Inventory had also identified that flashes of anger with his mother and some of his male peers at school contributed to the disputes he was experiencing. The therapist felt that Admir would probably benefit from developing his insight and understanding of anger management strategies. Rather than interrupt the present focus of the session, this was identified as an option for further discussion. The use of anger management techniques is discussed in Chapter 10: Interpersonal Gaps.

### Rehearse the social skills necessary to implement the approach

When an approach to dealing with the dispute has been chosen, therapy then focuses on preparing to put this option into action. This will require developing a plan and the necessary social skills for the young person to deal more effectively with the dispute. Some young people will need the therapist to first explain or model specific skills or techniques. For most young people, practising the necessary skills in session with the therapist will be essential. This can be followed by practice outside therapy, perhaps first with safe people, for example, a friend or family member not involved in the dispute, and ultimately with the other party(ies) in the dispute. Alternatively, as in the case of Jan, her parents were invited to a therapy session to work on dispute resolution with the assistance of the therapist. This latter option could include the therapist coaching and modelling for the young person, and possibly also the others involved in the dispute, to actively develop their skills and confidence in using conflict resolution techniques. Involving parents or others in therapy in order to address disputes is discussed later in this chapter.

Subsequent sessions will review progress in dealing with conflict in the real world and facilitate further skill refinement. A range of techniques can be employed according to the young person's needs and preferences, including discussion, brainstorming, role play, empty chair technique, and modelling.

For Admir, role play was used to experiment with different ways he could go about discussing the idea of timeout with his mother, including choosing the best time and how to introduce the conversation. As is often the case with young people, Admir was unsure about what was expected of him in role play and was initially nervous.

The therapist modelled a number of ways in which Admir could introduce the suggestion of timeout to his mother. The therapist and Admir discussed how his mother might respond and which approach might be most successful. Admir then played the role of himself and the therapist responded as his mother might respond. After this practise, Admir felt more confident and was keen to try out this conversation with his mother. In common with many securely attached clients, he was motivated for change and willing to work on issues outside therapy. The use of role play and other skill rehearsal techniques is discussed in Chapter 4: Clinical Techniques.

### *Integrate the approach in life*

Implementation of strategies in the real world is usually more complex and challenging than rehearsal in session. The therapist anticipated that this would be the case for Admir, in part due to his mother's psychosocial issues, which are discussed later in this chapter. An important part of preparing for implementation in the real world is assisting the young person to anticipate some of the challenges he may experience and think through options for dealing with these. Potential difficulties should be contextualised in advance in order to help guard against the young person framing these as failures, an all-too-common response for young people who are depressed.

Therapist:   *You seem more confident at the prospect of trying out some of these options for communicating with your mother. I'm not surprised, because*

| | |
|---|---|
| | *you've come up with some great ideas and thought carefully about how you might communicate with her. Am I understanding that correctly?* |
| Admir: | Yeah. I hadn't thought about some of this stuff before. |
| Therapist: | So understandably, you are keen to give it a go. I don't want to dampen your enthusiasm but, as you know, sometimes things don't go exactly to plan. We've been guessing how your mother might respond, but we can't know for sure. For example, you mentioned that your mother gets very stressed and you can be surprised by what she worries about. So let's think through what your options are if your mother doesn't respond as you hope. Also, when disputes don't readily change, often people feel that they have failed. I want to encourage you to be on guard for that feeling. Sometimes it takes a number of attempts to bring about change. We can learn a lot from interactions that don't go as we would hope. This can help us find a more effective approach. In fact, sometimes it's the only way we make progress with problems—trial and error. I'm sure you know the best way to learn a new skill is practice. Think back to your first time on your skateboard. Could you do it as well as you do now? No, and how did you get better? You practised. You kept getting back on when you fell off. It's the same with communication skills. What we're aiming for is not only to help the dispute with your mother and reduce your depression but also for you to come out of therapy with more ideas and confidence for dealing with other disputes or stressful times you might face in the future. This is something we'll explore in future sessions. Do you have any thoughts about what I'm saying? |
| Admir: | It makes sense but what if she doesn't change. She thinks it's all my fault. |
| Therapist: | You're right that it takes both parties to solve a dispute. You can't change your mother, but you can change the way you behave and that might bring about some change in her. For example, she doesn't like you swearing. If you rein that in, she might go a bit easier on you. That's just an example, and you can probably think of other ways you can give her more of what she wants. It doesn't have to be things that are going to be too difficult for you but it might be sufficient for her to back off a bit. If your mother doesn't respond, you and I can consider some other approaches. |

The therapist suspected that Admir's mother, Fatima, might have difficulty responding positively to Admir's initiative to change the dispute. Fatima appeared to be experiencing significant stress and possible mental health issues. The attempt to prepare Admir for a range of possible responses was well placed as, in fact, Admir wasn't able to make much progress alone with his mother. Following his attempt, he agreed to invite her to a therapy session. The therapist's approach to addressing Fatima's needs and concerns, including her mental health, is discussed below in the section entitled "Involving parents or others in working on Interpersonal Disputes".

Some young people will require additional specific dispute resolution techniques such as the two approaches outlined below: Conflict-Solving Styles and

Mapping. These techniques were not necessary for Admir. He may well have benefited from them but, given the time-limited nature of IPT, this was judged not to be the best use of time. If, however, Admir had not so readily displayed insight and identified alternative strategies for dealing with the dispute, then these techniques may be appropriate for him.

The dialogue above introduces the idea that if Admir were to yield to some things his mother wants, this may lessen the conflict. The therapist stipulates that this might be making concessions about things which are not too important to Admir but that might mean a lot to his mother. The notion of elegant currency, that is giving something to the other person that does not cost you a lot but is valuable to the other person, could follow on effectively from Mapping or a similar exercise which identifies the needs and fears of each party. The concept of elegant currency can be effective for both young people and their significant others.

*Interpersonal Disputes technique number 2: Conflict-solving styles*

The conflict-solving styles, discussed in Chapter 4: Clinical Techniques, comprises five styles: Withdrawal, Suppression, Compromise, Win/Lose and Win/Win. This model can assist the young person to deal more effectively with the dispute by:

- developing new insight into his or her own and the other person's responses to conflict
- identifying alternative responses
- depersonalising the conflict by normalising some of the responses to conflict as common styles and often an indicator that people are stressed
- increasing the young person's sense of agency that there are options he or she can try to improve the situation
- providing hope that this new information may enable more positive outcomes to occur

After determining that this might be a helpful activity for the young person, there are four stages to the technique:

A   Explain the model

   The model can be presented to the young person using a handout or clinical tool (see, for example, Figure 4.5), or through a verbal description. Alternatively, before introducing the model, the therapist might start with a conversation that initially invites the young person to reflect on what she has noticed about the ways in which she and other people deal with disputes. The advantages and disadvantages of each style of dealing with difficulties can be discussed, including the impact on the people involved in the dispute, on the relationship and on the conflict.

B   Apply the model to the young person's situation

   The therapist assists the young person to apply the styles to her own situation. Exploration of the pros and cons and potential outcomes for the styles at different levels of conflict is a useful aspect of helping the young person apply the model to her situation. Consider asking the following:

- *Which of these styles do you recognise in yourself?*
- *Think of specific examples of incidents when you were feeling stressed, tired, or overwhelmed. In those situations, which style are you most likely to use?*
- *Which of these styles do you recognise in other people, including the people you are in dispute with?*
- *What might be the pros and cons of different styles?*
- *What outcomes have you noticed when you or other people have used that style?*
- *Which level of conflict is that style most effective with?*
- *In relation to your current dispute, what might happen if you used some of the other styles (that you haven't tried)?*

This conversation reinforces the point that some strategies might be more or less effective depending on the level of the conflict and the approach of the other party. The therapist might refer back to the young person's Conflict Curve to aid application.

C   Reflection—the young person considers how the model might assist the dispute

   The realisation that there are a range of alternative styles of dealing with conflict can promote a hopeful outlook, for example, "Now I see there are some new ways to deal with the dispute, maybe we can get to a different outcome". It can be helpful for the therapist to return at this stage to the point made earlier that while the young person cannot change the other person, she can change her own behaviour and that may lead the relationship in positive directions.

D   Skills development—develop the skills and confidence necessary to use the model in real-life situations

   The approaches mentioned above can be used to develop the young person's social skills and confidence, including rehearsing skills in session and outside therapy. Additionally, the other parties in the dispute could be invited to a session if the young person elects for this.

The conflict-solving styles model won't be necessary for all young people, but it will be useful for those who have difficulty recognising alternative ways of responding to conflict, as discussed in the case of Tanya, in Chapter 4.

*Interpersonal Disputes technique number 3: Mapping*

Understanding the needs and fears of each party in a dispute can transform the conflict and deepen the relationship. This increased understanding aims to create mutual compassion and a realisation that the other person's behaviour may be based on his or her needs and vulnerabilities rather than on a lack of regard or respect. This realisation can change the attitude and approach of the people involved to dealing with the dispute. Furthermore, the increased mutual understanding and compassion can bring about positive changes in the way they relate to each other more generally.

Mapping is a strategy described by Cornelius and Faire (1989) that is useful for clarifying issues present in conflict. Mapping a dispute is a means for identifying the underlying needs and fears of each party. It can be introduced as a way of developing understanding that can help generate solutions to a dispute. It is a particularly useful technique when conflict has become stuck and the people involved see no way of reaching a mutually acceptable resolution.[2]

In attempting to deal with conflict, some people get stuck in the process of trying to find a workable solution and don't feel comfortable with addressing the associated emotions. They may try to avoid the emotions altogether. Other people get so caught up with the emotions that they don't engage with the process of finding a solution. These different orientations can lead to misunderstandings and assumptions that the other party is unwilling to find an effective solution, which can aggravate the conflict. Mapping helps ensure that a balance is struck between the two—that both the process of finding a solution and understanding the associated emotions are addressed.

Mapping a dispute clarifies issues, identifies the parties, elicits precise requirements of those involved, and enables the generation of possible solutions that meet the requirements of the participants.

The technique can be conducted with the client alone or with the other parties to the dispute present. The therapist asks the people involved to put aside blame, at least for the time being, and to try and understand the needs and concerns of the other party.

The components of Mapping (adapted from Cornelius and Faire, 1989) are the following:

- Find a nonjudgmental description of the problem
- List the major needs and fears of each party
- Generate solutions.

## Find a nonjudgmental description of the problem

The most important factor in referring to the dispute is to keep the definition as unemotive as possible, so that no one feels he or she is being victimised. The issue should be named in broad, objective terms that all parties would agree on, taking care not to label anyone as the problem. For example, although an adolescent may frame a dispute as "Mum's being a bitch", a less emotive definition that still preserves the crux of the matter, may be "Curfew times".

## List the major needs and concerns of all parties

When Mapping is used with just the young person, the therapist encourages the young person to step into the others' shoes and identify their needs and concerns or fears, as well as identifying his own, as in the case of Manu.

**Manu** is a 20-year-old student with a secure attachment style. He lived alone with his mother, who he claimed to be intrusive, overly involved in his life, and stifling of any romantic relationships he contemplated. Manu was angry at his mother and frustrated by her constant inappropriate "mothering", especially in front of his friends. He insisted that the only way forward was to move out of home. His mother was totally against this, which Manu interpreted as another attempt by her to run his life. He approached a college counsellor for assistance with financial matters related to finding a new residence. The therapist requested they undertake a Mapping exercise prior to exploring Manu's solutions. Manu agreed and had no trouble identifying his own needs (independence, to be treated like an adult, have his own space, get on with his studies, enjoy greater

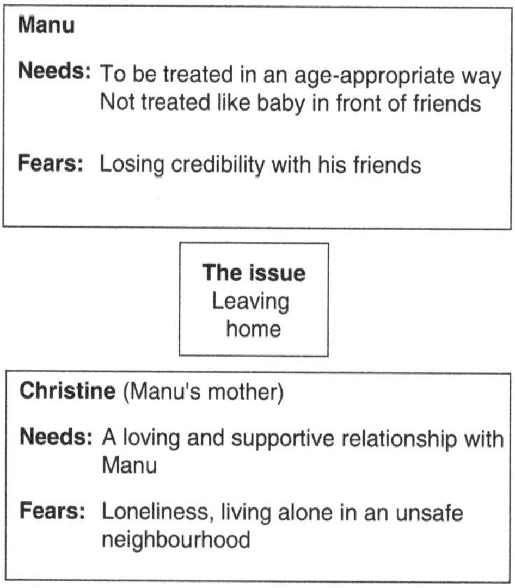

---

**Manu**

**Needs:** To be treated in an age-appropriate way
Not treated like baby in front of friends

**Fears:** Losing credibility with his friends

---

**The issue**
Leaving home

---

**Christine** (Manu's mother)

**Needs:** A loving and supportive relationship with Manu

**Fears:** Loneliness, living alone in an unsafe neighbourhood

---

*Figure 8.5* Manu's dispute map.

freedom) and fears (being seen by his friends as controlled by his mother, not being able to bring a girlfriend home, being "suffocated"). Manu recoded his responses in Figure 8.5.

Manu was then asked what he thought his mother's needs and fears were in relation to him moving out. It was clear to the therapist that Manu had not previously considered his mother's perspective. He realised that she most likely wanted what was best for him, as she had done since he was born, but she had not adjusted her expectations of him since he was small. Manu recognised that his mother probably feared loneliness, especially as she had very few friends of her own. Additionally, he realised that she may fear for her own safety if Manu moved out as it was a potentially unsafe neighbourhood. Although this shift in Manu's perspective did not provide a solution, it gave Manu a more comprehensive "map of the territory" for him to continue his thinking.

After some social skills practice with the therapist, Manu eventually moved out but was able to do so on good terms and in a way that minimised conflict with his mother. He stated that he no longer felt so angry towards her and that this had taken the heat out of their relationship. The therapist acknowledged Manu's success in achieving his goal of moving out and doing this in a way that was respectful and caring of his mother, which emerged as an additional consideration during the Mapping. The therapist assisted Manu to identify his strengths that helped him to use this technique so effectively, such as being able to think about someone else's needs, having compassion for others, his loving nature, and his ability to quickly get back in touch with this despite his anger, which had been overshadowing his concern for his mother.

The therapist pointed out that Manu's success in producing a good outcome to conflict in his current situation boded well for his ability to deal with difficulties in the future. The therapist recommended that Manu remember that techniques such as Mapping along with his above-mentioned competencies can be helpful and suggested that they return to think about this further in the last few sessions of therapy to help generalise the skills and reinforce the learning.

## Generating solutions

The process of identifying solutions is demonstrated in the case of **Gina**, aged 15, introduced in Chapter 5, who lives with her mother, father, and younger sister. She believes her position in her peer group is tenuous due to her parents not allowing her to do the things her friends are allowed to do. A major argument occurred when Gina told her mother she was getting her tongue pierced. Gina believed this would firm up her position in her peer group. Her mother, however, flatly refused.

Gina believed that nothing she could do would change her mother's stance. Gina was already ruminating about her position in the peer group and this intensified following the argument. Gina focused almost exclusively on perceived interactions that she believed were emblematic of her being rejected. Within this context, Gina developed symptoms of social anxiety including panic attacks at school and home. She began to miss school classes, and, when she did attend, she spent most of her time alone.

Gina was referred to her school counsellor by a teacher who had noticed that she had changed from being a reserved but capable student to become morose, insular, and half-hearted about her schoolwork. The therapist assessed that Gina was experiencing symptoms of depression and social anxiety and, together with Gina, identified the Problem Area as Interpersonal Disputes.

Gina conceded that if this conflict could be resolved she would be more able to reconnect with her peer group and her depressive and anxious symptoms would begin to abate. However, she could see no solution to her parents' intransigence and therefore no solution to her growing isolation.

The therapist first explored what attempts had been made by Gina and her parents to solve the conflict. After establishing that it seemed unlikely that the conflict would change without assistance, the therapist introduced Mapping in order to give Gina some realistic hope of finding a way of meeting her needs. This is a classic example of the connection between a young person's attachment needs not being met and her symptoms. In Gina's case, it is shown in her need for connection with her peers and also her need for her parents to be interested in understanding these needs.

*Therapist:* Gina, last week we talked about your depression and anxiety, and we agreed that it was about not feeling a part of your group of friends anymore. You feel you don't fit in because your parents won't let you get piercings like your friends. Have I understood correctly?

*Gina:* Yeah, it's not that I don't fit in—more like they see me as some kind of mummy's girl.

*Therapist:* If you and your folks could come to some sort of agreement about the piercings, would that make a difference?

*Gina:* As if that would happen .... Yeah, maybe.

*Therapist:* I want to suggest an approach that may give you and your parents a better chance of coming to an agreement—not just about this problem but also other problems in the future. Is that okay?

*Gina:* S'pose.

*Therapist:* It's called Mapping. It can help you and your parents understand the conflict better and what each person wants out of the situation. This in turn can make it easier to find a solution that is acceptable to all of you.

The discussion about needs and fears revealed that Gina's main needs were to feel that she was a part of the group and to feel good about herself. Her primary fears were that she would spend the rest of her high school years alone. She suggested her mother's needs related to having a daughter she could be proud of while her father's needs were for peace and quiet at home.

Gina believed her parents feared that association with her group of friends would lead her to not do as well as she could academically or even to drop out of school. Gina expressed anger about her parent's assumption that her peers were a bad influence. She was keen to go to university and pointed out that her schoolwork dropped after she stopped associating with these friends. She stated that her father feared that the expensive orthodontic work Gina had undergone in Year 8 would be compromised by a metal stud in her tongue. She suspected her mother's main fear was what other people might think of her as a mother if she allowed her daughter to have a tongue stud. Figure 8.6 represents the dispute map produced by this conversation.

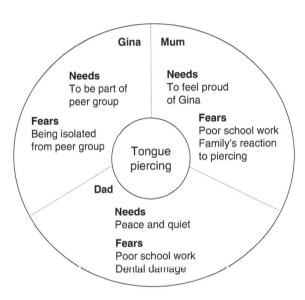

*Figure 8.6* Gina's dispute map.

*Therapist:* The next part of this process is generating solutions. Now, considering the needs and fears of all the people you have identified as being part of this problem, let's see if we can come up with solutions that meet as many needs and fears as possible. Do we have enough information to make a choice yet? I think you said your mum was "paranoid" about infection. Perhaps we could do some research so you can answer your mum's worry about infection.

The process of generating solutions included conversations between Gina and the therapist and between Gina, the therapist, and her parents. Although her parents would not give ground on the tongue piercing, they began to see how important this group of friends was to Gina and acknowledged her school grades were always good when she was associating with this group. Gina suggested that if she could get more ear piercings done, that may be enough. Her parents reluctantly agreed. As this decision addressed many of the needs and concerns of the three people involved, it was feasible and fair.

Solution implementation was straightforward, and Gina felt more comfortable about acceptance by her group of friends. Her mood began to lift and therapy then focused on how this dispute had contributed to her feelings of isolation and depression. The therapist fostered Gina's belief that now the conflict had been largely resolved and her isolation was less pressing, she could expect her symptoms of depression to continue to lessen. Markers of improvement were identified, including changes that Gina might notice first: spending more time with her friends, re-engagement with her studies, and improvement in mood.

The therapist drew Gina's attention to the potential of Mapping and similar processes for dealing with future challenges and discussed this further during the Consolidation Phase.

## Involving parents or others in working on Interpersonal Disputes

General considerations in assessing the capacity of parents or others to participate constructively in the Middle Phase of IPT-A are discussed in Chapter 6.

Therapy can provide an opportunity for the people affected by a dispute to address the conflict head on. While it is not the aim of IPT-A to evoke conflict between the young person and the other party, if conflict does erupt in session, this is not necessarily a bad thing. After all, it is unlikely to be new for either party. Conflict in the session will demonstrate relationship dynamics. This may afford clinical insights and provide an opportunity for the therapist to model and perhaps coach both parties in conflict resolution strategies.

### When a parent has mental health issues or other impediments

The person with whom the young person is in dispute may be affected by mental illness, drugs and alcohol, or other issues that limit his or her ability to effectively address the dispute or to support the young person in general. These factors may contribute to unrealistic expectations and inappropriate behaviour by the parent that triggers or maintains disputes.

### When the parent is amenable to addressing their impediments

In the case of **Admir**, the therapist suspected that his mother, Fatima, was experiencing symptoms of obsessive-compulsive disorder and possibly also post-traumatic stress disorder. The therapist hypothesised that these conditions were contributing to her apparently unreasonable expectations of Admir and fuelling conflict between them. With Admir's agreement, the therapist spoke with Fatima alone. Fatima acknowledged that she had significant symptoms of anxiety and recognised that this affected her relationship with Admir. Fatima came from a country where mental health services were rare and where symptoms of PTSD were common due to long-term exposure to war conditions and civil unrest. In this context, the notion of seeking specialist help for her symptoms was alien to her. Furthermore, Fatima disclosed that she feared stigma if it became known that she had mental health problems. This included concern that it would damage the marriage prospects of her extended family, including Admir. Her fear of stigma extended to Admir's depression, but Fatima stated that it was acceptable for him to see a counsellor because this was occurring at school and could be seen as educational support rather than mental illness.

Given that a mental health referral was unacceptable to Fatima, at least at present, the therapist decided to take a different tack to addressing Fatima's symptoms by addressing her social isolation. The therapist also made a mental note to consult a specialist in the Transcultural Mental Health Service[3]. Fatima disclosed that she had little meaningful social contact apart from with Admir and her daughter's family. In order to explore options for increasing social support that might be acceptable to Fatima, the therapist enquired about her favourite pastimes, which included her religion, gardening, and cooking. The therapist suggested that Fatima might enjoy joining a local community garden. The garden fostered social interaction between those involved, including pooling some of their produce for occasional community meals and regularly exchanging seed and cuttings for propagation. Fatima was pleased to hear that there were a number of other Muslim women involved in the project and this made the suggestion culturally acceptable for her.

*Therapist:* *Fatima, thank you for helping me to understand more about your concerns for Admir and about your own situation. As you know, conflict between teenagers and their parents can happen as young people want greater independence. Most parents find this difficult. It's hard when there is only one parent because all the responsibility falls on you and you don't have a partner to discuss it with. On top of this, you mentioned how you struggle with your anxiety. It makes many areas of your life difficult. Also, you don't talk with many people apart from your family. Have I understood that correctly?*

*Fatima:* *Yes, Admir makes me sick with worry, and I can't talk to anyone outside the family. I don't want people to think I'm a bad mother. People—sometimes they gossip.*

*Therapist:* *From talking with you and Admir it is clear that your arguments are making you both miserable and that you have both run out of ideas about how to improve things. As I mentioned a couple of weeks ago, the arguments are contributing to Admir's depression and they seem to be making your anxiety worse. I'm hopeful we can improve this as Admir seems committed to working with me and you are willing to look at things you can do to help. Just as Admir's depression is affecting his schoolwork and perhaps making him more irritable and cranky with you than usual, your anxiety and stress may be affecting the way you respond to him.*

> There are treatments that could help your anxiety. I know you don't want to see a professional service about your anxiety, but if that changes, I can help you find someone you can work with. There are other ways you could help your anxiety. At the moment, you're spending most of your time worrying at home. You might find that spending more time doing things you enjoy will give you a break from your worries and help you feel calmer around Admir and less stressed more generally. You mentioned a friend you haven't seen for a long time who you could get back in touch with. It's great that you are interested in visiting the community garden. You'd meet people with similar interests. Also, you mentioned that pottering in the garden at home helps you feel less anxious.

A time-limited intervention such as IPT-A does not provide sufficient opportunity to fully address parent issues such as Fatima's. The therapist did, however, support Fatima in seeking help for her symptoms and increasing her social support, in addition to developing her understanding of Admir's needs. This, together with increasing Admir's insight about his role in exacerbating the disputes with his mother and helping them both to develop and practice alternative strategies for managing disputes, significantly reduced the conflict between them. Admir's recovery from depression accelerated and Fatima reported feeling less stressed.

In the case of **Jan**, discussed above, her parents initially refused to participate in therapy, stating that her behaviour towards them, including being rude and disrespectful, was unacceptable. They felt they were being completely reasonable and generous as parents and it was up to Jan to see the error of her ways and take responsibility for her behaviour. They did not want to cloud this message by attending therapy, which might give Jan a sense that somehow the responsibility for change lay with them. They were not aware that Jan's irritability might be a symptom of her depression. This information and additional psychoeducation about depression challenged their assumption that Jan was being deliberately difficult and disrespectful and facilitated them to think about the conflict differently and consider participating in therapy.

### When a parent is not amenable to addressing their impediments

Where the parent or other party is unwilling to address ways they might be contributing to the conflict and they remain unresponsive to the therapist's best efforts to address this, therapy will focus on assisting the client to manage the conflict by taking responsibility for their side of the dispute and developing their conflict management skills. The loss of the relationship the young person hoped for should be acknowledged and some assistance with mourning the loss may be needed.

In situations such as these, the therapist's role as a transitory attachment figure is especially important. The therapist should also consider developing additional sources of support and nurture for the young person. In the case of **Admir**, if his mother had not been available or willing, the involvement of Admir's sister or brother-in-law may have been appropriate. They both know Admir and his mother well, they are familiar with the conflict and they play a significant role in Admir's life.

## Concluding the Middle Phase

By the end of the Middle Phase of IPT-A, progress will either have been made in resolving the dispute or in finding other ways of reducing the young person's symptoms. The latter may include ways to manage the dispute to reduce the distress caused and to develop other relationships that can meet the young person's attachment needs. The therapist will usually check progress by reviewing the markers of improvement that were identified collaboratively with the young person during the Initial Phase of therapy. Reviewing symptoms may occur several times during the Middle Phase (see Chapter 6). If any symptoms have not improved as much as would be expected, additional attention can be given to these in the next phase of IPT-A. The case of Kylie in Chapter 11 illustrates this. Parents or others will usually be updated about progress during and/or at the end of the Middle Phase, providing the young person is agreeable to this. They may be requested to support the young person in skills-practice exercises outside therapy.

## Summary

Despite some common perceptions, the years of adolescence and early adulthood are not universally ones that are fraught with conflict. Some young people do, however, experience disputes that have a negative impact on their future life trajectory and that contribute to significant distress and mental disorder. For these young people, if they can find ways to solve the dispute through improving their communication and their capacity to better understand their own needs and those of the other party, then the effect can be life changing. It may not only resolve the present dispute but also equip them with approaches that will help deal with future conflict and adversity. Even when a dispute cannot be resolved, a young person's wellbeing can be transformed by developing an attitude of trying to better understand the needs and concerns of the people involved, revising their expectations to make them more realistic, and developing alternative supportive relationships.

Furthermore, if young people model respectful and effective responses to the disputes they encounter in their future lives, this has the potential to benefit many people.

## Notes

1 In this chapter, the words dispute and conflict are used interchangeably to refer to this Problem Area.

2 Information about Mapping and other conflict resolution techniques is available at the Conflict Resolution Network: http://www.crnhq.org/.
3 Transcultural or Cross-Cultural Mental Health Services are available in countries such as Australia. They provide cultural consultancy both to therapists and mental health clients. This is distinct from language interpretation services, which might be necessary but not sufficient for effective cross-cultural therapy. These specialist mental health services employ clinicians from a range of cultural backgrounds with the aim of assisting the therapist to understand which part of a client's presentation may be related to cultural issues and, equally importantly, they can assist the client to understand the therapist's Western mental health framework and approach.

# References

Allen, J., Insabella, G., Porter, M., Smith, F., Land, D., & Phillips, N. (2006). A social-interactional model of the development of depressive symptoms in adolescence. *Journal of Consulting and Clinical Psychology*, 74(1), 55–65.

Arnett, J. (1999). Adolescent storm and stress, reconsidered. *American Psychologist*, 54(5), 317–326.

Branje, S. (2018). Development of parent–adolescent relationships: Conflict interactions as a mechanism of change. *Child Development Perspectives*, 12(3), 171–176.

Cornelius, H., & Faire, S. (1989). *Everyone can win: how to resolve conflict*. Brookvale, N.S.W.: Simon & Schuster.

Hadiwijaya, H., Klimstra, T., Vermunt, J., Branje, S., & Meeus, W. (2017). On the development of harmony, turbulence, and independence in parent–adolescent relationships: A five-wave longitudinal study. *Journal of Youth and Adolescence*, 46(8), 1772–1788.

Hall, G. S. (1904). *Adolescence: Its psychology and its relations to physiology, anthropology, sociology, sex, crime, religion, and education*. (Vols. I & II). New York: D.Appleton & Co.

Lam, C. (1997). A cultural perspective on the study of Chinese adolescent development. *Child and Adolescent Social Work Journal*, 14(2), 95–113.

Yap, M., Pilkington, P., Ryan, S., & Jorm, A. (2014). Parental factors associated with depression and anxiety in young people: a systematic review and meta-analysis. *Journal of Affective Disorders*, 156, 8–23.

# 9   Role Transition

**Contents**

| | |
|---|---|
| Introduction | 241 |
| Defining Role Transition | 242 |
| Assessing the Problem Area | 243 |
| Working on the Problem Area in the Middle Phase of IPT-A | 246 |
|     Step 1. Identify Role Transition as central to the symptoms | 246 |
|     Step 2. Review positive and negative aspects of the old role | 248 |
|     Step 3. Review positive and negative aspects of the new role | 253 |
|     Step 4. Identify role options to reduce symptoms | 257 |
|     Step 5. Plan, rehearse, and implement changes | 261 |
|     Involving significant others in assessment and treatment of Role Transition | 265 |
| Additional issues | 265 |
|     Role Transition in relation to sexuality or gender identity | 265 |
|     Integrating structural approaches to effectively address oppression within an IPT-A intervention | 276 |
| References | 277 |

## Introduction

Just as grief and loss are guaranteed in life, so, too, are experiences of transition. Adolescence itself is a transition, full of changes both small and major. In a relatively brief period of a few years, the young person is expected to transform from the role of a child to that of an adult. The adjustments required during this period of development may be especially difficult when challenging life events occur. For example, mood disorders and substance use problems in young people can be associated with common life stressors, such as the ending of a romantic relationship, family disruption, or interpersonal difficulties (e.g., Aliri et al., 2018; Low et al., 2012).

Similar to other Problem Areas, not all Role Transitions cause ongoing difficulty, require therapy, or lead to depression or other disorders. Therapy is indicated when the distress of the change in role progresses to symptoms of disorder. The work of this Problem Area then focuses on assisting young people to adjust to the new role. This usually involves helping them to develop a balanced view of the transition and then to find ways to function in the new role. Communicating their psychosocial needs to others in ways that maximise the likelihood of others responding positively is fundamental to enhancing young people's support in these new circumstances. This is a central theme running through all the Problem Areas, and, accordingly, many of the techniques for social skills development discussed in the other Problem Area chapters can also be considered for Role Transition.

Young people can have very different responses to apparently similar transitions. The young person's attachment style and the capacity of his or her social support system are key considerations in understanding the impact of a Role Transition.

This chapter defines Role Transition, discusses key assessment issues and then outlines a five-step approach to working on this Problem Area. The cases of two young people are discussed in some detail: Pippa's Role Transition relates to changes in her family structure, and Grant's involves his sexual orientation.

## Defining Role Transition

The term Role Transition in IPT-A refers to life changes that require the young person to play a new role, where she experiences difficulty adjusting to this change of role and where this difficulty is the major cause of her symptoms or distress. This will usually entail the young person experiencing one or more of the following characteristics:

- Not wanting to relinquish the old role
- Not choosing or wanting the new role
- Not feeling prepared for the new role
- Not seeing how he or she can meet his or her needs or other peoples' expectations in the new role

This Problem Area encompasses a wide range of transitions. The transitions may be normal developmental changes, such as from childhood to puberty; primary or junior school to high school; or high school to university, college, work, or unemployment. These changes are biologically, socially, economically, or culturally determined and are often expected. Other transitions result from critical life events and may not be expected, such as bereavement, pregnancy, illness, relocation to a different country or region, disability, parental separation, incarceration or incapacity, a grandparent developing dementia, or a treasured aunt or uncle being promoted so he or she no longer has as much time for the young person.

Role Transition   243

The unexpected nature of a life change may be the major reason why the young person is not prepared to take on the new role. Additionally, a lack of maturity, whether psychological, social, cognitive, or biological, may explain why the young person is not prepared for a change of role.

The young person may only experience particular aspects of a transition as difficult. For example, an older adolescent may cope well with her peer group changing and re-forming around romantic relationships rather than group affiliation and connections. Yet she may struggle with moving towards greater financial independence. Another young person might easily adjust to his emerging sexual attractions but be greatly perturbed by increasing academic pressures or expectations to take on greater family responsibilities.

A common characteristic of Role Transition is that the shift in expectations of the young person's role has major psychological and interpersonal consequences. The young person cannot see how he can negotiate his path through the change in ways that meet his own needs or other people's expectations. The resulting stress can create a range of symptoms.

## Assessing the Problem Area

There are several aspects to the assessment of Role Transition. A life change that potentially constitutes a Role Transition must be identified. It then needs to be confirmed whether the life change is the major Problem Area associated with the onset of symptoms. Further assessment will be necessary in order to understand the impact of the Role Transition on the young person and to identify effective pathways forward.

This section outlines these processes and highlights some common characteristics that may point to Role Transition being the major Problem Area.

### *Early indicators*

Sometimes indicators of Role Transition are apparent early in therapy, including during the holistic assessment (Chapter 2). During the Initial Phase of IPT-A, a combination of discussion and the timeline technique, discussed in Chapter 5, will usually be sufficient to clearly identify the major Problem Area. Role Transition is identified if the interpersonal history and review of life events suggest that the onset of mental disorder coincided with a life change that requires a change of role.

### *Self-esteem and social functioning*

This Problem Area is often associated with lowered self-esteem and impaired social functioning. Self-esteem is adversely affected because the young person is unsure how to function well in the new role. Young people may fear failure and letting down or disappointing people who are important to them. This will often be associated with feelings of embarrassment and humiliation, which negatively impact self-esteem. Adolescents may be unsure how to project their preferred image or persona in the changed circumstances. This can drive or be driven by a fear of rejection by their peers. Their lack of confidence in the new role frequently leads them to feel self-conscious and awkward, not only in relation to the changed role but also in their social functioning more generally. Sometimes this becomes a self-fulfilling cycle, whereby young people feeling pessimistic about their ability to make the new role work both for themselves and others undermines their confidence and performance, which in turn confirms their negative outlook and self-assessment. Depression or anxiety can exacerbate this bleak view of themselves and their prospects.

*Screening to identify life changes that may constitute a Role Transition*

As mentioned, early indicators that the young person has experienced potentially difficult transitions should be present during the holistic assessment stage and the Initial Phase of IPT-A. Some active screening by the therapist is usually required to ensure that changes that may constitute Role Transition are not missed. Questions such as those below can be helpful.

*Examples of questions that can help identify possible Role Transitions*

- Tell me about any changes you've been through over recent months. They might be big, or not so big.
- Have any of the people you're close to been through any changes recently? How have those changes affected you?
- Have there been any important changes at home, at school, with your friends, or in your sport or other interests?
- Have your routines or activities changed? What's that been like for you?
- How has your health been over the last year or two?
- Have you had any accidents or injuries recently?
- Have there been any recent changes to the health, happiness, or wellbeing of the people you're close to?
- Are you expecting any big changes for you, your family or friends in the coming months?
- Have your goals or dreams for the future changed recently?
- Were there any changes in the expectations other people have of you in the period before you became depressed?
- Have you noticed any changes in your confidence?
- Has the way you think about yourself or your abilities changed recently?
- Have there been any changes in who you find yourself attracted to romantically?

Some of these questions are broad, while others focus on specific areas of potential transitions. It can be helpful to use a combination of both. The broader questions may bring to light issues the therapist has not thought of, and the more specific questions can guide the young person to consider changes in areas of life that he or she might not otherwise mention. The therapist needs to tread carefully around sensitive issues but, at the same time, not avoid screening for issues that may be potentially embarrassing or awkward for the client to discuss. Some examples are included in the discussion of Role Transition in relation to sexuality and gender identity at the end of this chapter.

The above questions will help identify significant life changes, but these won't necessarily involve a change of role for the young person. Further exploration is often required to explore if these changes have in fact required the young person to take on a new role. Questions which ask about changes in responsibilities, expectations, identity, or the way the young person relates to others can be helpful in this regard.

### *Examples of questions to check if a life change constitutes Role Transition*

- *When your sister went away to university you became the oldest child at home. Has that meant extra responsibilities for you?*
- *Since your grandmother's death, have you been expected to do any of the things she did at home?*
- *How have your injuries affected the way people relate to you, and you to them?*
- *You've recently moved from junior school to high school: what has it been like for you? How has it affected your friendships?*
- *How have things changed for you since you began university?*
- *Has starting the new job brought about any changes you weren't expecting?*
- *What has leaving school been like for you? Has it turned out as you imagined it would?*
- *You moved home not so long ago, what was that like for you? How does this affect your relationships (with friends, family, etc.)?*
- *How has your diagnosis with this condition changed the way you think about yourself?*
- *What effect has your parent's separation had on your relationship with them?*
- *How has becoming captain of your team affected your relationships with your teammates and other people?*

Parents and others can provide valuable information when assessing Role Transition.

### *Confirming if Role Transition is the Problem Area*

Even when a transition appears to be a significant one, the therapist needs to confirm if it constitutes the major Problem Area associated with the onset of the young person's symptoms.

When more than one Problem Area appears to be associated with the young person's symptoms, the aim is to differentiate primary and secondary Problem Areas. Role Transition frequently co-occurs with significant feelings of loss and may be triggered by loss events. Role Transitions that are forced on the young person by changes occurring in the lives of their significant others may lead to Interpersonal Disputes. For example, parents becoming ill, disabled, changing jobs, or separating may not only change the young person's routines, resources, and access to that person but may also adversely affect the mental health and wellbeing of the parent. This can damage the quality of care the parent is able to offer the young person and can create or exacerbate conflict. When the Problem Area of Interpersonal Gaps coexists with Role Transition, it will usually be more difficult for the young person to communicate his or her needs effectively and adjust to the transition.

The process of deciding which Problem Area to address first when two or more are present is discussed in Chapter 6.

## Working on the Problem Area in the Middle Phase of IPT-A

This chapter presents a five-step approach for addressing Role Transition in the Middle Phase of IPT-A:

1   Identify Role Transition as central to the symptoms
2   Review positive and negative aspects of the old role
3   Review positive and negative aspects of the new role
4   Identify options that will lead to symptom reduction
5   Plan, rehearse and implement changes

These steps provide a generic model that can be utilised to address a wide range of Role Transitions. The approach helps to make abstract concepts concrete and provides activity-based learning and visual representations.

For many young people, an important part of this Problem Area is addressing feelings of loss, ambivalence, and other affect associated with the Role Transition. This can be achieved as part of this five-step process, as in the case of Pippa below. For some young people, it will be necessary before they can effectively participate in Steps 4 and 5, where options to reduce symptoms are identified and implemented. For other young people, including those who may be easily distracted by their affect, the therapist may decide that it is better to address this before or during the early steps of the process.

### Step 1. Identify Role Transition as central to the symptoms

This is the most abstract of the Problem Areas and therefore more attention may need to be given to explaining Role Transition and assisting young people to appreciate its relevance to their symptoms, compared to the other Problem Areas. Although more effort may be required to explain the concept, it has a wide range of applications and can be a particularly creative construct to work with. For some young people, finding analogies or metaphors that they can relate to will be the most effective way to help them grasp the concept of Role Transition.

Consider, for example, **Agi**, aged 13, who has acting experience. The therapist asked,

> Let's imagine that your director suddenly asked you to play a new part, without adequate time to prepare and learn your lines. What would that be like for you?

This may be sufficient for Agi to grasp the essence of Role Transition because she can easily imagine the impact of such a sudden change. Some prompting by the therapist about the consequences on her confidence, functioning, and feelings in such a scenario could further enhance her grasp of how the concept might relate to her symptoms.

The case of **Pippa** illustrates a relatively straightforward application of this Problem Area and unfolds in stages through the chapter, demonstrating each step of the process.

Pippa, aged 14, has a preoccupied attachment style and was referred to a Youth Mental Health Service by her mother. Pippa had been experiencing symptoms consistent with moderate level depression for three months. She lives with her mother and two younger siblings. Until recently, she had regular contact with her father at weekends and occasionally midweek. Her parents separated two years ago. The timeline revealed that six months prior to the onset of her depression, her father began living with his new partner, and the new partner's two daughters moved into that house one month prior to the depression.

Before the timeline activity, Pippa was not able to relate her symptoms to any particular life events or issues. Following the timeline, she began to see some connections and collaboratively identified Role Transition as the major Problem Area associated with her depression.

The therapist dialogue in Pippa's fourth session provides an example of how the process for addressing Role Transition might be introduced.

*Therapist:* Pip, you have told me about the changes in your family over the last two years, and we've discovered that this seems to be related to how miserable you have been feeling. I'd like to explore how these changes have affected you in more detail. I think this will put us in a good place to understand what will help you feel better and recover from your depression. Does that sound okay?

*Pippa:* Yeah.

*Therapist:* Can I check I've got things right? You've been through a number of changes. First, your parents weren't getting on, and then your dad moved out. He eventually found a new partner, and they moved in together about six months ago. Then very recently, his new partner's two daughters moved in. The timeline showed us that's when your depression increased. We discussed the four Problem Areas in IPT-A and we both felt that Role Transition best explained your depression. You probably remember Role Transition is when our lives change in ways that we wouldn't choose and we don't feel prepared for. I explained that this can leave us feeling unsure how to behave, how to

|  |  |
|---|---|
|  | meet other people's expectations, or how to get our own needs met in the new situation. This can have major negative impacts on the way people feel, and this seems to be what has happened for you.<br>You've had some time to think about this over the last couple of weeks. Do you think what I'm saying is correct? |
| Pippa: | Yeah, it made sense after you explained it. And from the timeline thing we did. |

### Step 2. Review positive and negative aspects of the old role

Once the young person has an adequate understanding of the concept of Role Transition, work on the second step of the process can begin: reviewing both positive and negative aspects of the old role and the associated affect. The young person's understanding does not need to be complete at this stage as her insight will develop as she progresses through the five steps.

As always in IPT-A, the therapist strives to make the therapy process transparent, including explaining activities and giving the young person choices so that she experiences therapy as a collaborative process.

The therapist dialogue with Pippa in session 5 provides an example of how the exploration of positive and negative aspects of the old role might be introduced.

|  |  |
|---|---|
| Therapist: | I'd like to explain what I have in mind for today and the next few sessions and check if that sounds okay to you. One way of working on Role Transition is to explore the old and new role in detail, the way things used to be and the way they are now, so we can really understand how the changes have affected you. |

(Therapist shows Pippa Clinical Tool 9.1: Role Transition.)

|  |  |
|---|---|
| Therapist: | You can see in this diagram a place to write down things that were good and not so good about the way things used to be and also about the current situation. I get the impression that you don't see much positive in the current situation with your family, and that's a big part of the problem. It feels to you the way things used to be was much better and the current situation is awful. I'd like to understand more of the details of that. This will then help us work out what your options are so that you can feel better and your depression improve. We can then do some planning to implement whichever options you choose and then we might need to spend some time developing your confidence and rehearsing ways you could talk to people about what would make things better for you. How does that sound? |
| Pippa: | I understand what you're saying, but I don't see how it can help. Mum and Dad aren't going to get back together. |

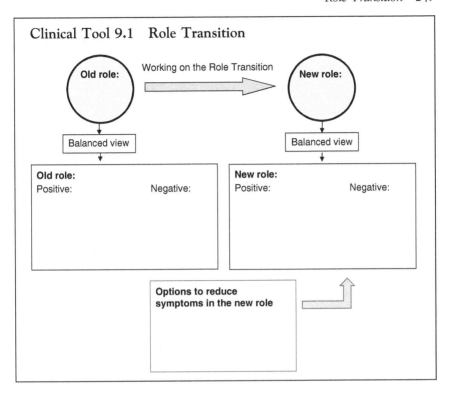

| Therapist: | We can't undo your parents separating, but if we can understand more about how it has affected you and if you can communicate that to your parents, they might be able to change some of the things you're not happy about. I know you feel sad, and probably other feelings as well, about your parents' separation. I get the impression you've bottled up a lot of your feelings and you haven't told your Mum and Dad, or even your friends, everything about how difficult you found it. Is that right? |
| --- | --- |
| Pippa: | They know I'm upset but not all of it. |
| Therapist: | When our feelings are bottled up, it can weigh us down and make us miserable. I think that is part of what is keeping your depression in place. So what I am suggesting is that we find ways for you to talk with me about how the changes have affected you. Then, if you want, we'll find ways for you to help the important people in your life understand how this has affected you and how they can best support you. What do you think about what I'm suggesting? |
| Pippa: | It sounds hard. |
| Therapist: | It certainly can be hard trying to figure it all out by yourself. My job is to help you with this. What I can tell you is that most people do start to feel better when they talk about these things. You've mentioned that you have |

|  | already noticed you have been feeling a little better, and I'd expect we will both notice that increase over the next few weeks. Are you happy for us to go in the direction I've outlined? |
|---|---|
| Pippa: | Yeah. I guess it is good to talk. |

*Exploring the old role*

In the dialogue above, the therapist has set the scene for the work that follows. The process and its rationale have been explained, and Pippa has been invited to play an active role. The dialogue that follows with Pippa, also from session 5, provides an example of how the old role can be examined and some of the associated affect explored.

| Therapist: | Why don't you draw a rough diagram on the whiteboard like on the page (Clinical Tool 9.1)? This format uses circles for the old role and new role. You could use the same or any shape and then underneath each role, a space to write a list of positive things and a list of negative things. |
|---|---|

Pippa draws a diagram on the whiteboard.

| Therapist: | Great. Let's start with the old role. That's back before Mum and Dad separated. Tell me as many things as you can think of about what was good about the old situation? |
|---|---|
| Pippa: | Things were normal. They were both there. I could talk to them. I didn't have to wait till I saw Mum or Dad. |
| Therapist: | Would you like to make notes about this on the board? |

Pippa writes

- normal
- there to talk
- no waiting

| Pippa: | Is that okay? |
|---|---|
| Therapist: | Perfect. Keep going. |
| Pippa: | I didn't have to plan ahead. I had all my stuff in the same place. |
| Therapist: | Anything else? |
| Pippa: | Before Mum and Dad started arguing, everyone was happy. |

The conversation continued in this manner with the therapist encouraging Pippa until she ran out of things to add to the list.

| Therapist: | This next question might sound a bit odd because I know you'd like things to be the way they used to be, but was there ever anything that wasn't so good in the old role back when Mum and Dad were living together? |
|---|---|

*Pippa:* (after thinking about this for a while): *They'd argue. And even when they weren't arguing, there was tension, like I knew they weren't happy. I was worrying they might split up.*
*Therapist:* *Do you want to jot this down?*

Pippa writes

- arguments
- Mum and Dad not happy
- tension
- worrying

(See Figure 9.1 Family structure Role Transition—Pippa old role.)

*Therapist:* *And is there anything else?*
*Pippa:* *I can't think of anything else.*
*Therapist:* *If anything else does come to mind, just add it in. Let's now think about the current situation, your new role, but before we do, is there anything you want to say about what you have come up with so far?*
*Pippa:* *I suppose I'd forgotten about the tension and worrying about them splitting up.*

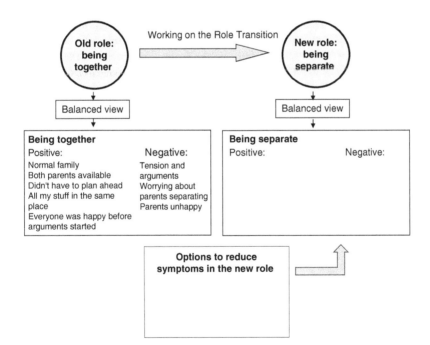

*Figure 9.1* Family structure Role Transition—Pippa old role.

*Therapist:* How much did that affect you?
*Pippa:* Quite a bit. I really stressed about it.
*Therapist:* When I asked you to rate your depression, you said it was about a two, with zero being the worst you've ever felt and ten being feeling great, no depression at all. What number would you give to how you were feeling when you were worrying about your parents splitting up?
*Pippa:* Maybe a four. But it was different to the depression. It wasn't all the time. Like I'd forget about it at school or with my friends.
*Therapist:* So when you were really worrying, you felt almost as bad as you have over the last few months, but you weren't feeling like that all the time. When you were away from home, you enjoyed yourself mostly?
*Pippa:* Yeah.
*Therapist:* What about when you were at home? How much of the time were you worrying there?
*Pippa:* Oh, it wasn't all the time. It just gradually got more and more before I knew they were definitely splitting up.
*Therapist:* What was the scariest thing for you about the possibility of them separating?
*Pippa:* Just not knowing what would happen—who I'd live with—if I'd get to see the other one.
*Therapist:* So the uncertainty, not knowing what would happen, and how it would affect your relationships with your parents was really worrying. As you know, IPT is about how changes in our lives affect our relationships and how that affects how we feel. So this is exactly what we will be talking more about. We'll come back to it but is it okay if we leave that left side of the board for the moment and think about the right side, the new role or your current situation?
*Pippa:* Sure.

The process of discussing positive and negative aspects of the role often identifies what has been lost or is missing in the new situation. Sometimes powerful feelings of sadness or anger are present. In exploring the old role, the therapist is alert to issues that may be relevant to attachment needs and how these have been affected by the Role Transition. The uncertainty Pippa described would be difficult for most young people and especially so for Pippa, given her preoccupied attachment characteristics. The therapist noted this for future exploration.

The approach outlined in the above dialogue is consistent with the technique of Motivational Interviewing, an evidence-based intervention for addressing substance use issues in adults and young people (Miller and Rollnick, 2002). Motivational Interviewing, as the name implies, works by building motivation for change. The principles can also be helpful in building Readiness for Change in relation to mental disorder (see Chapter 2).

## Step 3. Review positive and negative aspects of the new role

After exploring the positive and negative aspects of the old role, the focus turns to the new role. Usually, the young person will view the new role negatively, so it will often be more seamless if the therapist invites him to list the negative aspects of the new role before proceeding to the positive aspects. Care needs to be exercised in enquiring about positive aspects of the new role, especially if it has come about in difficult circumstances. For example, if the new role has resulted from illness, accident, or bereavement, asking about positives may feel quite jarring for the young person and lead him to wonder if the therapist has actually understood his distress.

The therapist dialogue with Pippa continues:

| | |
|---|---|
| Therapist: | I know there's a lot you don't like about this new situation—your dad living with Josie and her daughters. Let's come up with a list of the negatives. |
| Pippa: | (without pause and with feeling): I hate Josie and her kids are bitches. |
| Therapist: | What don't you like about them and can you write it down? |
| Pippa: | She thinks she can tell me what to do. She's got no right. She's not my mother. |
| Therapist: | Sounds like that really makes you angry? |
| Pippa: | She really pisses me off. |
| Therapist: | What are some of the things she tells you to do that pisses you off? |
| Pippa: | Lots of stuff. Like "Isn't it time to go to bed? You don't want to be tired for school tomorrow". |
| Therapist: | Anything else? |
| Pippa: | Even things like put a hat on, or sunscreen, or look after my sisters when I take them out. Of course I'll look after them! It's like she thinks I don't know that. And besides, she's got no right to tell me to do stuff! |
| Therapist: | Do you mean she's got no right because she's not your parent? |
| Pippa: | Yeah. And it feels creepy. She acts like she really cares, but she doesn't know me. She's only doing it to make a show in front of dad. |
| Therapist: | How do you mean creepy? |
| Pippa: | Like she is putting it on. It's not real. |
| Therapist: | Does she do anything else that pisses you off? |
| Pippa: | Plenty. She never gives me any time by myself with Dad. She's always there. Like she might be cooking, and I'll go and sit next to Dad while he's watching telly and she'll start asking him or me stuff, or coming in and fussing around. |
| Therapist: | When did you last get some time alone with your dad? |
| Pippa: | Not since she's moved in. |
| Therapist: | Wow, so that's eight months? |
| Pippa: | Well, I suppose there have been a few short times like when he drives me to netball. And I guess I do see him without her when he picks us up from mum's place, but my sisters are always there. |

254    *The Middle Phase of IPT-A*

| | |
|---|---|
| *Therapist:* | Sounds like getting some time alone with your dad is important for you. We'll come back and talk more about that and, if you want, about the ways Josie annoys you. You mentioned Josie's daughters. Could you tell me about them? |
| *Pippa:* | I guess Leah isn't too bad. Sometimes she is really annoying, but she can be okay. She's too young to understand. But Cindy should know better. She uses my make-up and stuff when I'm not there. She doesn't even ask! |
| *Therapist:* | That makes you angry as well? |
| *Pippa:* | Yeah. And she talks to Dad like he's her father or something. And how he loves her and she loves him and he loves her mum. Bitch! |

At this point the therapist decided to briefly diverge from simply continuing with listing the negatives in order to guide the exploration towards some of the underlying issues and feelings.

| | |
|---|---|
| *Therapist:* | Would I be right in thinking this gets you wondering where you and your sisters fit in this new arrangement and in your dad's affections? |
| *Pippa:* | How do you mean? |
| *Therapist:* | Well, sometimes when people we love form new relationships, we may wonder what that means for our relationship with them, for example, will they still have time for us, will the new people become more important than we are for that person? |
| *Pippa:* | I guess I have been wondering about that—if he still loves us as much? |
| *Therapist:* | Have you spoken with him about this? |
| *Pippa:* | No. |
| *Therapist:* | I suspect it is important for your parents to understand how these changes have affected you. We'll come back to focus on this, but I don't want to interrupt your flow with the list. You seem to be on a bit of a roll with more to say about what you don't like about the new situation. Is it okay to continue? |
| *Pippa:* | Yeah. There's lots I don't like. Like having to be super organised and think ahead all the time about what I'll need when I'm at his place. I forget things and sometimes can't finish assignments till I get back to mum's because I don't have all my school stuff with me. |

Pippa needed little prompting from the therapist to produce a long list of things she didn't like about the new situation. The therapist could have decided to leave the exploration of affect until after generating the list but judged that acknowledging Pippa's obvious anger would assist her in producing her list of negatives.

Initially Pippa found it difficult to identify any positives about the new situation; however, after a silence, she began to identify things that had improved. She mentioned that her parents argued less since they had separated. Pippa reflected that her parents now hardly spoke, and there was an upside in this for her, apart from less arguing. She was able to spend time with friends when her parents thought she was at the other's household and they

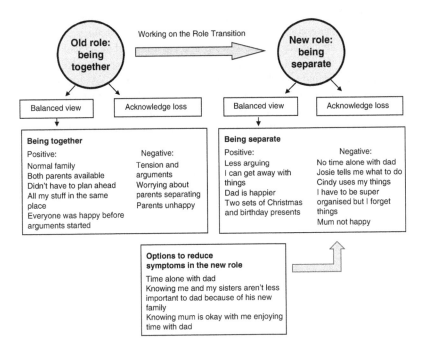

*Figure 9.2* Family structure Role Transition—Pippa.

wouldn't discover her whereabouts. Pippa recognised that her father was happier since the separation. She also thought that he felt guilty about the family splitting up and this benefited her when she wanted something from him. She added that he had been particularly generous with Christmas and birthday presents.

The more balanced view of the new role that developed during this conversation is summarised in Figure 9.2 Family structure Role Transition—Pippa. After completing these lists, Pippa reflected on the learning from this process.

Therapist: When you look at these lists, what do you make of them?

Pippa: How do you mean?

Therapist: Well, sometimes going through the process of writing down the positives and negatives of both the old and new situation and then looking at it all together can bring new thoughts.

Pippa: I suppose I hadn't really thought much about the positives of mum and dad splitting up. And that there were some negatives about when they were together.

Therapist: Does that have any implications for the way you view the changes?

Pippa: Not sure. Maybe this is like you were saying a few weeks ago, how depression can make you only see the negative stuff. Don't get me wrong, though, I would still rather they hadn't split up.

*Therapist:* Have I understood this correctly? You have been missing a lot about the way things used to be and remembering mainly good things about that. You weren't feeling anything positive about your dad living with his new family. When you look at the lists, however, you are noticing that there are things you like and don't like about both roles. As you said, the depression may be leading you to only see the negative side. These lists question that view and help us see a more balanced picture. But I do understand you wish things were the way they used to be. Have I got that right?

*Pippa:* Yeah.

*Therapist:* When you look at these lists, how do you feel about the changes?

*Pippa:* I suppose it doesn't feel quite so bad.

*Therapist:* It's something you can do yourself when you're feeling low about any situation, not just this one. Take a little time to consider if there are some positives that you're not seeing—to check if there is a negative bias going on. That's just the first part of this process. The next part I think might be particularly helpful for you. It's looking at what might help you feel better in the new situation. Is it okay if we think about that?

*Pippa:* Sure, but I don't see how things can change.

Pippa's lack of confidence about the possibility of positive change is directly addressed in the next stage of this process, Step 4: Identify role options that will reduce symptoms.

*When further exploration is needed*

When the process of identifying positive and negative aspects of both the old and new role is carried out in a detailed way, it may well provide a sufficiently thorough exploration of the Role Transition to guide the next step of identifying options that will lead to symptom reduction. However, if further information is needed, questions such as the following may assist in finding solutions.

- *How have you tried to deal with this transition?*
- *How have you coped with other changes or transitions?*
- *Think of someone you look up to or admire; it might be someone you know or have heard about, or it could be a character from online, a book, TV, or film. What might that person do in a situation like this?*
- *What do you most miss from the old role? Who might understand this best?*
- *If you had a magic wand, what would you change in the new role? Have you told anyone about this?*
- *If you were making a YouTube video about this, who would be in it? What would it look like?*
- *Tell me about how you have tried to let other people know what this transition has been like for you.*

- Who would you like to better understand this? What could you say to them to help them understand?
- How would you like them to respond? What could you say to them to help them understand what you need?
- What have you told your best friend about this?
- How did you feel about the way he or she responded?
- How could your friend best support you?
- In order for you to feel that your friend understood this, what would he or she be doing or saying?

*Addressing loss*

If Pippa had not responded well to the process described above, or if the therapist was still unsure about what the most significant aspects of the transition are for Pippa, she could be invited to use other techniques. This might include drawing or painting the old and new role, writing about them, making a You Tube video, sculpting clay models, making masks, or creating papier-mâché representations. The use of creative techniques is discussed in more detail in Chapter 7.

Techniques such as these may also be useful when further exploration of the affect associated with the Role Transition would be helpful, especially when the young person is not comfortable with verbal approaches. Role play and chair work (see Chapter 4) can also be effective ways to explore the impact of a Role Transition and the associated affect. For example, if using chair work, the old and new roles could be represented by two facing chairs. The young person might then be invited to have a conversation with herself speaking from the perspective of each role as she moves between the chairs. This could include discussing or debating the positive and negative aspects of each role, thus providing an alternative to the method outlined above for Steps 2 and 3. The focus could also be on the affect involved in the Role Transition by inviting the young person to give voice to the emotions, thoughts, and body sensations associated with each chair.

For many young people, in order to be able to effectively communicate their attachment needs to others, the therapist will need to first assist them to describe their feelings of loss and other affect associated with the Role Transition. For Pippa, discussion was sufficient to explore her feelings of anger and sadness and this took place in Steps 3 and 4.

*Step 4. Identify role options to reduce symptoms*

Having previously explored the detail of positive and negative aspects of the old and new roles, the therapist and young person will be well placed to formulate options to reduce symptoms. The most potent solutions tend to focus on addressing attachment needs that aren't being met in the new situation. It is often especially time efficient (an ongoing consideration in brief interventions) to start with issues that the young person most misses about the old role or something that most concerns her about the new role. As is frequently the case in IPT-A, the skills learnt and insights gained from addressing one or two particularly salient issues can often be generalised to other applications, avoiding the need for the same level of detailed work on the remaining difficulties in the new role. Choosing to focus on the issue(s) of most importance for the young person provides particularly effective learning. The relevance will be high and engagement is likely to be maximised. An exception to this might be if temperamentally the young person is "slow to warm up" (Chess and Thomas, 1999) or feels too daunted by tackling the biggest issues first. Building her familiarity and trust with the process by initially discussing something that is less daunting but also relevant will help her to approach more challenging applications. This is likely to be pertinent for clients with avoidant attachment style. For these young people, maximising their sense of control by offering choice and options is an important consideration to promote engagement.

In summary, the young person is invited to identify which issue she would like to focus on first. Once the focus has been determined, options to reduce symptoms are generated and explored.

Examples of therapist language for this next step of the process are included in the continuing dialogue with Pippa that occurred in session 6.

*Therapist:* Pip, you mentioned that you don't see how things can change. When transitions are forced on you, often people feel hopeless about changing things and that can feed depression. However, when there is good communication between the people involved, it's much easier to come up with arrangements that suit everyone. I don't mean your parents getting back together, but if we can help them understand more about what you need, they might be able to make some changes so that you get more of the things you're missing and less of the things you don't like.
When you look at the lists you've come up with, which one is your biggest concern? It might be something you miss about the old role, or don't like about the new role, or maybe it's something you haven't actually written down here.

*Pippa:* Josie telling me what to do.

*Therapist:* Is that what you'd most like to change?

*Pippa:* Probably the most important thing is not getting time alone with Dad.

*Therapist:* How about we start with that? Do you think he understands how important it is for you?

*Pippa:* Well, he should.

*Therapist:* Have you tried to tell him how you feel about this?

*Pippa:* Why should I? He's my father. He should know without me having to tell him!

*Therapist:* Sounds like you feel angry about this?

| | |
|---|---|
| Pippa: | *They're always there. It's like I've got to share him all the time and that's not fair. They've got him to themselves when we're not there.* |

Pippa's anger appeared to be mixed with sadness as she spoke. In session 7, the therapist invited Pippa to describe her feelings in more detail, the aim ultimately being to assist her to communicate her attachment needs in the new role to her parents.

As this discussion continued, Pippa was able to describe her feelings of loss in more detail, and this benefited the conversation that followed focusing on identifying options.

| | |
|---|---|
| Therapist: | *You know, some fathers have blind spots around feelings and relationships, especially when they're busy, and you mentioned he's working long hours. I'm not trying to make excuses for him, and I can understand that you feel angry and sad because this is really important to you. Sometimes we need to spell things out to the other person in the relationship to make clear our feelings and needs. Then, when they understand, they may be happy to do what they can to give us more of the things we need in the relationship. You're expecting or hoping your dad will figure out what you need. He may eventually do that but you could speed up his understanding by talking with him. Is there anything that's stopped you from trying to talk with him about this apart from thinking he should understand without you telling him?* |
| Pippa: | *I don't want to do it when they're around.* |
| Therapist: | *Fair enough. Anything else?* |
| Pippa: | *I'm not sure.* |
| Therapist: | *How do you think he would react if you told him how you feel about this?* |
| Pippa: | *I'm not sure now he has his new family.* |
| Therapist: | *What about before he moved out?* |
| Pippa: | *He'd probably make time for me if I really asked.* |
| Therapist: | *And now you're not sure. Can you tell me more about how the new family make you less sure?* |
| Pippa: | *(Looking and sounding sad) Maybe he is too busy with them and his job.* |
| Therapist: | *You are sounding different compared to before when you were angry. What are you feeling now?* |
| Pippa: | *Sad.* |

The therapist continued to explore Pippa's needs in the new role and her associated affect. In addition to discussing her sadness, Pippa also identified that she was scared to ask her father for time alone. She worried that sharing her needs and having them rejected would confirm her worst fears that she and her sisters were being supplanted in her father's affections by his new family. In her assessment, this would be more painful than not asking. The therapist assisted Pippa to weigh the pros and cons of discussing her needs with her father. Pippa's dilemma is common: dealing with the uncertainty of not knowing exactly how other people will respond when we ask for help and experiencing the potential pain of perceived rejection if other people do not respond in the ways we hope they will. Feelings of uncertainty can be magnified by preoccupied attachment. The therapist predicted that this might be affecting Pippa given her attachment style. A brief excerpt of dialogue is included below.

Many young people find it helpful to be reminded or taught about factors that might help predict the responses of others, such as how the person has behaved previously. Through this process, Pippa recalled that her father had usually responded well when she asked him for help and did the same for her sisters. She remembered seeing him also do this with extended family and friends. Pippa came to the view that it was more likely than not that her father would do his best to meet her needs. Although she couldn't be 100% certain about this, she decided it was worth trying to talk with him about what she needed in the new family circumstances. Next, Pippa needed to review how she might go about communicating her needs to her father and then practice options for doing this. These steps are discussed in Step 5 below.

*Therapist:* Pip, you mentioned how the uncertainty around all these changes has been one of the most difficult things for you. For example, in the old role, not knowing if or when your parents might split up and worrying about it. In the new role, you're wondering how important you are to your dad now he's living with Josie and her daughters. Am I right?

*Pippa:* Yeah.

*Therapist:* I think anyone would find that difficult. I suspect that something additional is going on for you. Back in our third session, when we were talking about how easy you find it to trust other people, we identified that sometimes you're not sure if people will be there for you when you need them. You don't feel that way all the time but when you do it can have a big effect on how you feel. Sometimes you won't dare to ask for what you need in case you feel rejected?

(Pippa nods)

Or if you do try to ask, you may be feeling anxious or angry and not get the message across as well as you want to?

(Pippa nods again)

And then the other person doesn't get it. I wouldn't be surprised if this unsureness about trust might be affecting how you communicate or don't communicate with your parents.

*Pippa:* Probably.

*Therapist:* If you are interested, next session we could look at how being aware of this aspect of yourself might help you to explain what you need to your parents.

Pippa's greatest concerns centred on her attachment needs. For other young people, the centrality of attachment may be less obvious in relation to their major concerns about the new role, at least initially. When this is the case, the therapist will need to assist the young person to relate her concerns about the Role Transition to its impact on relationships. Her concerns may focus on failing in the new role but she may be less aware of underlying fears regarding disappointing people who are important to her or feeling humiliated, embarrassed, or rejected if she cannot function well in the new role.

If time allows, it is often beneficial to explore the impact of Role Transition on more than one significant relationship. For example, in the case of Pippa, in addition to addressing her relationship with her father, the therapist was interested to understand how the Role Transition had affected her relationship with her mother and others in her Closeness Circles.

The things that most concerned Pippa about her relationship with her mother were a sense that her mother was unhappy and lonely and that because of this Pippa could not talk to her about how much she missed time alone with her father. Additionally, after Pippa began having regular time alone with her father, she felt unable to show her happiness to her mother due to a sense that she was somehow betraying her mother by enjoying her father. The therapist assisted Pippa to explore these concerns and then to identify options for communicating her needs to her mother. The therapist offered a joint session with Pippa's parents to help them understand Pippa's needs and framed this in the context of common needs and dynamics following parental separation. Pippa preferred not to invite both parents to the same session for fear of conflict occurring between them but was pleased to invite them to separate sessions.

### Step 5. Plan, rehearse, and implement changes

As with the other Problem Areas, a key aspect of operationalising the insights gained in exploring Role Transition is to assist the young person to communicate his needs to his significant others. A bridge must be built to enable the young person to move from discussing his needs in session with the therapist to an ability to communicate these needs effectively to the important people in his life.

Social skills development, confidence building, and trust in the therapeutic relationship are the components of the bridge. Some young people will need to develop new social skills in order to communicate effectively about the new role. Other young people may already have the necessary social skills but will require assistance to recognise and apply their existing competencies in the new situation. The young person's symptoms, including mental disorder, can make it difficult for him to recognise his coping abilities and positive attributes. Additionally, the novelty of the new situation, compared to his previous experience, may overwhelm his sense of competence. By definition, Role Transition is often characterised by the new role being thrust upon the young person unexpectedly. IPT-A provides him with some catch-up time to make up for some of the lack of preparedness.

Pippa has identified her primary needs in relation to her parents. She would like some time alone with her father. This is associated with a broader need for reassurance that she and her sisters are not being supplanted in his affections by his new family. In relation to her mother, Pippa wants to be able to talk about her father and say how important he is to her without being concerned that this would be disloyal or upsetting for her mother.

Beginning in session 7 and continuing in session 8, Pippa's therapy focused on planning and practising key communication with her father and then later her mother. An excerpt of the dialogue is included here.

*Therapist:* Pip, to summarise where we're up to, in our last session you mentioned that the most negative thing for you about the new role in relation to your father is that you are not getting time alone with him. I've been encouraging you to consider telling him how important this is for you, and I suggested you could have a think about it during the week, including what you might like to say to help him understand your needs, as well as when, where and how you might go about this. Did you have a chance to give it some thought?

*Pippa:* Yeah. I don't want to do it when they're around and they're always there. I thought maybe I could ask him to drive me somewhere like to a friend's place, and I could talk to him while we are driving.

*Therapist:* Great. Are there other reasons apart from getting him alone that you're thinking about the car?

*Pippa:* Before they separated, he sometimes would drive me to school, or we'd check out the surf after school. I'd tell him about things while we were driving and he would ask lots of questions, like he was really listening.

*Therapist:* Is there a chance some of his new family might be in the car, maybe tagging along for the drive, or to be dropped off somewhere else? Would you make it clear to him that you want it to be just him?

*Pippa:* Hadn't thought about that. I guess when I phone him to ask for the lift, I could say I'd like it to just be him because I want to talk.

*Therapist:* That sounds great. You're also setting up the conversation in advance by letting him know it's not just a lift you're after, you want to talk as well. How about we run over what you want to say and how you might say it? What are the main things you would say?

*Pippa:* I miss having time with him, just me and him.

*Therapist:* How often and for how long would you ideally like to have time with him alone?

*Pippa:* Maybe once a week or fortnight. If I have something I want to tell him, then sooner, but if I'm busy with assignments and netball, or don't have anything special to talk about, maybe not so frequent. It doesn't have to be for a long time. Like if I'm over at his place and they are all there, maybe we could just go out in the garden for a while or for a walk around *the block, or he could come up to see me in my room, like even for ten or fifteen minutes to check in.*

Therapist: I think you said that really well. You could say it just like that to your dad. It's clear and includes examples of what you'd like. What you're asking for seems very reasonable. You're saying even quite short chunks of time would help you feel connected to him and give you an opportunity to mention if something important is going on for you that you want him to know about. What about having longer periods of time, maybe a day or half day, with him occasionally. Is that something you'd like?

Pippa: That would be great, but he's pretty busy.

Therapist: Even though he is busy, from what you told me and from meeting him, it seems to me that he cares about you a lot. If you don't ask, you may not get what you need in relationships. As I said, your dad and other people can't magically read your mind, but if you can help them understand what you need, although there's no guarantee, it increases the likelihood that you will get at least some of what you want and sometimes you might get all of what you need. How about we practice? Let's set it up so that we can both experiment and try out different ways you could communicate with him. We could play around with this and even have some fun with it like trying out things that seem a bit left of field. This will help us find an approach that you feel comfortable with and that we think would be effective. Does that sound okay?

Pippa: Yeah. Is this what you mean when you talked about role play?

Therapist: That's certainly one way we can do it. We could start by me pretending to be your dad and you trying out different ways you could start the conversation, or if you prefer, I could be you and you could play the role of your dad?

Pippa: The second. You be me, and I'll be dad.

Therapist: So your role is to think about whether what I'm saying is clear and respond as you think your dad might. It sounds like there's two conversations you want to have with your dad. The first is setting up a meeting so that you'll be alone and then the second is telling him more about what you need. Which would you like to start with?

Pippa: The first.

The therapist used several variations of the language Pippa had just used such as "Hi, dad. Would you be able to drive me over to Sally's place sometime over the weekend? As well as needing a lift, there's something I'd like to talk with you about, just you and me". Pippa liked that this was simple and clear. It would be easy for her to remember and easy for her father to understand. She seemed to find it straightforward saying this with the therapist playing the role of her father. After a couple of practices the therapist, in the role of Pippa's father responded, "Sorry, sweetheart, I'm really busy this weekend". Out of the role, the therapist asked Pippa how she might respond to that.

*Pippa:* I guess it doesn't have to be this weekend. When could we get together to talk, just you and me?

*Therapist:* (in the role of Pippa's father): How about on Wednesday after school? I could pick you up and we could swing by the beach before I drop you home?

*Pippa:* That would be great.

*Therapist:* (Out of role): Well done. You invited him to suggest a time, which is a good strategy because you can't know everything about his schedule. You're sounding reasonably confident about this and able to think on your feet depending on how your dad responds. Is that correct?

*Pippa:* Yeah. I think I'm okay about setting up the talk, but having the talk is more difficult.

*Therapist:* So let's move on to that. Tell me more about it feeling difficult. You mentioned before about worrying that your dad might not respond as you want.

Pippa and the therapist discussed the potential difficulties and role played a range of ways she could communicate her needs to her father, including factoring in alternative ways he could respond.

Pippa's father responded in a way that exceeded her expectations. He immediately made a time the following weekend for them to meet and do whatever Pippa chose. He also apologised for not realising this was important to her. He acknowledged the difficulties for her and her sisters in the new family arrangements and asked her to let him know if there was anything else he could do to make it easier for her. He stressed that he wanted her to be able to talk with him whenever she needed to. Pippa felt reassured by these responses. Her concern that she and her sisters had been supplanted in her father's affections by his new family diminished, and this made it easier for her to discuss these concerns with him. Following this conversation, Pippa's symptoms improved significantly.

This was a powerful learning experience for Pippa, demonstrating that communicating clearly about what you need in relationships increases the likelihood of your needs being met in the ways you want. In the following session, Pippa planned and rehearsed some communication with her mother who also responded positively to her daughter's needs.

In summary, the processes employed during Step 5: Plan and rehearse changes, are the following:

- identify what needs to be communicated
- explore options and develop a plan for how it might most effectively be communicated
- practice and revise communication
- consider safety issues

The therapist initially leads a conversation about what the young person most wants to communicate to her significant others about her needs in the new role, then discusses options for how she might go about this. This is followed by identifying and rehearsing strategies for effective communication. As in the case of Pippa, the therapist's role often includes a significant coaching component to develop the young person's skills and insight while, at the same time, being alert to possible pitfalls. The therapist assists the young person to fine tune strategies to increase the clarity and effectiveness of her communication.

### Involving significant others in assessment and treatment of Role Transition

The young person's parents, carers, teachers, grandparents, siblings, friends, or others can provide valuable information when assessing the Problem Area and may also be a necessary part of the treatment, providing the young person agrees to their involvement.

These people may be a great source of help for the young person, and this capacity should be assessed so that it can be drawn upon to assist therapy.

If the support available to the young person is insufficient to meet his or her needs, the work of this Problem Area will involve enhancing existing relationships and/or augmenting them with new relationships. Sometimes the problem lies with the way support is provided. A minor tweak may be all that is required to better target this help. For example, Pippa's father thought he was being supportive, but it was only after Pippa communicated her needs clearly that he was able to provide exactly what she needed to begin to resolve her depressive symptoms. Enhanced communication and education about the concept of Role Transition and how this relates to the young person's symptoms often goes a long way to fine tune the support offered by the people who are important to the client.

## Additional issues

### Role Transition in relation to sexuality or gender identity

Adolescents may experience a range of difficulties in relation to sex, sexuality, and gender identity that can constitute Role Transition, including the following:

- early or late onset puberty
- unreciprocated or unwanted sexual or romantic interest
- commencing or ending a sexual or romantic relationship
- same-sex attraction
- gender identity issues

These changes may or may not constitute Role Transition, depending on whether the young person feels prepared for the change and, crucially,

266   *The Middle Phase of IPT-A*

whether she feels able to meet her attachment needs in the new role. Difficulties may be related to biological sexual maturity occurring before the young person has developed corresponding cognitive, emotional, or social maturity. The young person may experience confusion in relation to these issues and lack accurate information to help her understand her experience and guide her behaviour. Adolescents often turn to peers and the Internet to inform themselves, and these sources may be less than reliable. Competing messages or pressure from peers, the media, culture, or religion add additional layers of complexity. This multiplicity of complicating factors can make it difficult for young people to adjust to these changes and may lead to a range of symptoms, including mental disorder.

*Assessment*

Two general principles of assessment are especially important given the potentially sensitive nature of these issues. The therapist needs to

- show sensitivity but not avoid assessing these issues, even though they may be potentially awkward or embarrassing topics for the young person (see Chapter 2)
- clarify language and terminology to avoid misunderstandings

Some of the broad questions included in the assessment section of this chapter are designed to provide the young person with an opportunity to bring up issues of sex and sexuality if they are relevant. For example,

> *Have there been any issues or changes around who you find yourself attracted to romantically?*

Some young people will be comfortable with questions that are more direct, such as

> *Are you attracted to guys, or girls, both, or neither, or maybe you're not sure?*

An alternative question, which retains directness but states it in a way that may be less confronting, might be

> *Some girls are attracted to guys, some are attracted to other girls, some are attracted to both, and some aren't sure. Some people don't like talking about this. I'm wondering if there might be any changes or difficulties going on for you at the moment around this. Is it okay to talk about this?*

A general question such as the following may help to identify issues of gender identity:

*Has the way you think about yourself changed recently?*

However, more specific questions that directly name gender issues may be required to identify potential Role Transitions in relation to gender identity:

*Some girls don't feel right being a girl. They feel more like a boy. Same for some boys. Is there anything like that going on you?*

It may be helpful for the therapist to explore and clarify the meaning that the young person associates with different descriptors, especially language or labels that he chooses to describe himself or others. For example, some young people like terms such as gay, lesbian ,or bisexual, while others prefer descriptors that they see as being more inclusive, such as same-sex attracted or queer. The latter two refer to orientations other than heterosexual and the term queer is also often used in ways that include gender identity issues.

Young people define sex and sexuality in a range of ways. Three significant components are (1) sexual orientation, or the direction of one's attractions; (2) sexual identity, which is basically what one tells oneself about one's orientation, for example, "I'm lesbian, bisexual, or heterosexual"; and (3) sexual behaviour, which encompasses whether or not one acts on one's attractions and in what ways. Congruence between these components has been associated with mental health and wellbeing and incongruence with distress and disorder (Annor et al., 2018). An example of incongruence would be a young person who is attracted to her own gender but is strongly attached to a heterosexual identity. The ensuing repression and possible overcompensation in maintaining a heterosexual identity may have adverse effects on the young person's physical and mental health (Bremner and Hillin, 1993).

*Psychoeducation to assist Role Transition*

Young people experiencing difficulty in relation to sex, sexuality, or gender identity often require some psychoeducation including about Role Transition, as in the case of Grant below. Accurate information can help reduce a young person's confusion and promote self-acceptance.

Psychoeducation is also often essential for the young person's parents or others, both in terms of addressing their own concerns and in order for them to support their young person effectively. Information about risk and protection may galvanise parents to support the young person's adjustment to a Role Transition. For example, this might include understanding that, compared to other young people, girls experiencing early onset menarche are at elevated risk for a range of psychosocial problems including depression and substance use (e.g., Graber, 2013) or that same-sex attracted young people experience increased risk of suicide, depression, and substance use problems as do transgender young people (e.g., Corboz et al., 2008; Ross et al., 2018;). Furthermore, balancing information about risk with knowing that the majority of same-sex attracted young people move through adolescence without experiencing psychopathology (Corboz et al., 2008) and that the love, support, and acceptance of parents and others will have a powerful protective effect (e.g., Taliaferro and Muehlenkamp, 2017) may also help inform their relationship with the young person.

*Step 1. Identify Role Transition as central to the symptoms*

The case of Grant illustrates how the use of a metaphor might be introduced to explain the concept of Role Transition and to identify options for symptom reduction.

**Grant**, aged 15, was taken to his school counsellor by his sister, aged 16. Grant presented with severe symptoms of anxiety and moderate depression. His symptoms had increased significantly three weeks prior to this meeting. This occurred after Grant disclosed to his best friend that he thought he was gay. The friend told another student, who, in turn, passed the information on to other students. Within a few days, Grant was ostracised by the boys at his school and was subjected to harassment, including violence.

Grant's parents had separated five years ago. Grant and his sister lived with their mother and had occasional weekend stays with their father. Grant had been reluctant to disclose the harassment and his sexual orientation to his mother, in part because he felt protective towards her due to her previous history of mental disorder. Following persistent questioning about his recent cuts and bruises, he eventually disclosed what had been happening and why. His mother became tearful and attempted to reassure him by saying that he was still her son and she loved him. Despite his mother's reassurance, Grant was convinced that she was disappointed in him. Additionally, Grant worried that his father would reject him if he knew he was gay. This was based on numerous negative comments his father had made about gay people.

At the first meeting with the therapist, Grant discussed his recent experiences at school and concerns about his parents. He disclosed that he believed that homosexuality was incompatible with his religion. Grant stated that he wished he wasn't gay but suspected it wasn't possible to make himself "straight". Grant's holistic assessment summary is included in Figure 9.3.

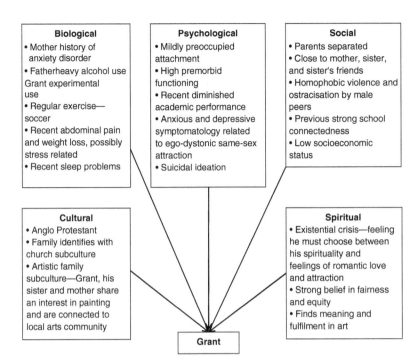

*Figure 9.3* Grant—holistic assessment summary.

During the Initial Phase of IPT-A, the therapist and Grant collaboratively identified Role Transition as the Problem Area associated with his symptoms. The timeline activity revealed that in addition to a clear escalation in his symptoms over the last three weeks, Grant was well aware that his symptoms had been building over the previous year as he had struggled with his growing awareness of his sexual orientation. The therapist assisted Grant to understand this adjustment to his sexual orientation as Role Transition and briefly explained the five-step model outlined above. Some dialogue from Grant's fifth IPT-A session is included below.

*Therapist:* *If your coach asked you to stop playing goalkeeper and play forward, how would you feel about that?*
*Grant:* *I wouldn't want to. I like being goalkeeper.*
*Therapist:* *What do you like about it?*
*Grant:* *I'm kind of good at it.*
*Therapist:* *Your sister said you're brilliant.*

Grant smiles.

*Therapist:* *I can understand that it's enjoyable doing something you're so good at. Is there anything else you like about being goalkeeper?*

| | |
|---|---|
| Grant: | I like being at the back and being able to see everything that's happening on the field. And I can hear my sister and her friends behind me talking to me and joking and Mum or Dad cheering me. |
| Therapist: | Is there anything you don't like about being goalkeeper? |
| Grant: | I don't like if I miss the ball or if I cop it in the face. |
| Therapist: | So there are some things you don't like but mainly you really like it? |
| Grant: | Yep. |
| Therapist: | What would it be like playing forward? |
| Grant: | I wouldn't want to. |
| Therapist: | Why not? |
| Grant: | I might not be very good; I might really screw up. |
| Therapist: | What would that be like? |
| Grant: | Embarrassing. People might give me a hard time. |
| Therapist: | Anything else? |

Grant shakes his head.

| | |
|---|---|
| Therapist: | Is there anything that might be good about playing forward? |

Grant shrugs.

| | |
|---|---|
| Therapist: | (after a pause) Well, tell me what would being a forward involve? What would you actually do? |
| Grant: | Run around a lot passing the ball, tackling and trying to score. |
| Therapist: | Would you enjoy any of that? |
| Grant: | It would be a lot different to being in goal. I guess it might be interesting. Like, even though I like being goalkeeper, sometimes I get bored, or I feel a bit left out, especially when we're playing a team which isn't so good and all the action is up the other end of the field. |
| Therapist: | How would it be if, rather than the coach suddenly telling you to stop being goalkeeper and be a forward, the deal was that you could just try it out during practice sessions? Maybe you could have some special coaching or training so you'd feel more confident; maybe have a chance to talk with some other people who have had a lot of experience as forwards and ask them questions about how they do it? |
| Grant: | That wouldn't be so bad. |
| Therapist: | Grant, it's quite common that when people are faced with taking on a new role, like if your coach asked you to stop being goalkeeper and play forward, they don't want to make the change for the reasons you mentioned. But some changes don't have to be an all-or-nothing, like a complete, sudden change. It could be trying out, or experimenting with a new role in safe situations, or maybe practicing and developing skills for a new role. What do you think about what I'm saying? |
| Grant: | It makes sense. But I'm not sure what it means about me being gay. |

In the above dialogue the therapist has discussed Role Transition using a metaphor drawn directly from Grant's life that is engaging and nonthreatening for him. Some key aspects have been introduced that may assist him to adjust to a possible transition that he finds much more threatening, i.e., in relation to sexual orientation. These aspects include timing, preparation, and choice. These issues are further articulated in the dialogue that follows. The process of exploring the positive and negative aspects of the old and new role is also elaborated to help Grant realise that he has some options that will reduce his distress.

*Therapist:* It is a bit of a leap from what we're talking about with soccer to how you feel about being gay. You were telling me that the change to playing forward would feel very different depending how it happened. For example, if you had some time to practice off field, you might then feel more confident. If the decision about whether to make the change was yours rather than the coach's, you would feel more in control. You might even enjoy the change. Would you agree?

*Grant:* Yeah.

*Therapist:* You've probably realised where I'm heading with this. I was wondering if what happened to you around being gay is similar to what it would be like if the coach suddenly wanted you to play forward. You told Peter, and then suddenly it was all around the school, and you were getting a really hard time from some of the guys and you didn't know what to do. This came on top of you already worrying about what people would think of you if they knew, including your parents' reaction and your church's attitude. You were thrown in the deep end before you'd worked out how to handle all this. Not surprisingly you see being gay as completely negative. You want to be back in the role of being straight or "normal" as you say. Is that right?

*Grant:* Yeah. But there's no cure.

*Therapist:* No, there isn't. Being gay's not an illness. But I'm thinking, if we consider this as a potential Role Transition for you, just like changing positions in soccer, it might not seem quite so bleak. I'd like to talk with you some more about the positives and negatives you see in both trying to be straight and in this potential new role of being gay. It will put us in a great place to think about things that might help maximise positives and minimise negatives. It would include finding ways for you to be less worried about the things you are fearing at the moment, such as how to fit in. Would you like to give this a go?

*Grant:* Yeah, I'm interested but can I ask you something? You're saying if I choose to play the role of being gay. But everyone knows now.

*Therapist:* Everyone?

*Grant:* Everyone at school.

*Therapist:* Tell me if I'm wrong but from what you said, you feel you've been, in your sister's language, "outed", before you are ready and you see no going back in terms of people knowing. But maybe you do have some options. I'm not exactly sure how this might work for you but what if you were to say "Ha ha, fooled you all. Sucked in!" and not confirm whether you are gay or not?

> I'm thinking, who says that at 15 you have to decide if you're gay or straight? And who says you have to go public about it? What if you were to leave the decision for another year, what would that be like? Or what if you were to leave it until you finish school? Another option would be to keep private whatever you do decide or just share it with a few safe people?
>
> Grant: I hadn't thought about it like that.
>
> Therapist: What I'm saying here is that I think you may have more options than you've realised. I think anyone who's been through what you have would find it difficult to see options. This has all happened before you are ready and while you're still trying to think it through.

(Grant nods)

> You've felt completely stuck with the situation and this goes a long way to explaining your depression. As we saw with the timeline, you were already feeling stressed and worrying a lot of the time before this happened, and your symptoms have increased dramatically over the last three weeks. Yours is a very common response when people feel trapped in situations they don't want. But, on the positive side, if we can find some options to improve things, then your depression and anxiety will improve. I wouldn't be surprised if you start to feel a lot better once you have figured out what to do.

In the dialogue above, the therapist has helped Grant to understand the concept of Role Transition, its connection to his symptoms, and how it might provide a way forward for him. The next steps have been explained briefly to Grant and are elaborated below: exploring the positive and negative aspects of the old and new role and then using them to identify options to reduce symptoms. Helping the young person recognise that he has options can be highly therapeutic, especially if he feels trapped in a no-win situation. In order to further sow seeds of hope, the therapist mentioned working with a number of same-sex attracted young people using this approach; that they benefited significantly; and that, even if this wasn't the case for Grant, there were other approaches that they could explore until they found something that would make a real difference for him.

*Cautions in identifying same-sex attraction as a Role Transition*

Conceptualising same-sex attraction as a possible Role Transition may not be as clearly relevant for all young people as it was for Grant. There are potential positives and negatives in referring to same-sex attraction as a choice. This way of framing the new role may help avoid the young person feeling that the therapist is pushing them towards the new role rather than inviting them to consider it as an option. At the same time, the therapist should also be aware that the young person may be hyper-alert to judgmental attitudes. He may not view his sexual orientation as a choice and, if so, may experience such conceptualisations or assumptions as dismissive and an indication that the therapist has not understood his experience.

*Step 2 and 3: Develop a more balanced view of the old and new roles*

The process outlined below assisted Grant to develop a more balanced view of his old and new role. It took place in session 5 and 6 and is summarised in Figure 9.4 Same-sex attraction Role Transition—Grant. Grant readily produced a list of positive aspects of the old role and of being heterosexual—or, more precisely, of being someone people assumed to be heterosexual. This included being seen as "normal", which for him meant fitting in and being like everyone else; not experiencing violence and harassment; having the ideal future he imagined for himself and which he was sure his parents wanted for him, i.e., getting married and having children; and being included by the boys at school in regular social interactions.

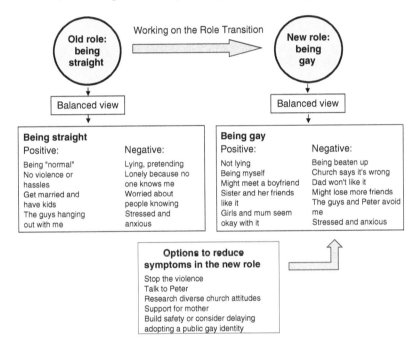

*Figure 9.4* Same-sex attraction Role Transition—Grant

It took Grant longer to identify negative aspects of this role, but he eventually listed several significant concerns. They included lying and pretending to everyone, which left him feeling dishonest and lonely even when he was with people who loved him because no one knew who he really was; worrying about people finding out he was gay; and feeling stressed and anxious most of the time. Grant was also able to recognise that the nausea and stomach pains he had been experiencing may be related to this stress.

The therapist then explored the negative side of the potential new role of being gay. Grant quickly listed a number of concerns. These included physical violence; feeling that being gay was incompatible with his church, which viewed homosexuality as sinful and leading, according to his minister, to "eternal damnation"; worrying that his father would reject him; continued ostracism by the boys at the school; and continuing to feel stressed and anxious.

Grant initially struggled to think of anything positive about being gay. After some time he mentioned that he might feel better about himself if he was being honest with people who were important to him. Grant also recalled that his sister, her friends, and the girls at school not only didn't mind him being gay, but some of them seemed to think that it was "cool". Additionally, he mentioned that his mother was keen to reassure him that she loved him regardless of his sexuality.

When invited to contemplate these lists, Grant agreed that the roles were not as starkly binary as he had previously viewed them.

*Step 4. Identifying options that will lead to symptom reduction*

As part of the process of identifying options to reduce symptoms, ways were explored to support the new role by reducing its negative and increasing its positive aspects.

In sessions 6 and 7, the therapist addressed each of Grant's major concerns, commencing by repeating a clear statement that Grant had a right to feel safe.

Therapist: *The violence and harassment you have experienced is outrageous, and it must stop. Schools have a responsibility to ensure the safety of all students and staff. I know you haven't wanted to tell the teachers because you're worried that it may make things worse. There are things the school could do to make things safer for you, and everyone else, in a way that no one has to know it's about you.*

Grant agreed to the therapist addressing safety issues with the school. He preferred this option to his mother being asked to intervene as he was concerned that this would be additional stress for her. The school took the matter seriously and strengthened its whole-of-school approach to bullying and harassment. This included education for students and staff, as well as ensuring safe spaces were available to students, such as the library or gym, and providing additional staff supervision across the school premises during breaks and when students were arriving and leaving.

In relation to Grant's concerns about his religion, the therapist provided brief information about there being elements of acceptance and judgment in all major religions regarding homosexuality and other issues. The therapist offered to help point Grant and his mother in directions where they could explore this further. This was something of a revelation for Grant. He and his mother met with a progressive minister from another church in the same faith tradition. This helped Grant realise that he didn't have to choose between his spirituality and his feelings of love and attraction.

Simply understanding that he had some options in relation to these issues had a powerful impact on Grant. He began to see a way forward, and he reported improvement in his symptoms at session 7. This was further enhanced when the therapist assisted him to identify options in relation to his father. The therapist offered to be involved in the discussions with his father and provided education about common patterns of parental adjustment to learning that their child is same-sex attracted, including initial feelings of shock, grief, denial, anger, rejection, or acceptance. This was framed as an adjustment process that many parents move through to arrive at a point of acceptance.

The therapist continued in this manner, addressing each of Grant's concerns, including pointing out that many gay couples marry and some have children.

*Step 5. Plan, rehearse, and implement changes.*

During sessions 7 and 8, plans were made to implement changes and communication strategies were rehearsed.

Regarding his best friend, Grant assumed that Peter was avoiding him because he no longer wanted to be friends. After some discussion, Grant agreed that there may be other explanations for Peter and some of the other boys at the school avoiding him. His sister had already suggested that it was because they were scared people would think they were gay by association. After considering a number of options, Grant decided to ask his sister to act as an intermediary and sound out a meeting with Peter. When they met, Peter apologised and confirmed that he still wanted to be friends. After this success, Grant elected to use therapy time for considering options to restore other friendships.

Grant became more optimistic about the possibility that being gay might be compatible with his attachment needs. His symptoms continued to decrease as he took action that addressed his concerns about the new role. Grant's mother, sister, and friend assisted him with some of the steps, and each action involved Grant rehearsing communication skills with the therapist.

As Grant felt more accepting of his sexual orientation, he became interested in learning about other same-sex attracted young people, including how they deal with challenges such as coming out and coping with parent and school concerns. He began attending a peer support group for same sex-attracted young people during the final week of the Middle Phase of therapy. Initially he was nervous about going to the group, but this was resolved as he quickly made friends at the group and the conversations with other young people helped him understand his recent negative experiences in the context of homophobia. His internal narrative transformed from one of being a helpless victim to feeling more empowered and socially connected. He became interested in social activism over the ensuring months, and this provided ongoing opportunities for positive social support. On learning of the existence of Parents and Friends of Lesbians and Gays (PFLAG), a support group for parents and friends of lesbians and gay men, Grant suggested his mother attend and she derived considerable benefit from the group, further enhancing her ability to support Grant.

It is important to note that young people whose same-sex attraction is egodystonic, i.e., they do not want to be gay, lesbian, or bisexual, may not want to attend a peer support group because it is not congruent with their current identity. Despite knowing that Grant would not yet want to attend such a group, the therapist brought its existence to his attention several weeks earlier. The therapist felt it would be helpful for Grant to know some same-sex attracted young people are not only comfortable with their sexuality but they are also seeking out and enjoying a social world of mutual support.

As well as reducing his symptoms, this process developed Grant's competence and capacity to deal with these and future challenges. The Consolidation Phase reinforced these gains and assisted Grant to generalise his learning.

## Integrating structural approaches to effectively address oppression within an IPT-A intervention

The case of Grant, described above, illustrates an example of an intervention that combines typical IPT-A techniques, such as social skills development, with the systemic understanding and actions necessary to effectively address oppression and abuse. Grant's symptoms were related to his experience of homophobia. Key aspects of Grant's Role Transition that stemmed from this perspective are summarised below. The approach outlined can be readily adapted to address the impact of other forms of oppression on the young person's symptoms, such as sexism, racism, negative attitudes towards disability, etc. The therapist's role included the following:

- Clearly identifying and naming oppression
- Unequivocally stating that the mistreatment was unacceptable, that the abuse was not Grant's fault, and that he had a right to safety and respect
- Advocating for the responsible agency to implement strategies to stop the abuse
- Contextualising action to stop abuse of an individual student within a broader framework for making schools safe for all students and staff
- Assisting Grant to recognise the associated affect and other impacts of the abuse: many young people, including Grant, find the concept of internalised oppression helpful in this regard (Bremner and Hillin, 1993)
- Identifying self-help strategies, including accurate information about same-sex attraction, in order to counter misinformation. This can be targeted for the young person, parents, or other significant people
- Facilitating accessing social support from other young people and families with similar experiences, which can foster the development of coping strategies and empowering internal narratives

Grant's school addressed the bullying he was experiencing and this was a crucial aspect of his Role Transition and symptom reduction. Some schools may not respond as appropriately to oppression or abuse. If a school or other agency is not amenable to taking appropriate action, the therapist may need to exercise some advocacy, either directly with the agency concerned or by supporting the young person and their significant others in this role. Raising concerns about duty of care and legal liability may be sufficient to challenge resistance or inertia and motivate change. Where necessary, these concerns can be backed up by quoting research about harassment and abuse being risk factors for a range of adverse outcomes including mental disorder, suicide, and poor academic achievement (e.g., Taliaferro and Muehlenkamp, 2017; Ullman, 2015).

## Summary

The concept of Role Transition may be more difficult for some young people and significant others to understand compared to the other Problem Areas, but this is balanced by its wide range of potential applications. Role Transition can be used in innovative ways to creatively guide young people to actions that effectively reduce their symptoms.

In common with the other Problem Areas, a key aim is to enhance the young person's ability to communicate his or her needs for closeness and support within existing relationships and also potentially in future relationships. The work of internalising the gains and generalising the benefits is pursued in some detail during the Consolidation Phase of IPT-A.

## References

Annor, F., Clayton, H., Gilbert, L., Ivey-Stephenson, A., Irving, S., David-Ferdon, C., & Kann, L. (2018). Sexual orientation discordance and nonfatal suicidal behaviors in U.S. high school students. *American Journal of Preventative Medicine, 54*(4), 530–538.

Aliri, J., Muela, A., Gorostiaga, A., Balluerka, N., Aritzeta, A., & Soroa, G. (2018). Stressful Life Events and Depressive Symptomatology Among Basque Adolescents: The Mediating Role of Attachment Representations. *Psychological Reports, 122,* 789–808, 10.1177/0033294118771970.

Bremner, J., & Hillin, A. (1993). *Sexuality, young people and care: Creating positive contexts for training, policy and development.* Lyme Regis, UK: Russel House.

Chess, S., & Thomas, A. (1999). *Goodness of fit: Clinical applications from infancy through adult life.* Ann Arbor, MI: Edwards Brothers.

Corboz, J., Dowsett, G., Mitchell, A., Couch, M., Agius, P., & Pitts, M. (2008). *Feeling queer and blue: A review of the literature on depression and related issues among gay, lesbian, bisexual and other homosexually active people.* Melbourne: La Trobe University, Australian Research Centre in Sex, Health and Society.

Graber, J. A. (2013). Pubertal timing and the development of psychopathology in adolescence and beyond. *Hormones and Behaviour, 64,* 262–269.

Low, N., Dugas, E., O'Loughlin, E., Rodriguez, D., Contreras, G., Chaiton, M., & O'Loughlin, J. (2012). Common stressful life events and difficulties are associated with mental health symptoms and substance use in young adolescents, *BMC Psychiatry, 12,* 122–138.

Miller, W. R., & Rollnick, S. (2002). *Motivational interviewing: Preparing people for change* (2nd ed.). New York: The Guilford Press.

Ross, L., Salway, T., Tarasoff, L., MacKay, J., Hawkins, B., & Fehr, C. (2018). Prevalence of depression and anxiety among bisexual people compared to gay, lesbian, and heterosexual individuals: A systematic review and meta-analysis. *Journal of Sex Research, 55*(4–5), 435–456.

Taliaferro, L., & Muehlenkamp, J. (2017). Nonsuicidal self-injury and suicidality among sexual minority youth: Risk factors and protective connectedness factors. *Academic Pediatrics, 17*(7), 715–722.

Ullman, J. (2015). *Free2Be?: Exploring the schooling experiences of Australia's sexuality and gender diverse secondary school students.* Penrith, N.S.W.: University of Western Sydney.

# 10 Interpersonal Gaps

**Contents**

| | |
|---|---|
| Introduction | 278 |
| Assessing the Problem Area | 281 |
|   1  *Confirm the Problem Area* | 282 |
|   2  *Identify the specific gaps in social skills* | 284 |
| Working on the Problem Area in the Middle Phase | 285 |
|   3  *Recognise the connection between Interpersonal Gaps and distress* | 287 |
|   4  *Develop social skills to fill or compensate for the current gaps* | 287 |
|   5  *Enhance social support by maintaining, expanding, and/or deepening social networks* | 303 |
| Working with significant others | 308 |
| Summary | 311 |
| References | 311 |

## Introduction

The term Interpersonal Gaps refers to gaps in social skills and behaviours that adversely affect the young person's ability to initiate and maintain relationships. This Problem Area has been elsewhere labelled Interpersonal Deficits (Mufson et al., 1993; Mufson et al., 2004). This term is accurate as it refers to deficits in the young person's abilities to initiate and maintain relationships. However, as IPT-A is a transparent intervention and the Problem Areas are collaboratively chosen, the term "deficits" may further negatively impact on an already sensitive sense of self. The term "Gaps" conveys the same meaning but is less pejorative.

The effect of these missing social competencies can be profound. They have been demonstrated to be associated with poor mental health (e.g., D'Zurilla et al., 1998; Lasgaard et al., 2011; Segrin, 2000). Interpersonal Gaps may prevent the young person from effectively communicating his needs for closeness and support. If the young person lacks the ability to create and sustain effective relationships, he will miss crucial age-appropriate interpersonal experiences as well as the accompanying social and emotional learning and insight. Some of these young people crave the connection that they see their peers enjoying in their relationships. They may experience increasing loneliness and isolation as they move through adolescence. Interpersonal Gaps is identified as the Problem Area when the young person's distress or disorder is linked to his inability to initiate or maintain relationships.

From early adolescence onwards, social interactions become increasingly sophisticated and nuanced. Young people who lack these competencies tend to be conspicuous and may be shunned. They often have a sense of missing out as they see their peers connecting in new ways. They may realise that they don't fully understand social interactions, that they are missing subtle layers of communication, being bypassed, left behind, or sometimes actively excluded. Often they won't know exactly what they're doing wrong but will be aware that they are somehow lacking and perhaps feel unattractive or unworthy as a result, thus impacting on their sense of self.

Interpersonal Gaps can be global or specific. Some young people's limited social competencies permeate and adversely affect their ability to communicate and relate across most contexts, topics, and relationships. Other young people may only be held back in specific areas. They may generally function well in social situations but lack skills or confidence with particular aspects of communication. For example, some young men may be comfortable relating to other males but may lack confidence relating to females. Although these specific gaps are limited, they can nonetheless have significant negative impacts. They may relate to the expression of emotion, level of interest or involvement in the lives of others, expression of sexual or romantic interest, or ability to understand the needs and responses of others. Other factors that may be related to gaps in social learning include inappropriate use of humour, choice of clothing, sensitivity to criticism, and feeling overwhelmed when with others. The impediments related to these gaps may be caused by under-expression, over-expression, or inappropriate expression. For example, a young person who under-expresses her emotions may be perceived by others as cold, aloof, robotic, or uninteresting. An overexpression of emotion may be experienced by others as overwhelming, exhausting, or inauthentic. It could also be dismissed as the young person exaggerating or being a "drama queen". The young person who readily experiences anger, irritation, or aggression may express these in ways that others find threatening or off-putting. Over-sensitivity to criticism may lead the young person to withdraw or react in other ways that undermine her relationships. On the other hand, a lack of social sensitivity can lead the young person to misunderstand those she relates to and for other people to find her, at best, socially inept and, at worst, selfish, dismissive or rude.

Appropriateness of communication is a relative concept and will vary with context, including social and cultural norms. It includes notions of timing, pace, and depth of disclosure. The young person who discloses detailed personal information immediately on meeting a new person may drive some people away. Conversely, the young person who never discloses personal information is likely to experience only shallow interactions with others. He or she may be lonely and longing for deeper connection among a sea of superficial communication.

There is a range of reasons why young people develop distress or disorder driven by Interpersonal Gaps. It may be that the young person is highly intelligent in other areas of life but his social intelligence is not highly developed. Gaps in social learning may be intrinsic to the young person, for example, related to his attachment style, temperament, or personality. Gaps can also be related to external factors such as no one teaching the young person how to communicate effectively rather than intrinsic factors holding them back. Fortunately for these young people, as they get older, their social circles tend to widen and they encounter a broader range of social interactions. In time they may encounter more appropriate modelling, and this will be all that is required for some of them to catch up in their social skill development. Unfortunately, however, this catch-up may occur several years in the future and won't help them to deal with their present depression or other difficulties related to their Interpersonal Gaps. Gaps that have originated in both intrinsic and external ways may also be longstanding and persist unless the young person receives an effective intervention.

Gaps in interpersonal skills can also arise in a reactive way resulting from experiences such as depression and other disorders. Mental disorder and some physical health conditions often adversely affect social functioning, and a developmental interplay occurs between these factors. The social impairment may prevent new social learning due to isolation and lack of social support. This can in turn not only create and reinforce Interpersonal Gaps but also increase vulnerability to stress and future episodes of depression, which often creates further isolation. The good news is that, especially in adolescence, these reactive gaps will often be relatively recent and amenable to change, especially as the young person's depression lifts. There is an additional early intervention bonus in addressing gaps in young people. The sooner the gaps are identified and managed, the less damage will be done to young people's life trajectories, the quicker they will achieve healthy functioning, and the more resilient they will be to future challenges.

Interpersonal Gaps tend to be self-maintaining because they limit social interaction and prevent the learning that can be gained from these experiences. The negative impact of Interpersonal Gaps on normal adolescent development is also mediated by attachment. A common thread running through Interpersonal Gaps, regardless of their specific nature, is that not only do they impair the young person's ability to communicate but also often lead to an adverse response in others. This creates a double and rebounding disadvantage. The young person struggles to communicate his attachment needs to others and simultaneously may create a negative reaction in other people, which further undermines the young person's ability to meet his needs for closeness and support.

The primary aim when working with this Problem Area is to identify the gaps in the young person's social skills and substitute more adaptive communication behaviours so that she can experience more satisfying relationships, including enhancing her capacity to effectively elicit support and communicate her needs. As with all the Problem Areas, because IPT-A is time limited, only a certain amount of progress can be achieved. If the young person's Interpersonal Gaps are many, varied, and longstanding, progress may be slow. The adage of straws on the camel's back is particularly pertinent. The camel can get back on its feet by lightening its load a little. It may not be necessary to remove the whole load. Similarly, teaching only a few social skills can make a significant difference to the young person. As she starts achieving more success in social interactions, her confidence can gradually increase, which in turn tends to generate further success. As the momentum of the young person's life trajectory changes in the directions she longs for, she has new reasons to be hopeful and her depression or other disorders will tend to improve.

The steps for working on Interpersonal Gaps are the following:

1. Confirm the Problem Area
2. Identify the specific gaps in social skills
3. Recognise the connection between Interpersonal Gaps and distress
4. Develop social skills to fill or compensate for the current gaps
5. Enhance social support by maintaining, expanding and/or deepening social networks.

In discussing the steps, this chapter sets out key issues to be considered when identifying and assessing Interpersonal Gaps and then describes a number of approaches to address the gaps that have been identified. Brief case examples are included to illustrate a range of approaches and techniques. Additionally, the case of Crystal, introduced in Chapter 5, also demonstrates this Problem Area. Crystal was able to begin relationships but had difficulty maintaining connections due to a lack of insight about her own behaviour and how it impacted others.

## Assessing the Problem Area

The two primary tasks in assessing Interpersonal Gaps are first to confirm that this is the major Problem Area and second to precisely identify the nature of the gaps, including whether they are specific or global. It isn't necessary to identify the causes of the gaps, although sometimes this will become apparent. Because IPT-A is a time-limited intervention, the focus needs to be on understanding how the gaps are affecting the young person and then addressing these gaps by teaching new skills or adapting existing competencies.

## 1 Confirm the Problem Area

The Problem Area is identified during the Initial Phase of treatment. It is not sufficient to identify only the presence of gaps in the young person's social skills, or even that these gaps are causing difficulties. In order to confirm Interpersonal Gaps as the major Problem Area, it must be established that a gap in social skills is the primary contributor to distress, depression, or other disorder. It is essential that the young person understands this connection so that he or she can appreciate the rationale for the work that will follow during the Middle Phase. This insight will promote key ingredients for a successful recovery, i.e., engagement and hope. As with the other Problem Areas, the timeline (see Chapter 5) or similar techniques are key in determining an escalation in difficulties related to Interpersonal Gaps in the lead up to the onset of depression. This may suggest a causal relationship or close connection.

Psychoeducation is often an essential aspect of developing the young person's understanding and creating a positive framework to help him or her accept this conceptualisation. The latter is important because the young person will often feel shame and embarrassment at her lack of social success. Interpersonal Gaps may be associated with humiliation, including being ostracised, teased, or bullied. These feelings can add to the young person's distress and can be an impediment to effective therapy if they make the young person reluctant to own and explore her gaps. Helpful strategies include assisting the young person to recognise the affect associated with Interpersonal Gaps and providing information to reframe the gaps in a non-self-blaming way. Psychoeducation may include information that

- assists the young person to recognise his or her strengths as well as areas needing development
- points out that other people have things they need to work on
- normalises the need to develop social skills as an essential part of adolescence and movement towards adulthood
- encourages a non-judgmental, matter-of-fact approach that doesn't take setbacks too personally
- provides reassurance that success comes from trying things out and learning from failures
- suggests that conversation is an art and the skills can be developed
- listening and taking turns are necessary and this doesn't come naturally for some people, especially when the urge to dominate is strong
- gives encouragement that social skills can be learned and practised within session and through activities outside therapy
- reflects that experiences of ostracism or rejection may not always or solely be related to the young person's Interpersonal Gaps; they may also stem from other people's insecurities about fitting in and being accepted
- suggests feeling unsure or nervous in social situations is common and can even be interesting and attractive to others
- validates diversity and difference

Many of these messages will also be helpful for young people experiencing shame or embarrassment in relation to their inability to function well in relation to the other Problem Areas, particularly Role Transition.

Not all young people will need all of these messages. If the young person has few social competencies, the messages may need to be delivered carefully, in separated ways, perhaps one at a time and with frequent repetition.

The formula is Progress = small steps + multiple presentation + constant revision.

If the gaps seem to be chronic, then education can be framed in a way to take account of the likely slower rate of progress, whereas when gaps are recent and reactive, and therefore likely to be relatively more amenable to change, expectations about the rate of progress may be raised.

When Interpersonal Gaps coexist with other Problem Areas, it may be possible to work on more than one Problem Area. Work on Complex Grief, Interpersonal Disputes, and Role Transition usually involves developing and practising social skills so that the young person is more able to effectively communicate his or her needs to others. There will be many ways to teach social skills that address the young person's Interpersonal Gaps in terms that apply them directly to coexisting Problem Areas. For a young person experiencing Complex Grief, this might involve learning ways to communicate the experience of the loss and his or her need for support. Similarly, young people experiencing Interpersonal Disputes usually need to develop conflict management skills, including communicating their needs and eliciting the needs of other parties in the dispute. The difference when Interpersonal Gaps coincide with other Problem Areas is that some of the social skill development required is likely to be quite basic and the pace will probably need to be slower than when these Problem Areas occur without Interpersonal Gaps being present.

Information about the nature of the young person's Interpersonal Gaps is often readily available to the therapist as these gaps may be apparent in the therapy room. For example, inappropriate humour or disconcerting eye contact are clues. This won't always be the case as some gaps may be specific to situation and context—for example, difficulty starting a conversation with a peer, talking with someone of the opposite gender, talking with someone of the same gender, classroom behaviour, etc. In these situations, information may be gained from discussion with the young person. Exploring recent concrete examples in the form of Interpersonal Incidents and communication analysis often yields key information about Interpersonal Gaps. Discussion with informants who have directly observed the young person's communication difficulties is likely to be particularly helpful. This may include parents and other family members, teachers, coaches, or peers. As always, the young person's consent must be obtained before consulting other parties. Where possible, the young person can be present and directly involved in these consultations.

The process of confirming that Interpersonal Gaps is the major Problem Area, along with psychoeducation, helps to set the scene for the work that will follow.

## 2 Identify the specific gaps in social skills

The exact nature of the gaps must be determined in order to effectively focus the social skill development required to help bridge these gaps. This second step draws on the young person's expertise in her own life experiences and involves her in collaboratively identifying the specific gaps in her social skills.

A social skills inventory (discussed below) provides a comprehensive map of the young person's communication competencies. This includes identifying areas of strength, weakness, and good-enough functioning. The areas of weakness become the focus of therapy. Strengths and areas of good-enough functioning aren't ignored, as they may be adapted to help bridge gaps or to give the young person clues about other ways to address the gaps.

The sheer number and wide range of social skills required for effective communication can be daunting. Even relatively simple social skills are made up of numerous micro skills including oral and nonverbal components. A social skills inventory will explore those verbal and non-verbal aspects of communication.

Oral communication, for example, requires choices, both conscious and unconscious, about a wide range of factors, including voice modulation, clarity, pitch, volume, and speed. Nonverbal communication, such as body language and visual cues, is often key to interpreting oral communication. Nonverbal components can reinforce verbal communication and may carry meaning of their own.

Often what *isn't* said is as important as what is actually stated. Sometimes, it is more important. Similarly, the way things are said can completely change the meaning of the statement. Nuances are subtle and can be easily missed if the young person is not familiar with and alert to these complexities of communication.

Body language includes posture, movements, and gestures such as a shrug or pointed finger. Facial expressions, such as raised eyebrows, a smile, or a frown, can communicate specific feelings. Indications of approach or withdrawal, such as eye contact, proximity, and touch, convey additional layers of meaning or intent.

Even small gaps in the young person's grasp of just one facet of communication can have major negative impacts on his ability to relate to others. The gaps may be either in relation to the young person's ability to recognise and interpret these components of communication in others, to utilise them appropriately in his own communication, or both. Eye contact is a good example of the power of a single aspect that can make or break communication. Used appropriately it can be inviting and a way of showing interest in others. Too much eye contact can be uncomfortable and may be intimidating. Conversely, people who avoid eye contact can give a negative impression, perhaps of lying, being nervous, or wishing the other person would go away. However, in some cultures, for example, Australian Aboriginal culture, avoiding eye contact may be a sign of respect. Too much or too little eye contact can sabotage an otherwise adequate, or even excellent, set of social skills.

A social skills inventory can be carried out by systematically evaluating the young person's competencies against a list of key social skills or in a less structured way through discussion. Specific gaps may have been identified through the methods mentioned in Step 1: Confirming the Problem Area, e.g., general discussion, exploring Interpersonal Incidents, and communication analysis. As always in IPT-A, regardless of the approach taken to identifying the specific nature of Interpersonal Gaps, transparency is key. This provides an opportunity to educate the young person and to invite him to evaluate his skills and competencies. IPT-A clinicians have found the list of skills in Clinical tool 10.1 Social skills list to be a helpful reference point. The list comprises skills for initiating and maintaining relationships. Additional skills for handling emotions and stress as well as for preventing and managing interpersonal difficulties are included, as these skills are also crucial in maintaining relationships. A list such as this, or an adapted version, can be shared with and explained to the young person and, with consent, his significant others. Young people can be invited to rate their skills as (A) good, (B) good enough but not great, and (C) needing attention.

Social skills inventories are available as psychometric instruments that include scoring information, such as Social Skills Inventory (Riggio and Carney, 2003), Social Problem Solving Inventory (Revised) (d'Zurilla et al., 2002), Social Skills Improvement System Rating Scales (Gresham and Elliott, 2008), and Social Skills Inventory for Adolescents (Del Prette and Del Prette, 2009). These instruments can be administered as a formal assessment tool producing precise scores. Such precise assessment, however, is often not necessary for the purposes of IPT-A. Alternatively, it may be more helpful to use these tools in an informal way to guide discussion with the young person and his significant others to identify areas of strength and weakness. The reader may prefer to use a social skill inventory that he or she is already familiar with. A generic list is provided below that could be easily augmented or abridged to focus more effectively on a young person's particular competencies and needs.

Sometimes, it is not a lack of social skills that is creating and maintaining a young person's Interpersonal Gaps. An inability to function well in social interactions may be related to feelings such as anger, fear, rejection, embarrassment, or awkwardness. Emotions such as these can block the young person from remembering and utilising her competencies. The therapist should be alert to this dynamic; when it is present, it can be addressed in the steps that follow. The strategies discussed for dealing with difficult emotions in the chapters on the other Problem Areas can be integrated into work on Interpersonal Gaps.

## Working on the Problem Area in the Middle Phase

It should be noted that Step 2 Identify the specific gaps in social skills is included under the heading of Assessing the Problem Area as it is primarily about assessment. It occurs in the Middle Phase of IPT-A, although often some relevant information will come to light during Step 1: Confirm the

### Clinical Tool 10.1  Social skills list

This list can help identify your social skills. It can be used to inform a discussion about your skills, or you may find it helpful to rate your skills as (A) good, (B) good enough but not great, and (C) needing attention.

#### Skills for initiating relationships

- listening
- beginning and continuing a conversation
- asking questions
- introducing oneself and others
- joining an existing conversation or activity

#### Skills for maintaining relationships

- expressing thanks
- giving and receiving compliments
- asking for help and receiving support
- supporting other people
- dealing with conflict and difference
- assertiveness
- making complaints
- apologising
- preparing for a difficult conversation—planning, gathering information, deciding what to say or do, staying focused, listening to the other person
- being a good friend
- awareness of self and others

#### Skills for handling emotions, dealing with stress, and avoiding trouble

- identifying, expressing, and managing feelings, including fear, sadness, anger, embarrassment, affection, and love
- understanding other people's emotions, including empathy and seeking clarification
- dealing with stressful situations, including teasing, bullying, social exclusion, and criticism
- avoiding trouble, risky situations and fights, including dealing with pressure from individuals and groups

Problem Area, which occurs in the Initial Phase. Once the specific gaps in social skills have been identified, further work may be required before beginning to fill the gaps so that the young person understands the impact of the gaps on her well-being.

### 3 Recognise the connection between Interpersonal Gaps and distress

It is essential that the young person recognises the way in which gaps in his social functioning are adversely affecting his relationships and his well-being in general. This understanding provides the rationale and motivation for the work that follows and a reason to be hopeful of positive change. This link cannot be taken for granted even when the young person has participated in identifying and discussing the specific features of his Interpersonal Gaps. Although he might recognise that there is a connection between his communication problems and depression or other difficulties, this awareness may be vague and unsophisticated. His insight will inevitably increase as he develops and practices social skills in Step 4: Develop social skills to fill or compensate for the current gaps. However, when comprehension is particularly low, some brief education before embarking on the next step will be helpful.

### 4 Develop social skills to fill or compensate for the current gaps

When the specific nature of the Interpersonal Gaps has been identified and the young person has some comprehension of the impact of the gaps on her relationships and distress, she will be well-placed to address the gaps. This may involve developing new social skills and confidence or adapting existing skills to help bridge the gaps.

The young person is involved in deciding which gaps to prioritise and the order in which they will be tackled. Although there may not be time to address all the young person's gaps, this is fortunately often not necessary in order to bring about significant improvement in his or her symptoms. All that may be required is to experience more success in relationships. With realistic aims in mind, the goal is usually to achieve good-enough communication rather than perfect or high-level communication skills.

Examples of a range of approaches to improving young people's interpersonal functioning are included below:

- The art of conversation
- Using questions
- Social skills training and self-esteem programs
- Apps, bibliotherapy, and media-enhanced therapy
- Checking for intended meaning
- Support materials, including skill reminders and practice reports

- Rehearsing skills outside therapy sessions
- Managing emotions that adversely affect social interactions

This is not an exhaustive listing. If the reader is familiar with other approaches to developing social skills, it may well be appropriate to use these within an IPT-A intervention providing they address the aims of Interpersonal Psychotherapy.

Role play and chair work (see Chapter 4) are particularly helpful techniques for developing social skills and can be used in the approaches mentioned above.

*The art of conversation*

Appropriate conversation skills can reduce social isolation and rejection, which can drive depression-associated Interpersonal Gaps. As mentioned previously, conversation is an art, in the sense that it relies on skills and sensibilities that most of us develop over time. It involves resisting the natural urge to dominate. Some people have an affinity for social interaction and may develop their conversational skills unconsciously. They absorb them as if by osmosis from the people around them. Others make a conscious effort to notice how other people behave in social situations and find ways to assimilate these competencies into their social repertoire without assistance. Young people experiencing Interpersonal Gaps, however, are likely to require both conscious effort and assistance in the form of teaching, instruction, modelling, rehearsing *in vivo* and *in vitro*, and mentoring in order to develop their conversational skills. As noted, this may involve acquiring social skills and insights for the first time, or, if the Interpersonal Gaps are more recent, it may be sufficient for them to rediscover and connect with their previous social competencies.

In previous eras, conversation skills were often taught more commonly and deliberately than they are today. In some cultures, this was particularly so for young women. The custom of sending young women of particular social classes to the "finishing" schools of Europe and elsewhere is a notable example. One of the aims of these institutions was to produce competent social hostesses. The skills taught included the ability to initiate and maintain conversation, to put people at ease in social situations, and to draw people out using a wide range of means such as questions, anecdotes, and stories. Regardless of their social station, young men and women were inculcated in the social skills associated with their position and role, albeit within the context of the more constrained gender roles of earlier times. This was achieved through formal and informal teaching and modelling by parents, family members and communities. It is less common for conversation skills to be formally taught today, and this may be precisely what young people with Interpersonal Gaps need. It can be provided in therapy, and the young person's significant others, if able, may be able to take on an instructor role outside therapy.

For some young people, texting may have reduced face-to-face contact and impacted conversation skills. For these young people, social media may have a greater influence than conversation.

*Using questions*

For many, there is much pleasure to be enjoyed through good conversation. Part of the pleasure is discovering the intrinsically interesting aspects of other people. Our capacity to enjoy sharing and receiving information from others is part of our heritage as a highly social species. Our need to seek proximity in times of difficulty is hardwired into us, generation after generation over aeons of time (see Chapter 3). The capacity to communicate effectively helped our species survive and has thus been favoured by evolution.

Conversation is more than just asking questions, but questions can be a key part of conversation and are a good place to start in teaching conversation skills. The basics of conversation need to be pointed out to some young people:

- If someone dominates interaction, talking constantly about him- or herself and showing little interest in the other person, a monologue occurs rather than conversation.
- When we don't ask questions, we miss out on learning about the other person, including details we might find charming or riveting. Conversely, we may find that we do not want to spend any more time with them.
- We can learn a lot about human nature and ourselves from others, and when we don't converse in ways that invite information, we miss crucial learning.
- Questions are a way of turn-taking, of explicitly passing the baton to someone else and inviting them to speak.
- Questions elicit information. They are a way of showing interest in another person and can lead a conversation in a particular direction.

Some young people have never learnt how to ask questions in order to start or continue a conversation. Other young people become nervous and can't think of anything to say or ask. Learning and practising ways to employ questions in social interactions can greatly assist these young people. The advantages of open-ended questions compared to closed questions should be explored, followed by strategies to help young people remember and appropriately utilise questions. The following poem can be used to teach young people about questions and to help them remember a wide range of ways to enquire and invite a social exchange.

> *I keep six honest serving men*
> *(They taught me all I knew)*
> *Their names are What and Why and When*
> *And How and Where and Who*
>
> Rudyard Kipling

In addition to what, why, when, how, where, and who, the young person can be encouraged to generate other questions he would feel comfortable asking. Examples of other ways of initiating or continuing a conversation include

- *Tell me about…*
- *Tell me more.*
- *What do you think about…?*

It will be beneficial for many young people to demonstrate how questions can be combined with other social skills, such as self-disclosure, to steer a conversation in a particular direction and deepen the relationship. For example, after the young person discloses something about themselves, they might invite reciprocal sharing by ask a question such as

- *How do you feel when things like that happen?*
- *What do your parents do then?*

Some young people will need guidance around judging appropriate levels of self-disclosure and how, when, and with whom to share information about themselves.

### Social skills training and self-esteem programs

Many different social skills training programs for young people are available for individual and group training. Broader social skills programs can provide a valuable adjunct to IPT-A. Aspects of these skills training programs could be included in individual IPT-A sessions, or the young person could attend group skills development programs to complement the work of individual therapy. Groups can provide potent learning for adolescents, allowing them to practice with and receive feedback from their peers. Some programs target particular age groups, such as Skillstreaming the Adolescent (McGinnis et al., 2011) (http://www.skillstreaming.com).

Assertiveness skills training provides an effective repertoire of social skills and is linked with the notion of self-esteem. Self-esteem and a sense of rights are central to creating satisfying relationships and maintaining appropriate boundaries and limits in social interactions.

Additionally, programs are available to teach social skills to young people with autism or attention-deficit/hyperactivity disorder (ADHD). Elements of these programs may be beneficial for young people experiencing Interpersonal Gaps. Although young people with autism or ADHD are not necessarily depressed, many of their social skill gaps mirror those experienced by young people with symptoms of depression or anxiety that are driven by Interpersonal Gaps.

### Apps, bibliotherapy, and media enhanced therapy

Apps can be a helpful aid to therapy, using game formats and other approaches to provide psychoeducation and social skill practice. Examples include the following:

- Let's be social: https://itunes.apple.com/au/app/lets-be-social-social-skills-development/id1140153485
- 10 Ways: https://itunes.apple.com/au/app/10-ways-a-social-skills-game/id1116372204?mt=8
- ADDITUDE: https://www.additudemag.com/slideshows/educational-apps-for-kids-with-adhd-social-skills/

Books, YouTube, film, and television provide a rich source of material for teaching social skills, and this can be an engaging approach for some young people. Young people can be invited to reflect on communication between characters they are familiar with. For example, some young people grew up with Harry Potter books and films and still enjoy the stories. They could be asked to think about how Hermione, Harry, Ron, Professor Dumbledore, or other characters might communicate or behave. Other young people may respond well to analysing the communication of a favourite character from a YouTube or television serial. Questions might include how a particular character starts or deepens a conversation, asks for help, or deals with a disagreement or difference. The discussion can be focused on global communication skills or specific skills, depending on the nature of the young person's Interpersonal Gaps.

**Jacob**, aged 14, felt shy in social situations, even with people who he knew fairly well. He particularly hated situations where he might need to start a conversation, stating that he felt so nervous he did not know what to say. This left him feeling increasingly isolated at school. He also dreaded gatherings with extended family, worrying that he would not know what to say and that relatives would be watching him and be concerned about his social awkwardness.

*Therapist:* Jacob, you were telling me that you have read all the Harry Potter books and have seen the films. Which would you say is your favourite book or film in the series?
*Jacob:* Probably Philosophers Stone.
*Therapist:* And what do you like about it?
*Jacob:* Well, it was the first one. I loved the whole thing about Hogwarts and Harry discovering magic and mystical stuff.
*Therapist:* Would you be willing to dip into it during the next week and look for examples of how one or two of the characters start conversations? For our next session, try to bring three examples of communication that you like, or you think worked well. Also, try to find an example or two of what looks like an attempt to start a conversation that didn't go so well. If you have time, you could have a think about why those pieces of communication either worked well or not so well. Then we can discuss next week what's going on in these examples and see if there's anything there that might give you some ideas of how you can start a conversation with the sort of people you meet, either at school or at those family gatherings you worry about.

*Checking for intended meaning*

Wallen (1967) developed a model of communication called The Interpersonal Gap. It describes a common communication problem whereby the communication and actions of one person are misinterpreted by another person. The intention of person A is different from the effect on person B. Person A knows what is meant, but person B's interpretation in response is quite different from that intended by person A. According to Wallen, this incongruence lies at the heart of many communication problems, including most conflict. Wallen's model can help the young person to understand, recognise, and prevent this common form of misunderstanding.

A frequent response when someone experiences another person's communication or actions as hurtful, insensitive, or in other ways negative is to identify the other person's behaviour as the problem and to respond accordingly, e.g., to expect them to change or to withdraw from them. Unlike much communication theory, Wallen placed the emphasis on the role of the receiver in preventing and remedying communication problems by clarifying the other person's communication and the intention behind it. The skills required to do this have been described by Crosby (2015) and have much in common with Emotional Intelligence (EQ) skills. They can be paraphrased as the following:

1. provide a description of the other person's communication or actions without judgement or interpretation
2. describe your own feelings about the other person's behaviour
3. clarify the feeling, intention and meaning the other person is experiencing
4. check you have correctly understood the other person's feeling, intention and meaning , e.g., paraphrase.

The resulting dialogue would be something along these lines:

> *When you said you didn't want me to come around after school, I felt sad and I wondered if you might not want to hang out with me so much anymore.*
>
> *Is that what you meant?*
>
> *Sounds like I got that wrong—the reason you didn't want me to come round after school is because you have an assignment overdue. You're saying you still want to hang out with me as much as before. Have I got that right?*

Chair work (see Chapter 4) can be a helpful way of addressing this area of misunderstanding and is used extensively in this Problem Area.

*Support materials–skill reminders and practice reports*

Support materials to assist with social skills development will be attractive to some young people and readily embraced. The materials may be in paper or electronic format. They can be informal notes developed by the young person or therapist during a therapy session or a more formal handout provided by the therapist. They can be a useful aid for memory, facilitate reflection and practice outside therapy, and may also be shared with the young person's significant others so that they can better understand and support the young person's skill development. Additionally, therapy can be an intense experience. The young person can feel assailed by a wide range of thoughts and emotions and afterwards may find it difficult to recall suggestions or instructions for skills practice. If he or she is concerned about remembering details from a session, his or her attention and participation may be affected. Knowing the important points are written down will assist some young people to be more fully present and involved in therapy. Some young people will use their phones for this.

Skill reminders briefly outline the skills being developed. Depending on the complexity of the skills and the young person's requirements, reminders or tip sheets may comprise a sentence, several paragraphs, or a series of bullet points that itemise the micro skills involved. They may be especially appreciated by young people who welcome visual learning aids and concrete reminders. These materials are likely to be most effective when developed by the therapist and young person together. They can be adapted from examples found on the internet and in social skills programs, but the process of tailoring generic materials to meet the client's individual needs adds value. This process familiarises the young person with the materials and may increase the likelihood that she will use the resource. It also further reinforces the young person sense that the therapist cares about her and is thinking about her needs.

**Jacob** placed a note on his phone. It simply stated:

*What Why When*
*How Where Who*
*Tell me about*
*Hermione*

Jacob's attachment style appeared to be preoccupied and, characteristically of this style, he was very concerned about other people's opinion of him. One of Jacob's biggest fears was to experience what he referred to as a "mind freeze" or mental blank when he wouldn't know what to say in social situations. This fear had caused him considerable distress and led him to avoid many social interactions. Initially, he carried his reminder with him at all times and found it greatly increased his confidence and ability to interact with others. The first three lines reminded Jacob of questions he could ask. "Hermione" was a prompt to remember his favourite Harry Potter character, whom he admired, in part, for her intelligence and calm demeanour that allowed her to avoid panicking and therefore figure out a solution to most problems.

Jacob found he only needed to refer to his reminder before encounters and having it with him helped him relax. He discovered he could enjoy conversations and finding out about people. Over time he felt less need to refer to his prompt. He discovered that the questions and other ways to converse seemed to form naturally in his mind now that he felt more relaxed in social situations.

**Liu**, aged 17, also derived particular reassurance from writing down prompts to help her in social interactions. She added reminders on her phone during therapy sessions. These were brief notes, sometimes a single word. Liu found it reassuring to capture an idea while the material was fresh in her mind. Liu appeared secure in her attachment. She was highly motivated to change and without prompting from the therapist would often embellish her notes in more detail immediately after a session, stating that writing helped her remember. Like Jacob, she only occasionally referred to her notes but commented that the process of typing it up helped her remember and this was a technique she had used with considerable success in her schoolwork.

*Rehearsing skills alone outside therapy sessions*

In addition to modelling and practising social skills with the therapist in session and ultimately practising with safe people outside therapy, the young person can be encouraged to practice alone. This might involve, for example, looking in a mirror, using a smart phone selfie video, or audio recording. Homework activities can be tailored to the young person's particular areas of discomfort or difficulty with social skills.

**Valentina**, aged 14, spoke in a monotone voice and showed little facial expression during social interactions. At the conclusion of a session spent practising voice inflection and facial expressions the therapist suggested she practice alone at home. Valentina found it helpful to record and view conversations with herself. The therapist encouraged her to bring her reflections and questions to their next session. Not only was she completely relaxed when alone, she also found she reflected in a different way compared to practising with the therapist. Valentina commented that she was surprised to find that she enjoyed experimenting with her facial expressions and tone of voice. Her older sister became curious about what she was doing and joined her for an extended practice session. They had fun "being silly" and laughed a lot. She gained some helpful tips and encouragement from her sister.

**Caleb**, aged 15, appeared to have an anxious avoidant attachment style. He had difficulty making eye contact in all his social interactions. He also had a tendency to look more serious than he intended and rarely smiled with people that he did not know well. As an adjunct to the work in session, his therapist suggested that he practice eye contact with himself using a mirror. The practice activity included an element of mindfulness to increase Caleb's awareness of his responses to eye contact. Conscious that Caleb would find this challenging, the therapist spent some time preparing him for this assignment.

*Therapist:* Caleb, I'd like to sum up a few of the things we've been discussing about eye contact and suggest something you can do to practice by yourself. As

Interpersonal Gaps 295

we were saying, eye contact can be a great way for connecting with people but, unfortunately, a lot of people find eye contact difficult. When used well, it can be attractive and a way of showing we are interested in others. Some people are unsure how much eye contact to make, or they feel really uncomfortable with eye contact, as you do. Other people make too much eye contact, which can feel creepy and push people away. However, if we avoid eye contact, it can also put people off. We can give the impression of not being interested or even of lying. So the bad news is the difficulty you have making eye contact seems to be having a major impact on your ability to make friends and may be affecting your interactions with the adults you need to interact with, such as some of your teachers. Better news is that it's not just you. Many people find eye contact difficult. Even better news is that with practice you can improve. I'd like to suggest a way you can practice. Is that okay?

Caleb: Yeah. I'd like to know.

Therapist: This assignment may feel strange and uncomfortable. It is an odd thing to do, to stare at yourself in the mirror. But the reason for doing it is the more you practice looking at people's eyes and get used to it, the more comfortable it will feel. You may notice some other benefits as well, like being more aware of your face and how you use it. The ultimate goal here is for you to be able to create the impression you want with others—that you are approachable, friendly, and good to get to know. This will help you have more success in your relationships. As we discovered, your depression seems to be related to the lack of success in making friends. So, as that improves, we can expect your depression to improve. Is this sounding okay?

Caleb: Yeah.

Therapist: There are three things I'd like you to practice. We can write them down to help you remember if you want when I've explained them:

1. Look at yourself in the mirror and hold your gaze as long as possible. While you're doing this, notice what you experience. It could be thoughts, feelings, or body sensations. It might be feelings of discomfort, or it could be other things. I'd like you to repeat it three times in a practice session and take a minute as a rest between each practice. If it's too uncomfortable to maintain eye contact, even looking yourself in the eye for a few seconds would be good.
2. The next thing I'd like you to try is again to make eye contact with yourself in the mirror, but this time look away briefly when it starts to feel uncomfortable and then look back at your eyes. Do this several times, noticing how you feel.
3. And then the last thing I'd like you to practice is the same as number two but this time, after you look away and then look back and make eye contact with yourself, I'd like you to try

> adding a smile or a frown. Again, be curious and notice what you experience: thoughts, feelings, or sensations in your body.
>
> It would be great if you could repeat each of these tasks three times every day this next week. Don't worry if you miss a day or two. Just do it as often as you can fit in. I'll be really interested to hear how you get on and we can discuss it at our next session. Can I check if you are interested in giving this a try and do you have any questions or concerns about it?

The therapist's hypothesis about Caleb's anxious avoidant attachment style suggested that he would engage in homework as he was motivated to change and that practising alone would be more acceptable to him than practising with others. This would be a helpful step in preparing the way for practising with others.

The mindfulness element of this practice activity is aimed at helping Caleb discover a new relationship with his discomfort during eye contact. By drawing his attention to observing his experience of eye contact, he may notice that his feelings of discomfort shift and change and that he can endure them. This will encourage a sense of curiosity and awareness of opportunities for change so that the discomfort has less power and influence over him. His discomfort may decrease through this practice but this is not the actual aim of mindfulness. Rather, mindfulness aims to build his awareness that he is more than his feelings of discomfort. In this way, he has the ability to change his relationship to the discomfort so that he can function despite it.

Depending on the young person's interests and presentation, the rationale for mindfulness practice may be explained before or after an activity such as this; however, this is not essential in order for him to benefit from the awareness that develops. In the case of Caleb, the term mindfulness was not even used. The use of mindfulness is discussed in Chapter 4.

Three practice sheets are included at the end of this chapter:

- Clinical tool 10.2 Practice sheet for a single skill
- Clinical tool 10.3 Practice sheet for a conversation or complex interaction
- Clinical tool 10.4 Practice sheet for a specific social skill

*Managing emotions that adversely affect social interactions*

For some young people, their Interpersonal Gaps comprise difficulty managing particular emotions and this negatively impacts their social interactions. We have included some approaches to managing anger as examples of ways to address these gaps.

Psychoeducation is often necessary so that the young person understands the rationale for addressing this issue and to help her identify and implement strategies to manage her anger in more constructive ways.

> **Clinical Tool 10.2  Practice sheet for a single skill**
>
> Make notes for yourself, with your therapist's assistance, to help you remember what you will be practising. This will help you prepare for your practice activity.
>   After the practice has occurred, make notes about what happened and bring these to your next session to discuss with your therapist.
>
> **Planning the practice**
>
> 1  Which skill I am practising?
> 2  What are the components I need to remember?
> 3  Who I can practice with?
> 4  When might be a good time and place to practice?
>
> **Reflecting after the practice on:**
>
> 1  What the outcome was
> 2  How the other person responded
> 3  How I felt about the interaction
> 4  What I did well
> 5  Something I'd like to improve

*The Anger chart*

Figure 10.1 outlines the common trajectory for angry outbursts and provides a helpful focus for education. An example of how the Anger Chart may be used to increase insight and inform anger management strategies is included in the following dialogue with **Ava**, aged 16, who appears to have an avoidant attachment style.

*Therapist:*   *From what you've told me about your anger, it sounds similar to this graph. There is a period of build up when you feel low-level stress. This builds and then there's a rapid escalation (the therapist points to relevant parts of Figure 10.1). You used the word "explosion" when you do or say something, which you often regret later. When you're in this explosion, it feels automatic or out of your control. No matter how much you later wished you hadn't said or done whatever it was, at the time you're so angry you feel unable to do anything else. Have I understood that correctly?*
*Ava:*   *Yep.*
*Therapist:*   *You feel like you can't change this part of yourself, but if you could, it*

> **Clinical Tool 10.3  Practice sheet for a conversation or complex interaction**
>
> **Planning the practice**
>
> 1. What is the issue or difficulty to be discussed?
> 2. Who is involved?
> 3. What do I need in this situation?
> 4. What do I suspect the other person/people might need?
> 5. What outcome would I like (based on everyone's needs)?
> 6. What are the key things I want to communicate to the other person?
> 7. What is an example of how I might say this?
> 8. What are the components or steps for this conversation that I need to remember?
> 9. When might be a good time and place to have the discussion?
>
> **Reflecting after the practice on:**
>
> 1. What I said and did
> 2. How the other person responded
> 3. How I felt about the interaction
> 4. What I did well
> 5. Something I'd like to improve about my side of the interaction
> 6. What the outcome was
> 7. How satisfied I am with the outcome on a 1 to 10 scale
> 8. How satisfied I think the other person might be with the outcome on a 1 to 10 scale

|  |  |
|---|---|
|  | sounds like it would make your life a lot easier. For example, you might not get into fights at school, your maths teacher might go a bit easier on you, and things might be calmer at home? |
| Ava: | I guess so. |
| Therapist: | I'd like to explain a bit about anger to see if you think that might help you understand what's going on in your relationships and help you figure out how you might reduce the explosions that are causing so many problems for you. It's not just you who finds it difficult to do something different when you are in the "explosion" stage (therapist points to this area of Figure 10.1). Many people experience that. It's difficult to think clearly when feeling such strong emotion. The good news is that it is possible to make changes when we are in the build-up period to prevent an explosion happening. The key is to recognise our |

## Clinical Tool 10.4  Practice sheet for a specific social skill
Preparing to ask for a date—finding common interests

### Description of the skill:
One aspect of preparing to ask someone for a date is to first identify interests that you share with the other person. Talking about each other's interests, hobbies, or pastimes may help you discover things you have in common. Additionally, this conversation will give you more of an idea about what the other person is like and whether you would like to ask him or her for a date.

### Steps
Step 1: Say hello and introduce yourself
Step 2: Ask the other person about the interests, hobbies, or pastimes he or she enjoys
Step 3: Share something about your interests and hobbies or pastimes
Step 4: See if you can find things in common with the other person
Step 5: Decide if you would like to ask the other person for a date

### Planning and preparation—when, where, how
Develop a brief plan of when and where you might have the conversation, what might you say, and how might the other person respond to what might you say.

### Dialogue
Develop an example of what you might say at each of the steps above.
Step 1:
Step 2:
Step 3:
Step 4:
Step 5:

### After the practice
**What actually happened**—a brief summary of what occurred

### Reflection
**How well did you do?** Rate how effective you were in using this skill on the following 1–5 scale:

| 1 | 2 | 3 | 4 | 5 |
|---|---|---|---|---|
| not effective at all | | | | extremely effective |

### Learning
In hindsight is there anything you have learned from this practice or you would do differently?

> early warning signals. These are things that tell us we are getting angry. They let us know that we need to do something different to prevent an explosion. How about I give you some examples of what I mean by signals, and then you tell me if you experience any of these or other things that you think might be a sign that your anger is building up?

Ava nods.

Therapist: It might be signs in the body like clinching fists or teeth, tightening in the throat, stomach churning, going red in the face, sweaty palms, or tightness in the chest. Do you ever notice any of that or other things in your body?

Ava: I get a dry mouth. My throat does get tight. Sometimes it does feel a bit difficult to breathe.

Therapist: It's great you've been able to notice that. This ability you have to notice these things will help us figure out some strategies you could try. I'd be interested to hear if you think of any other signs. Let me know if anything comes to mind. I'll explain a bit more. Some people notice they have particular thoughts going on in their head that make them angrier, like "this isn't fair" or "they always pick on me". Many people find they can't think about how to stop things escalating when they get to the point where they are really angry. Have you noticed anything about what goes on with your thoughts when you are angry?

Being conscious of Ava's avoidant fearful attachment style, the therapist chose to discuss anger management in a way that would not put Ava on the spot by using too much direct questioning. The aim was to provide education and gentle invitations for Ava to identify aspects of her own experience of anger. The therapist attempted to increase Inclusion, i.e., the importance of therapy

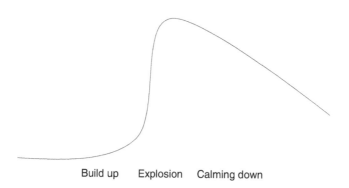

Figure 10.1 Ava's anger chart.

for Ava, (see Chapter 4) by linking the conversation to issues that motivated her, e.g., people at school and at home giving her "an easier time".

The therapist discussed body sensations and cognitions before addressing emotions, knowing that Ava finds it difficult to identify emotions and is often uncomfortable discussing them.

After listing a range of emotions that are commonly associated with angry outbursts, Ava was able to acknowledge that she sometimes felt threatened or rejected and this often preceded her angry "explosions". Following further discussion, Ava offered that feeling alone might be a common thread in triggering her angry behaviour.

Ava was involved in a mindfulness program at her school and this seemed to increase her ability to recognise her early warning symptoms. Mindfulness is discussed in Chapter 4.

Using behavioural chain analysis, the therapist encouraged Ava to identify options that might interrupt the escalation of her anger. This included options to temporarily remove Ava from the situation and reverse the physiology of anger. Ava liked the suggestion of walking away from the situation to take a drink of water, especially when the therapist explained that the sensations in her throat during a long drink can help to relax her muscles. Preparing Ava to use this strategy included practicing mindfulness while drinking to increase her awareness of the relaxing physiological sensations. Additionally, Ava was not aware that simply walking off to get a drink with no explanation to the other party might seem odd or rude. Her attention had to be drawn to this and time given to practising how she might explain this behaviour, e.g., "Excuse me, I'll be back in a minute. I just need to get a drink of water".

*Education about life stress*

Drawing the client's attention to the connection between anger and times of high stress can help her recognise when she needs to be particularly alert to the early warning signs of anger.

*Therapist:*     *Ava, many people find that when they are stressed they are more likely to get irritable and angry. It's a bit like a pot on the cooker. When the heat is turned up, the pot is more likely to boil over. So, too, when stress levels are high, there is a greater chance anger will erupt in damaging ways. Let's have a think about things that add to your stress levels.*

Ava found that education about potential stressors assisted her to monitor her stress levels. This included learning to differentiate different types of stressors:

- Major life events: these are acute stresses such as bereavements, a relationship ending, assault, or geographical relocation.

- Enduring life stress: these are ongoing stressful factors such as chronic illness, disability, parental mental illness, poverty, or substandard housing.
- Daily events: these may be of low intensity but are irritating or frustrating. Examples might include missing a train, a disagreement, or distressing demands of others.

It is helpful to balance building the young person's awareness of stressors with identification of positive factors that serve to increase resilience and uplift the young person. These might include nurturing and enjoyable activities that have been identified during the holistic assessment, such as recreation, positive aspects of relationships, exercise, good sleep, time in nature, etc.

Some young people can relate to the metaphor of stress scales. When the balance is weighted in the direction of stress, they need to be more alert about monitoring their early warning signs in order to prevent angry outbursts. They may be able to take action to reduce stress and build de-stress factors. Even when a particular stress factor is beyond the young person's power to change it, his responses to the stressor may be changeable, for example through mindfulness.

*Blind spots*

Interpersonal Gaps can be related to the young person's lack of awareness of how his communication style affects others. Providing a brief discussion of the Johari Window (Luft and Ingham, 1955) can be a helpful way to introduce discussion and contextualise these gaps in a nonjudgmental way. The window identifies issues as known or unknown, both to oneself and others, forming four quadrants (see Figure 10.2).

- public: known to self and others
- hidden: known to self but unknown to others
- unknown: unknown to self and others
- blind: known to others but unknown to self

The blind quadrant is an obvious focus for work on Interpersonal Gaps. Through feedback, the blind self grows smaller as the young person learns

1. How her behaviour is viewed by others
2. How her behaviour makes others feel
3. How her behaviour shapes the opinion others have of her
4. How 1–3 impacts on her view of herself
5. Strategies to change 1–3

Some young people may benefit from being introduced to the Johari Window, such as in the case of Ali, discussed in Chapter 4. Ali's blind self was reduced

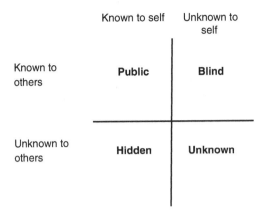

*Figure 10.2* Identifying blind spots.

through feedback from the therapist. The therapist might seek permission to provide feedback to reduce the young person's blind spots with dialogue such as the following:

> *During our sessions, I may notice things about the way you relate to me or other people. It might be helpful if I let you know so you can use this in your relationships, including after our therapy finishes. Is it okay if I share this with you?*

This transparency and explicit permission seeking can be helpful for all clients, especially those with insecure attachment. It is one of many ways in which the therapist can explain the process of therapy and provide the young person with opportunities to choose his level of participation.

### 5 Enhance social support by maintaining, expanding, and/or deepening social networks

In addition to developing social skills in therapy sessions and outside therapy, many young people with Interpersonal Gaps will need direction to develop their social support networks. Some will have limited or virtually non-existent social connections. Others may have extensive social networks, but these relationships are shallow because the young person lacks the skills to move beyond the superficial and so the connections provide little in the way of support.

The therapist and/or the young person's significant others need to assist these young people to identify ways to interact with new people and to deepen their existing relationships. Many young people will be able to identify helpful strategies through discussion, brainstorming, or the activities mentioned in

Step 4 above. If these approaches fail to help the young person to see potentially productive avenues, it will be appropriate and time efficient for the therapist to make suggestions. Often, existing activities can be adjusted to increase social interaction, for example changing a part-time job for one that involves greater interface with other people, as discussed later in the case of Hannah. As an added bonus, some of these activities can have antidepressant effects apart from their social benefits, for example, combining an interpersonal element with exercise routines, or sharing a pleasurable pastime with others. Early on in efforts to extend the young person's social network the therapist may need to play an active and even directive role. As the young person then begins to experience increasing social success, his confidence tends to build and he becomes more proactive and better able to recognise opportunities to engage with others.

Therapist dialogue such as the following helps to set the scene for this work during the Middle Phase of IPT-A.

> *In addition to the work we do in session, it will be important for you to practice skills outside therapy. We'll discuss which people might be good to do this with. It might be people in your family or others you know and feel comfortable with. One of the things we learned from your Closeness Circles was that you don't have many interactions with people outside your family. You mentioned you'd like to change this but you weren't sure how to do this. When you have tried to talk to other people, you've felt it hasn't gone very well. We'll find opportunities for you to practice talking with new people and developing friendships. It could be interests, such as your sport or gaming, that you can share with others or it might be looking at a different job for you because your current one doesn't give you much opportunity to interact with others.*

The cases of Matt, Hannah, and Arjun, discussed below, illustrate ways to extend young people's social networks and practice social skills outside therapy.

**Matt**, aged 20, commenced university 18 months ago but made no new friends there. He also lost touch with his school friends although they were never particularly close in the first place. By the time Matt came to therapy he was socially isolated, felt lonely, and was despondent about the prospects of this improving. During the first session, the therapist noted that Matt had an abrupt manner that seemed unfriendly and could easily be interpreted as aggressive or rude. Through social skills practice activities during the Middle Phase of IPT-A, Matt developed an increased awareness of social cues and discovered ways of making a more friendly impression when practising with the therapist. He had little idea, however, about how to apply this in his life. He welcomed the therapist's suggestion that it would be appropriate to talk to people in his tutorial groups. His practice assignments outside therapy consisted of speaking with other students during or after tutorials. His progress was reviewed each week and the learning was applied to fine tune his skills. Initially Matt relied on the therapist to help him identify appropriate next steps in initiating and deepening these relationships. After several successful interactions, he invited some other students for coffee and, after that went well, he invited them to a movie. The therapist also suggested that Matt consider joining the student photography society as this was an interest of his. At this point, his progress developed a momentum of its own powered by a sense of relief that he was finally understanding (1) what had been getting in the way of forming connections and (2) how to do things differently to effectively connect with people. The therapist also encouraged Matt to think about whether there were any of his school friends with whom he wished to reconnect. During the Consolidation Phase, Matt re-established friendships with two of his school friends and continued expanding his friendship network at university.

**Hannah**, aged 17, felt shy and anxious in social situations. She never initiated conversation with people she did not know well. Her social inhibition was related to beliefs that she was boring and uninteresting to others. When she moved with her family to a new city, she felt trapped in her isolation and loneliness. In addition to working on her conversation skills and self-esteem, the therapist suggested that she consider changing her part-time job from stacking shop shelves after closing time to a position that would involve more social interaction. Hannah's current job gave her little opportunity to practice social skills. It involved only minimal interactions with her supervisor and a couple of colleagues. She was able to find a job at the local cinema selling tickets and refreshments. This required constant interaction with the public. She felt daunted by this but was encouraged by a family friend who also worked at the cinema. Hannah was surprised to find that after a few shifts at her new job, she felt fairly relaxed when interacting with customers. Several factors contributed to this rapid change. The new role required Hannah to interact with people in a way she would normally avoid. Through this exposure, she learnt that she not only survived but also enjoyed situations that she had previously feared. The clearly delineated nature of the role gave her confidence. She quickly mastered the limited range of interactions required by the job and, rather than needing to hide her feelings of self-doubt behind this work persona, these feelings seemed to dissipate and were replaced by a newfound confidence. Hannah was pleased to find that the customers were almost universally in a good mood, as they were looking forward to their entertainment. She discovered that she liked the cinema's activity and sense of mild excitement, especially as people arrived for each showing. As her confidence built, she found herself interacting with customers more than was actually required. The therapist encouraged this and they practised questions and comments she could use at work to enhance her conversation skills. Hannah was aware of the need to limit conversation during busy times when a queue developed but found there were ample opportunities to chat with customers at slow times. Her job required her to ask questions such as "What would you like to see?",

"Which session time?", and "Would you like some refreshments?" The therapist assisted Hannah to identify additional questions that seemed to her to flow naturally from the more strictly work-related topics. Examples included "What sort of day have you had?", "What's the weather like outside?", and "You're a bit early for your session, would you like me to tell you about the cafes nearby?"

Hannah had overwhelmingly positive responses from cinema-goers. Despite these successes, her anxiety about dating, or even showing interest in people she was attracted to, continued. The therapist suggested she could practice paying small compliments to customers and work up to including people she was attracted to. In session, she identified a range of possible compliments she could offer that wouldn't be too threatening for her. Examples included: "I like your T-shirt", "That's a really nice necklace", and "They're cool sunglasses you've got". During the next therapy session, Hannah reported that her practice at work had gone well and she felt ready to focus on more personal compliments, which she would find challenging. Hannah practised giving a range of compliments in session, including statements such as: "I like your hair", "You look good in that", and "You look like you've been working out". After the therapist drew Hannah's attention to her body language, she added some eye contact and a smile to her practice of giving compliments. Hannah felt some security practising social skills in the role of the cinema job, feeling that she had permission to be friendly and would be able to hide behind this role in case she received a negative response.

The therapist also explained that part of the art of giving compliments was knowing how to receive them. Hannah agreed that she would like to be able to respond graciously if someone complimented her rather than dissolving into embarrassment and silence, which was her usual response. An additional part of Hannah's preparation for practice at work was to consider the appropriateness of making personal compliments in the workplace. Hannah was aware she needed to put some boundaries around this at work. She didn't want customers or her manager to think she was being inappropriate. Given her manager had recently commented positively on her friendliness and the way Hannah welcomed customers, she thought she could get away with being a little bolder. However, her natural caution made her reluctant to do so. Instead she opted for practising gentle flirting with someone she occasionally saw at sports games. This fitted Hannah's criteria of being relatively "safe" as she could easily avoid that person in the future if the interaction hadn't gone well. Hannah was intrigued and pleased to discover that she could interact in ways she had never dared to before.

Towards the end of the Middle Phase, the therapist encouraged Hannah to reflect on how she had been able to make so much progress. This included transparently discussing the "small steps, multiple presentations, constant revision" equation (discussed above). This was revisited in the Consolidation

Phase to help reinforce the gains and to give Hannah a strategy for addressing challenging social situations in the future.

The case of **Arjun,** aged 15, illustrates how his interest in exercise was used to extend his social network. Arjun's depression was related to coexisting Problem Areas. His major Problem Area was Complex Grief, and he was also experiencing Interpersonal Gaps as a secondary Problem Area. Arjun had been a successful athlete when he was younger but curtailed his sporting activities due to a medical condition. As he moved into early adolescence he gained considerable weight and felt unattractive. He also missed the social kudos he had derived from his athletic success. The therapist hypothesised that Arjun was mildly anxious avoidant in his attachment style but he also displayed some elements of secure attachment. His lack of confidence combined with Interpersonal Gaps prevented him from developing friendships and that left him feeling socially isolated outside his extended family. Arjun experienced several significant losses when he was 14 years old, including bereavements. These losses also had a major impact on his family and adversely affected the attention and support available to him from his parents.

Arjun made considerable progress during the Middle phase of IPT-A as he addressed his multiple losses. This included improving his communication with his family about his experiences of loss so that he felt more connected to and supported by them. The focus of therapy then turned to developing Arjun's social network with peers. The aim was to help him make friends and then, towards the end of therapy, some attention was given to eliciting and providing support in a friendship.

Arjun had recently become interested again in exercise after a new medical procedure made this possible for him. He particularly enjoyed his return to jogging and he was also easing into lifting weights. Arjun was open to the therapist's suggestion of using his interest in exercise to extend his social network but initially had no idea how to do this. After some discussion, he mentioned that he occasionally saw a neighbour out jogging. They had been friendly when they attended primary school together but had lost touch when they went to different high schools. The therapist correctly predicted that given Arjun's attachment style, the idea of reinitiating a friendship that might be based around a practical activity would not be too uncomfortable for him. Arjun practiced different ways he might invite his neighbour to join him jogging. He worked on this, both in session and with his older sister at home. The neighbour welcomed Arjun's invitation and they began running together regularly. Arjun immediately felt less isolated.

Work on extending Arjun's social network continued during the Consolidation Phase. The neighbour was also quite shy but had a couple of friends whom he introduced Arjun to. One of these friends had a garage, which was well equipped for weights training, and the four of them began meeting for workouts. The interactions between these four young men revolved primarily around exercise and sport. This suited Arjun initially. He was relieved that he didn't need to say much to feel part of the group and was delighted that it seemed to be sufficient for him just to turn up in order to feel included. In the final two therapy sessions the therapist briefly explored with Arjun how he might go about deepening his interactions with his peers. Arjun began to do this with one of his exercise friends, who had also experienced a recent bereavement, by talking about how their families had responded to their losses. At the end of the Consolidation Phase, Arjun identified his sister as someone who could support him to further develop his social skills, stating that he admired her ability to talk to people and draw them out.

For Arjun, most of the Middle phase of IP T-A was taken up with addressing Complex Grief. However, before the end of treatment, opportunities were also found to assist Arjun with his Interpersonal Gaps and to extend his social network. There wasn't time to address all of his communication issues, but the gains made transformed his sense of self from someone who was unattractive and isolated from his peers to someone who had friends and was likeable. His new experiences of connection set him on a trajectory of increasing confidence and openness to further extend and deepen his social network. As for all IPT-A clients, a crucial insight for Arjun was understanding the connection between his depression, the Problem Area(s) and his ongoing need to proactively seek connection with others.

## Working with significant others

With the young person's consent, the involvement of people who are important can streamline assessment and treatment.—parents, carers, teachers, grandparents, siblings, friends, and other people who are important to the client, know the young person well, and see her functioning in the day-to-day reality of their lives. The young person's significant others can play an important role in identifying Interpersonal Gaps, understanding the impact of the gaps on social functioning and determining how best to fill the gaps. In addition to providing helpful information, others may be actively involved in therapy sessions and assist the young person with skills practice activities outside therapy.

The perspective of the young person's significant others can provide a rich vein of information about his or her difficulties and strengths to extend or reinforce the therapist's hypothesises about the young person's social competencies and the most productive directions for therapy.

During the Initial Phase of IPT-A, parents, and sometimes other people, may be given information to help them understand the young person's difficulties and also the process of therapy. When others are to be involved in the Middle Phase of therapy, these earlier discussions can be briefly revisited. The rationale and parameters for this involvement will need to be explained and agreements sought. The therapist's updated hypothesis can also be discussed and the views of the others elicited. This will assist parents or others to understand the rationale for the work that will follow, motivate their support for the therapy, and place them in an informed position to assist the young person with skills practice. Consultation with parents and others may occur in session with the young person present, during separate meetings with the parent, or by phone. The involvement of other people is discussed in the chapters on the other Problem Areas. Some examples of therapist questions are included in Clinical tool 10.5 Questions for a young person's significant others about social competencies.

General and open-ended questions can be helpful in eliciting a broad range of information from people who are important to the young person regarding the young person's social skills. It can be helpful to ask about strengths as well as gaps. Requesting specific examples can assist the therapist in interpreting the information that is offered.

As with all lists of questions, they should be tailored to the individual's circumstances and used to guide discussion rather than create an experience resembling an interrogation. Some therapists may prefer to provide the young person's significant other with a copy of the list. Having the questions in front of them can facilitate a more equitable exchange and empower the other person to choose issues he or she would like to discuss. It may also help prevent a feeling of being grilled. Clinical tool 10.5 could also be adapted and utilised as a rating scale to be completed by the other person.

The capacity of the parent, or others, to play a supportive role in the young person's social skill development should be assessed. When they have an appropriate level of insight and sensitivity, they may be recruited to play the role of co-therapist to support the young person's skills practice activities outside therapy. Even people who are naturally very supportive will benefit from some brief education about how to perform this role well. Parents and others may benefit from the handout materials discussed above, including skill outlines and practice reports. Recommendations might include the following:

- provide teaching, coaching, and modelling to reinforce the specific work of therapy
- give positive feedback
- frame critical feedback in an encouraging manner

Sometimes the young person's Interpersonal Gaps are adversely affecting family dynamics. When this is the case, these issues can be directly addressed in therapy with parents or others. This is best done by keeping the focus on the young person's social skill development rather than on particular content issues. This approach is more likely to foster positive and collaborative discussion, whereas content issues may be partisan and tend to get bogged down in details, recrimination, and blame.

### Clinical Tool 10.5 Questions for a young person's significant others about social competencies

**General questions**

- How would you describe the way the young person interacts with other people?
- Please tell me about any concerns you have about the way the young person communicates?
- Have you observed any recurring patterns in the way the young person relates to others that seem to cause difficulties?
- What would you say are some of the strengths in the way the young person communicates with other people?
- What skills does the young person have in relationships?
- Could you give me an example of an interaction when you thought he or she communicated well?
- Can you recall a time when you could see he or she was struggling to communicate effectively?
- Does a situation come to mind where you could see he or she was misunderstanding someone else?
- Have you noticed times when you thought he or she was creating an impression in someone else that he or she did not intend? Can you give me an example?
- Have you observed any factors that seem to improve or reduce the young person's success in relationships? It might be things such as being tired, annoyed, or unsure. It could be things about the other person or about the situation.

**Specific social competencies**

How would you rate the young person's ability to do the following:

- tell other people when he or she is upset?
- help other people understand how he or she feels?
- help other people understand what he or she wants or needs?
- tell a story in an interesting way?
- show interest in others?
- understand other people's needs?
- ask for clarification?
- ask for help?
- speak up when being treated unfairly?
- make an appropriate amount of eye contact when talking with someone?
- introduce him- or herself to someone new?
- initiate a conversation?
- join an existing conversation?
- give compliments?
- receive compliments?
- respond to negative feedback or criticism?
- give negative feedback or criticism constructively?
- accurately perceive other people's emotions?

## Summary

For young people experiencing Interpersonal Gaps, their adolescence can be a litany of social failure. They are often baffled by their lack of success in their interpersonal communication and their isolation can be reinforced by experiences of social exclusion, humiliation, and bullying.

Although progress in helping young people with Interpersonal Gaps can be slow, gaps in social competencies during adolescence tend to be more amenable to change compared to when these gaps occur in adults. Given the time-limited nature of IPT-A, it is particularly important that work on this Problem Area is guided by thorough assessment so that it is effectively focused on where it will achieve most benefit. It is encouraging to note that for most of these young people even modest increases in their social skills can change the momentum of their lives, bringing a sense of hope for further improvement. This is often sufficient to improve their symptoms. Early intervention brings further good news. The sooner the gaps are identified and plugged, the less damage will be done to young people's life trajectory, the quicker they will achieve healthy functioning, and the more resilient they will be to future challenges.

## References

Crosby, G. (2015). *Fight, flight freeze: Taming your reptilian brain and other practical approaches to self-improvement*. (2nd ed.). Seattle, WA: Crosby OD Publishing.

Del Prette, A., & Del Prette, Z. A. P. (2009). *Inventory Social Skills for Adolescents (IHSA-del-prette): Application manual, apuração e interpretação*. Brazil: Psychologist's House.

D'Zurilla, T., Nezu, A., & Maydeu-Olivares, T. (2002). *Social problem-solving inventory—Revised (SPSI-R): Technical manual*. North Tonawanda, NY: Multi-Health System.

D'Zurilla, T., Chang, E., Nottingham, E., & Faccini, L. (1998k). Social problem-solving deficits and hopelessness, depression, and suicidal risk in college students and psychiatric inpatients. *Journal of Clinical Psychology*, 54(8), 1091–1107.

Gresham, F., & Elliott, S. (2008). *Social skills improvement system: Rating scales*. Bloomington, MN: Pearson Assessments.

Kipling, R. (1900). *The elephant's child, Ladies Home Journal*. http://www.kiplingsociety.co.uk/rg_elephantschild1.htm

Lasgaard, M., Goossens, L., & Elklit, A. (2011). Loneliness, depressive symptomatology, and suicide ideation in adolescence: cross-sectional and longitudinal analyses. *Journal Abnormal Child Psychology*, 39(1), 137–150.

Luft, J., & Ingham, H. (1955). The Johari window, a graphic model of interpersonal awareness. *Proceedings of the Western Training Laboratory in group development*. Los Angeles: University of California, Los Angeles.

McGinnis, E., Sprafkin, R., Gershaw, N., & Klein, P. (2011). *Skillstreaming the adolescent: A guide for teaching prosocial skills*. Research Press.

Mufson, L., Moreau, D., Weissman, M., & Klerman, G. (1993). *Interpersonal psychotherapy for depressed adolescents*. New York: The Guilford Press.

Mufson, L., Dorta, K., Moreau, D., & Weissman, M. (2004). *Interpersonal psychotherapy for depressed adolescents (2nd Edition)*. New York: The Guilford Press.

Riggio, R., & Carney, D. (2003). *Manual for the Social Skills Inventory* (2nd ed.). Redwood City, CA: MindGarden.

Segrin, C. (2000). Social skills deficits associated with depression. *Clinical Psychology Review, 20*(3), 379–403.

Wallen, J. (1967). *The Interpersonal Gap*. Mimeographed paper, Portland, Oregon: Northwest Regional Educational Laboratory.

# Part IV
# Consolidation Phase of IPT-A

# 11 Conclusion of Acute Treatment

| Contents | |
|---|---|
| The Consolidation Phase of IPT-A | 315 |
| The four primary tasks of Conclusion of Acute Treatment | 316 |
| *Stepping back from the role of transitory attachment figure* | 316 |
| *Facilitate independent functioning* | 320 |
| *Recognise early warning signs of relapse* | 326 |
| *Assess the need for further treatment* | 329 |
| Summary | 329 |
| References | 329 |

## The Consolidation Phase of IPT-A

The American Academy of Child and Adolescent Psychiatry published its *Practice Parameters for the Assessment and Treatment of Children and Adolescents with Depressive Disorders* in 2007 (Birmaher et al., 2007). Recommendation 10 of these parameters suggested "in order to consolidate the response to acute treatment and avoid relapses, treatment should always be continued for 6 to 12 months" and "to avoid recurrences, some depressed children and adolescents should be maintained in treatment for longer periods of time" (Birmaher et al., 2007, pp. 1517–1518). Clinical practice as well as these practice parameters suggest that IPT-A should be conceptualised as a two-staged treatment, in which the acute stage of treatment focuses on the resolution of immediate symptoms and distress and a subsequent Continuation and Maintenance Phase follows with the aims of preventing relapse and maintaining gains made in interpersonal functioning. The Consolidation Phase was originally called the Termination Phase (Mufson et al., 1993; Mufson et al., 2004). However, treatment does not normally terminate at this juncture. Whilst IPT-A remains a time-limited treatment—the notion of an end point theoretically drives both client and therapist to work more rapidly on resolving symptomatology and improving interpersonal skills—the end of the acute phase does not mean the end of treatment. Chapter 11 of Section 4 describes the Conclusion of Acute Treatment. Chapter 12 outlines the factors that need to be considered prior to making decisions about future treatment and then describes Continuation and Maintenance Therapy within an IPT-A context.

In the Consolidation Phase, the therapist has five primary tasks:

1   To step back from the role of transitory attachment figure
2   To facilitate independent functioning through assisting the young person to internalise and generalise the psychosocial goals made in treatment to date
3   To prepare the young person and the parents or caregivers to recognise early warning signs of relapse or recurrence and build a plan to deal with this, should it eventuate
4   To assess the need for and implement Continuation and Maintenance Therapy
5   To implement Continuation and Maintenance Therapy when indicated.

The first four of these tasks are addressed in Chapter 11, Conclusion of Acute Treatment; Task 5 is addressed in Chapter 12, Continuation and Maintenance.

## The four primary tasks of Conclusion of Acute Treatment

### Stepping back from the role of transitory attachment figure

It has been noted throughout this book and elsewhere (e.g., Mallinckrodt and Jeong, 2015) that during therapy with young people, the therapist takes on the role of transitory attachment figure. During the Consolidation Phase, the therapist begins the process of stepping back from this role and collaboratively begins to identify significant others in the young person's life who could, over time, take on some of the roles the therapist has played during the intervention. That is, if the therapist played the role of nurturer or listener, who in the young person's Closeness Circles could be enlisted to perform these roles? Secondly, what steps can the young person take to initiate this process?

In the example below, **Erin,** a 16-year-old (who was introduced in Chapter 4), recognized that the therapist played the roles of listener and clarifier. Erin and the therapist together explored her interpersonal world in attempt to identify others who could take on at least some of these roles.

*Therapist:*   Erin, while we've been working together, you've shared some pretty personal things about your thoughts and feelings after you found out about your colour blindness. We're getting towards the end of our time together now—only three sessions after today—and you've been telling me you are quite a bit better. I'm just wondering what you've found most helpful in our time together.

*Erin:*   Don't know really. Maybe just that someone finally took me seriously. And maybe also seeing the depression as a tunnel I could eventually

Conclusion of Acute Treatment 317

*come out of. Although I didn't believe you at first.* (Erin paused for a while and the therapist allowed the silence to continue.) *Also I think just being able to talk about stuff cleared some things up for me. Like I told you I was lonely and that sucked but I just didn't have the energy to talk to people. And they were opposites really. And maybe just talking that through made me see that I wouldn't be lonely forever.*

*Therapist:* Let's have another look at your Closeness Circles. Now that you are feeling a bit better, are there people there who you think would take you seriously and also would talk things through with you? Like we've been doing?

*Erin:* Yeah, of course. Dallas. Plus Mum, really.

*Therapist:* When you first drew up your circles, Mum was in your centre circle and Dallas was in the next one out. And you told me both of them were in the centre circle before you got depressed. Have there been any changes over the last few weeks?

*Erin:* Well Mum's still there, and I am actually talking to her more now. And Dallas is heading that way as well. He's almost there, come to think of it.

*Therapist:* I'm really pleased to hear that Erin. So let's pick one of them and think of a conversation you could possibly have with either Dallas or Mum, where those two things happen: you get taken seriously and you talk things through.

In the above dialogue the focus returned to Erin's interpersonal resources via the Closeness Circles. She saw her mother in the centre circle, noted they had resumed meaningful conversations, and noted also that Dallas was returning to his former central place in her life. Erin also conceded that both Dallas and her mother had begun taking her seriously and could talk things through with her. This reflects a significant shift in therapy that occurred during recent sessions. In the Consolidation Phase, these shifts are consciously marked and embedded into the client's interpersonal repertoire. While this is happening, the therapist is deliberately identifying other people who can provide the things the client found helpful in therapy. In Erin's case, the therapist explicitly steps back from the role of being the only person who was taking her seriously and talking things through with her, whilst helping Erin enlist Dallas and her mother to take on these roles.

Erin's affect in relation to these changes should also be acknowledged and monitored as this role transfer occurs. In the above dialogue, the final statement heralded a staged conversation in the therapy room where Erin engaged either Dallas or her Mum in role play conversation (or empty chair). The aims of this are the following:

- to give Erin more confidence in identifying and making her attachment needs known
- to familiarise her with feelings she might encounter in this process
- to hypothesise about the thoughts and feelings Dallas and her mother might experience during the encounter.

| | |
|---|---|
| Therapist: | We've used the empty chair a few times before. So maybe you picture your Mum on the chair this time? |
| Erin: | Yeah, she's wearing those 1990s jeans she had on last time she was here and a red top. She looks more disorganized than usual. |
| Therapist: | That's great Erin. You're becoming an experienced empty chairer! So could you swap chairs and be Mum for a bit? (Erin swaps chairs.) |
| Therapist: | (To Erin playing Mum.) Thanks for being here, Julie. Erin's doing so much better than she was when you were here last. |
| Erin: | (As Mum.) About time! I've noticed some differences. She's having dinner with us more now and seeing more of her friends. I suppose that's good. |
| Therapist: | Erin, how do you think Mum might be feeling now? |
| Erin: | Mostly relieved, but maybe a bit suspicious it's only temporary. |
| Therapist: | What do you want to say to Mum? |
| Erin: | (Changes chairs.) I hope you finally get how depressed I was before and that I didn't want to live anymore. |
| Therapist: | How's Mum feeling now? |
| Erin: | I'll ask her. (Changes chairs.) |
| Erin: | (as Mum) God, Erin, I didn't know it was that bad! |
| Therapist: | So how is Mum feeling? |
| Erin: | (Out of role.) I think she's feeling pretty guilty she didn't get it earlier. And she's crying again. I think she's beginning to get it. I feel sorry for her. |
| Therapist: | You feel sorry for her. Anything else? |
| Erin: | I guess it feels good to know she's beginning to realise how bad it was. |
| Therapist: | Okay, let's forget about the chairs for a minute. A couple of things there. You were able to tell Mum how bad things were for you and that you are feeling a bit better now. You think Mum is understanding that more now and it feels pretty good to be understood. You suggested Mum might even feel guilty for not getting it earlier. And you felt sorry for Mum. Now these are the kinds of things we have been having conversations about over the last few weeks, the kinds of things that have helped you feel better—being taken seriously and talking stuff over. But this time it was a conversation with Mum, not me. What are your thoughts? |

This dialogue transparently introduced the notion that conversations with her mother about Erin's depression could contain the same ingredients as conversations with the therapist: ingredients that contributed to Erin's improvement. The therapist has paved the way to step back, encouraging Erin to allow her mother to take over some of the attachment behaviours previously utilised by the therapist.

Whilst Erin's attachment style was secure, 19-year-old Ali (introduced in Chapter 4) demonstrated avoidant dismissive characteristics, and, as indicated previously, the pace of interpersonal change was managed accordingly.

By Conclusion of Acute Treatment, Ali had moved two friends from her outer circle to the middle circle.

*Therapist:* Ali, we've had eight sessions together and after today we have three left, before we decide what to do next. So we're reaching that time where we focus more on putting what we've done together in therapy into day to day practice outside therapy. First, though, you've told me your depression is quite a bit better now—you're sleeping better, your mood has improved from about 2/10 to about 6/10 on average, and you're seeing a bit more of your friends. I'm just wondering, from our time together, what have you found most helpful?

*Ali:* I think I've learnt to look at the evidence rather than rely on my feelings all the time. Especially around my friends. I used to think they all hated me, but when I looked at it there was no reason for me to believe that. But it's been like a battle between my feelings and my thoughts.

*Therapist:* So exploring that battle has been helpful?

*Ali:* Well, I'd never considered looking at the evidence before, so yeah, it was like the other side of the coin.

*Therapist:* I remember numerous conversations we've had about feelings and thoughts—we often called them the heart versus head dilemma. I'm glad you found that way of looking at things helpful, and I think it might be useful if those conversations continued.

*Ali:* Me, too.

*Therapist:* Remember a couple of sessions ago you were surprised to find after you let Bree into your life a bit more that not only did she call you a few times, but you also felt closer to her? Have you reached that level in your relationship with her where you could have conversations about the heart versus head dilemma?

*Ali:* Well we already have, sort of. She really gets it. She's a lot like me, only more so. She overthinks everything; she lives in her head. I was telling her about evidence and when she's overthinking, to look at evidence for and evidence against what she's stressing about. We started over the phone, but we had coffee last week and talked for hours.

*Therapist:* How was that for you?

*Ali:* Good, really. I think I helped her see things more realistically.

*Therapist:* You said "good". Can you help me understand that a bit more?

*Ali:* Well, it's pretty simple. We talked for a while. I enjoyed the conversation and Bree found it helpful.

*Therapist:* That's great, Ali. Help is a two-way street. You helped her and you felt good about it as well. That's a win-win. Are you going to see more of Bree?

*Ali:* Guess so. And Sophia as well. And I'm working up the courage to phone Mark.

Ali had already begun to use her friends to meet some of the attachment needs her therapist had previously been meeting. In the above dialogue, the therapist recognised this fact and then planned to continue to monitor Ali's progress with her friends session by session, whilst himself deliberately staging a withdrawal from fulfilling this role. As Ali's attachment behaviours are dismissive, the aim of this stage of treatment acknowledges her primary self-reliance but acknowledges also that her depression was related to ruptures within her interpersonal world. Being hated by one's friends may be noxious even to the most compulsively self-reliant young person. For Ali, the shift from being hated by to being helpful to her friends felt "good" and was emblematic of a shift in her depressive symptomatology.

Therapist: *We've talked quite a bit about how important it is for you to be emotionally self-sufficient—I think your words were you like to be a solo traveller. And we also worked out that even though being a solo traveller is important to you, there are times when having others around is very important in your life.*

Ali: *That seems to be a contradiction. But yeah, sometimes even solo travellers need company.*

Therapist: *I think we agreed your depression began at a time when you did need that company, but it just wasn't there. And over recent weeks you discovered two things: one, there are times in your life when having others around is really important, and, two, you discovered, or you're in the process of discovering, how to make that happen.*

Ali: *Looking at the circles, Bree and Sophie have already moved from there to there* (Ali pointed first to the outer of the three Closeness Circles, then to the middle circle) *and once Mark shifts in from out there* (Ali indicates a point outside the circles altogether), *that will make a difference.*

The second Primary Task of Conclusion of Acute Treatment is facilitating independent functioning.

## Facilitate independent functioning

Mufson et al. (2004) identify several tasks the therapist completes during what they term the "Termination Phase" prior to evaluating the need for Continuation and Maintenance Therapy. These tasks are aimed at assisting the young person to incorporate the psychosocial gains made during therapy into his or her behavioural repertoire (internalising). The therapist will assist the young person to apply these gains when confronted with psychosocial challenges in his or her interpersonal world that occur outside the therapy room (generalising). These tasks are accomplished while still focusing on the Problem Area(s) identified in the Initial Phase.

*Task 1. Elicit feelings in the young person about ending therapy*

In general, IPT-A sessions are held weekly (or as close to weekly as possible) during the Initial and Middle Phases of therapy but are titrated out during the Consolidation Phase. For example, if the young person has responded to therapy and there has been a significant reduction in depressive symptoms, in the Conclusion of Acute Treatment sessions may be scheduled at two-weekly, then three-weekly, monthly, or longer intervals during Continuation and Maintenance. There are several reasons for this, but perhaps the most salient is that the longer time frame between sessions gives the client extended opportunities to incorporate more of the psychosocial skills into his or her behavioural repertoire. Also, the longer intervals between sessions decreases the reliance of the client on the therapist and paves the way for more independent functioning. IPT-A is a transparent intervention and, consistent with this, this process is discussed with the client and the time-spacing of sessions is worked out collaboratively. As part of this, the client's feelings about the imminent end of the intervention are canvassed. The therapist will remind the young person that the acute phase of therapy is coming to an end before long and enquire how the client feels about this.

For example, **Ethan**, aged 16, was nearing the end of treatment. He had been referred by his parents after he seemed "more withdrawn than usual" and his parents had noted significant depressive symptomatology. His attachment behaviours indicated an avoidant style, with characteristics from both dismissive and fearful dimensions. His Problem Area was quite clearly Interpersonal Disputes, and he typically defaulted to a Withdrawal style when confronted with social problems.

*Therapist:* Ethan, this is our ninth session, and after today we have three sessions left, then we decide what to do next. I think you've come a fair way in our time together, but we do have to end soon. How do you feel about that?

*Ethan:* Dunno.

*Therapist:* I seem to remember that not wanting to talk about how you were feeling had a pretty big impact on the problems you were having with your folks and also on your depression. You might leave here today thinking there were things you wanted to say.

*Ethan:* Maybe.

*Therapist:* We talked about paying attention to how you were feeling—then trying to put that into words. So taking a bit more time to think, how do you feel about ending our time together?

*Ethan:* Dunno. (Pause). Maybe glad not to have to come anymore ... but maybe a bit worried this new stuff won't work.

In this dialogue, the therapist gained some understanding about two matters. First, Ethan is ambivalent about ending treatment; second, although Ethan tends to revert to his default position of noncommunication, he has developed some capacity, when encouraged to do so, to connect with and communicate feeling states. Both of these issues would become foci in the remaining weeks of the intervention.

Eliciting feelings about the end of treatment will also assist the therapist in the process of stepping back from the role of transient attachment figure. In cases like Ethan's where the attachment style is avoidant, this task often involves identifying other people who may be able to offer the kind of instrumental assistance the therapist has offered the young person during therapy. For these clients, the therapist has often been a source of relationship information, assisting the young person through direct techniques, modelling, and coaching to learn interpersonal strategies that help the client achieve relationship outcomes. Who else can provide at least some of this and how can the young person enlist significant others in this process? These questions would be transparently addressed during this phase of treatment.

In the case of young people with preoccupied attachment style, their response to enquiries about therapy approaching the end often indicates a developing dependence on the therapist (or on the process of therapy), which must be addressed more assertively. With these young people, rather than a focus on the help others may provide, the focus becomes identifying others who may provide the affective support they experienced during the intervention, while the therapist strategically retreats from this role. To accomplish this retreat, it is helpful for the therapist to return to the Affiliation, Inclusion, and Dominance paradigm described in Chapter 4. The focus would be on reducing Affiliation, keeping Inclusion high, and managing the power dynamic of the Dominance dimension so that the young clients build appropriate power in their interpersonal lives and concede power in the therapeutic alliance as the therapist gradually but deliberately reduces affective support.

For all clients, irrespective of attachment style, the therapist will be on the lookout for the young person's reaction to ending treatment. The therapist should acknowledge these thoughts and feelings (for example, apprehension, fear, sadness, anger, gladness) and ask for feedback from the client about what he or she has found effective and what hasn't worked as well. The therapist explains to the client that a return of symptoms sometimes occurs around ending acute treatment and isn't necessarily a sign of relapse.

*Task 2. Review remaining symptoms*

Depression is a recurring phenomenon in adolescence. Some estimates are that if untreated, depression returns about 45% of the time within two years and about 73% of the time within five years (Rey and Birmaher, 2009). These recurrences will be addressed later in the chapter. The purpose of the present task is to review the signs or symptoms of this particular episode that have not abated during the intervention and place them within the context of improvements that have occurred. This will help the young person focus on the gains made whilst alerting the therapist and the young person to further work that might be needed.

In the example that follows, **Kylie**, aged 14, was referred for therapy following a suicide attempt. She endorsed significant depressive symptomatology that was associated with moderate to severe distress and impairment in both social and cognitive functioning. A trigger for her depression was losing two friends in a motor vehicle accident. Kylie's Problem Area was identified as Complex Grief. She was securely attached.

*Therapist:* *Kylie, can you try and remember how you felt when we first started together? I mean, do you remember the reason you came here for therapy?*
*Kylie:* *Well, I'd taken those tablets and I was crying all the time.*
*Therapist:* *Yeah ... and do you remember any of the other symptoms we talked about?*
*Kylie:* *Not sleeping, doing crap at school, and some other stuff.*
*Therapist:* *Okay. And I remember the bad time you were having with your Mum and some friends ... do you remember that?*
*Kylie:* *Yeah.*
*Therapist:* *We worked out all these things seemed to start or at least got much worse after that car accident where Johnny and Mel died. We worked out that a lot of your depression was linked to losing those friends who were so important to you.*
*Kylie:* *(Silent)*
*Therapist:* *So since we started meeting together, how have things changed for you?*
*Kylie:* *(Pause) Well, I can think about Johnny and Mel now without tearing up all the time. And I'm not as irritable with my teachers at school. Or Mum. But I'm still not sleeping too well—better, but not good yet.*
*Therapist:* *And you were sad most of the time?*
*Kylie:* *I'm still sad, but not all the time now.*
*Therapist:* *So as time goes on, some of the symptoms of your depression seem to be lessening a bit. You're not as sad all the time, you're sleeping a bit better and you're not as irritable with your teachers. I'm wondering what's happening to some of the other thoughts and feelings. Most weeks I ask you about the thoughts you had about killing yourself and they don't seem as strong now ... and last week we talked about the trouble you were having concentrating on your schoolwork? How's that now?*
*Kylie:* *I still can't concentrate. Especially on my homework. It's still like I'm trying to think through a fog.*

In this dialogue, the therapist began to identify symptoms that had ameliorated and then explored symptoms that were still problematic. Following this, the therapist and young person would collaboratively construct a list that identifies symptoms that have significantly improved and those that need more work. This has the dual purpose of highlighting for the client that improvement has occurred but also acknowledging there was still a way to go. This task sets a path for the remainder of sessions that is clear to both therapist and young person, but within the context of markers of improvement: positive changes that have already occurred.

## Task 3. Recognise interpersonal competencies

Next, the interpersonal competencies that have been associated with symptom reduction are identified. The therapist reviews (1) the initial goals of treatment and (2) the progress made and strategies learned with a view toward independent application of these strategies by the young person in the future. Interpersonal competencies will vary from client to client and can be influenced by symptomatology, Problem Area, attachment style, and the young person's social network.

In the following example, **Rachel**, a 19-year-old university student with preoccupied attachment was referred by her general practitioner following family breakup. Rachel was the eldest of three children and prior to her parents separating had been mainly left to her own devices at home. Her only responsibilities, apart from some household jobs, were to take care of her younger sisters when her parents were at work. Following the breakup, Rachel continued to live with her mother and sisters and had accepted some extra babysitting responsibilities. She visited her father on average about twice a month and took phone calls from him at least weekly. She developed anxious-depressive symptoms that she attributed to listening to both parents criticise and belittle the other and often having to act as a mediator or arbitrator between them.

*Therapist:* Rachel, the Problem Area that we identified at the beginning of therapy that seemed most closely linked to your anxiety and depression was Role Transition. You started feeling sad and anxious not long after Dad left home, and you suddenly found yourself having to act like a referee between your Mum and your Dad. That was a new job for you and it seemed an impossible one, and one that you didn't like much at all. We both believed your depression and anxiety were linked to this. Do you remember what our goals were for the IPT-A?

*Rachel:* I remember we had to work out how to get from the way things were, when Mum and Dad were together, to the way things are now. Like a journey.

*Therapist:* Yeah, we had to work out how you could best let go of some of the things from before—like all the family being home in the one place—and then learn some things that would help you adjust to the new situation with your Mum and Dad living separately. Can you tell me some of the things that you've tried that have helped with this?

*Rachel:* Well, I told Mum I didn't want her to criticize Dad all the time. I told Dad the same. That's a bit better now.

*Therapist:* How did you tell them that?

*Rachel:* I just said to Mum I wish she wouldn't say that stuff about Dad. I think she stopped because she knew it was making things worse for me. Same with Dad.

Conclusion of Acute Treatment   325

*Therapist:*   So talking to Mum and Dad directly made a difference. That's great, Rachel. Can you think of another situation where telling people about things that are hard for you might make a difference?

In this exchange, the therapist affirmed Rachel's use of a strategy they had discussed in therapy and, in asking about other situations where this strategy may also be helpful, began the process of helping Rachel to identify how she might use this skill in other interactions. In this phase of therapy, the therapist first attempts to make the newly learned strategies a natural part of the client's behavioural repertoire (that is, to internalise these strategies) and, second, helps the young person explore other situations where this strategy may also be effective—that is, to generalise these newly learned interpersonal strategies. As the new role of being a member of a separated family becomes less daunting for Rachel, the therapist continues the process of linking the use of these strategies in everyday life to a reduction in the symptomatology of Rachel's anxiety and depression.

Another example that illustrates this task is the case of **Meg**, a 16-year-old whose Problem Area was Interpersonal Gaps. Meg had a brittle sense of self, and although she craved the attention of others, she was never certain about their availability. Her attachment style was avoidant fearful. Meg had become increasingly anxious about being rejected by her peers. It transpired that Meg had little difficulty initiating relationships, but these tended not to last long as she became quite angry and aggressive when people disagreed with her. As a consequence, friends and family reportedly stopped wanting to be with her and some actively avoided her. Until therapy, Meg had not recognised this characteristic that was quite obvious to others in her interpersonal world. Although Meg could initiate relationships, she had great difficulty maintaining them.

During the course of therapy, Meg had begun to recognise that her aggression was driving people away. Her therapist had used role play and the empty chair technique to demonstrate the effect of Meg's behaviour on others, to model more appropriate responses, to teach her strategies that would help her catch her anger early, and then to choose a more appropriate response. Meg was encouraged to rehearse these new strategies in session, attend to and discuss her affect with the therapist, and then practice the responses with "safe others" (usually her mother and brother) between sessions. The following dialogue took place in the ninth session of treatment.

*Therapist:*   At the beginning of our time together, we worked out that at least part of your anxiety was linked to feeling angry and aggressive when someone disagreed with you. Over the months before you started therapy, you had become quite anxious because you felt no one liked you anymore. One of the things we practiced during the last few sessions was how to be in a situation where someone didn't agree with you and for you not to get angry. You learned really well how to stay calm. Now, I want you to pretend it is me who is the one getting angry. I want you to teach me how to stay calm. Is that okay?

Following this role reversal, the therapist and Meg had a conversation that included identifying the steps Meg had used in order to teach the therapist how to stay calm. These steps were listed and typed up for Meg to take away. The conversation then turned to eliciting real-life examples where Meg had found this strategy effective and also situations where she was less successful. The effective examples were examined to identify how and why they were successful, and the less effective examples were also examined to discover what went wrong and what could be done differently to secure a more optimal outcome. The empty chair technique was used to help Meg explore her own affect and the likely affect others experienced for both the unsuccessful and the successful examples. In the following session, Meg was encouraged to consider other situations in her interpersonal interactions where this strategy of staying calm might produce desirable outcomes. Meg was surprised to discover she had developed such a powerful and transferable interpersonal competency.

*Task 4. Markers of improvement*

In the early sessions of acute treatment, the therapist will have alerted the young person to be looking for markers of improvement.

*Therapist:* *During our time together, we'll be constantly looking for signs that your depression is improving. You might notice signs such as improved mood, better sleep, being able to think a bit more clearly, getting on better with friends and family, that sort of thing. There'll be things that you notice, things your parents notice, things your friends notice about you, and things that I notice as well. We'll be paying special attention to these. They are signs of change.*

The attention to markers of improvement shifts the focus from the negative life experiences of depression to the fact that change is occurring. Often small variations are easily overlooked, but the continued focus on these markers clusters them together. By the Consolidation Phase, there should be sufficient markers to clearly demonstrate to the young person that his or her depression and associated improvements in interpersonal competencies have both shifted in the direction of independent functioning. The Consolidation Phase offers the opportunity to examine and celebrate these changes and, as noted above, to continue the process of assisting the client to internalise and generalise these interpersonal competencies in order to reduce the distress and impairment associated with depressive symptomatology now and into the future.[1]

### Recognise early warning signs of relapse

With the young person's consent, it can be helpful to invite the parents or caregivers in for a session or part of a session towards the end of Conclusion of Acute Treatment. (A further session can also be scheduled towards the end of the Maintenance Phase, with similar aims.) The aims of these sessions are, first, to summarise gains made in symptom reduction and interpersonal competencies, and, second, to assist the young person and his or her parents or caregivers to be alert for changes that may indicate a recurrence and make plans about what to do if this happens. Both of these conversations will have been discussed with the young person first, so he or she won't be taken by surprise or even feel betrayed by the therapist, who has previously indicated that therapeutic conversations are confidential.

The summary of symptom reduction and gains in interpersonal competencies will reinforce these improvements for the young person and also help the parents or caregivers understand and recognise changes that have occurred in order for them to reinforce these changes at home. In addition, parents or caregivers will then be more prepared to notice reversions to depressed behaviour, should this occur.

The construction of Care Maps will assist young people and their parents watch for changes indicating that depression may be recurring and make plans about how to address this. This is a collaborative process between the young person and their parents, with minimal input from the therapist. The therapist can begin the process by introducing the Care Map in the following way:

**Bill**, aged 15, has an avoidant dismissive attachment. His Problem Area is Interpersonal Disputes. For Bill, increased stress was accompanied by increased conflict with others. Stress progressed into a major depressive episode.

Therapist: *We've just been talking about how well Bill has done over the last few months, and we're all looking forward to that continuing. Depression does come back for some young people, though, and I'd like to make some plans for what to do if this happens. It's really important to recognise the early warning signs so we don't have to wait for things to get as bad as they were for Bill before we began therapy together.*

*We're going to construct a Care Map. A Care Map is two lists. On one, I'm going to ask the three of you to write down all the early warning signs you can think of: things that were going wrong for Bill when his depression began, including any triggers you are aware of that may have made his depression worse. Then make another list of anything you can think of that has helped in the past or may help in the future. Bill and I have had lots of conversations about things he finds helpful, and some of those things will be on that list. Is that okay? So, thinking back to when Bill was unwell, what do you think may have triggered his depression, and what changes did you first notice?*

The conversation between Bill and his parents identified triggers and changes in his behaviour that alerted them to the fact that Bill was becoming depressed. These are recorded on the left column of Figure 11.1.

The conversation then turned to things that may help if the depressive signs and symptoms returned. Figure 11.1 records (1) early warning signs and (2) things that will help, developed in session by Bill and his parents.

It is important to note that as Bill's attachment style was dismissive, many of the items in the "Things that will help" column are functional rather than

| Early warning signs | Things that will help |
| --- | --- |
| • Trouble getting to sleep | • Catch my negative thoughts early and |
| • Overthinking everything | don't let them keep them going |
| • Fighting with Angela | • Listen to music when I can't sleep |
| • Not wanting Angela to touch me | • Have short breaks from Angela, but tell |
| • Fighting with Mum and Dad | her I still want to hang out with her |
| • Fighting with teachers | • Mum and Dad not to fight back |
| • Not wanting to go to football training | • Tell Mum and Dad that things are not |
| • Being irritable | going well |
| • Feeling there's no point in anything | • Check my meds with my doctor |
| • Hating school more than usual | • Take a few days off school |
| • Just wanting to be alone | • Catch stress early and go to the beach |
| • Feeling lonely and no one cares | • It's okay to miss footy training from time to |
| • Stressing about everything | time, no need to feel guilty |
| • Sick of everything | • Go back to therapy |

*Figure 11.1* Bill's Care Map.

relational. He did, however, identify several relational factors as potentially helpful: the importance of having short breaks from his girlfriend Angela, requesting Mum and Dad not to be combative, talking to his Mum and Dad when things were not going well, and returning to therapy. These strategies represented for Bill a huge shift in the direction of independent application of interpersonal competencies, things that were clearly missing at the beginning of therapy.

Bill and his parents constructed the above Care Map with the plan of taking it home, filing it in a drawer, and doing no more about it. But if Bill started to show any signs of stress that lasted more than a few days, he and his parents agreed to take the Care Map out to see if it offered any help in identifying early warning signs and, if so, plan appropriate action.

*The letter*

Clinical practice suggests that it is beneficial in the penultimate session of Conclusion of Acute Treatment, (that is, following the meeting with the parents or caregivers) for the therapist to request the client write a letter to the therapist that she will read aloud at the beginning of the final session. The therapist makes it clear that this is not a letter of thanks, but a register of the changes the young person has noticed in herself since therapy began. The therapist then tells the young person that he also will write a letter to the young person, noting what changes the therapist has noticed over the same time period. The final session then begins with the young person reading her letter out loud, followed by the therapist reading his. The remainder of this session is taken up discussing issues that arise from these letters. Typically, this activity provides another occasion to make interpersonal gains concrete and transferable and reinforces to the young person her capacity for independent functioning. The client gets to keep both letters.

### Assess the need for further treatment

The therapist's final task in Conclusion of Acute Treatment is, in collaboration with the young person, to plan for future treatment in order to consolidate the gains made to date and to prevent relapse. Chapter 12 describes Continuation and Maintenance therapy and suggests some parameters that may be helpful in this determination. The therapist and young person will discuss a new treatment agreement to accommodate this final stage of treatment.

## Summary

The Conclusion of Acute Treatment offers the therapist the opportunity to:

- address any dependence the young person may have developed on the therapist (or on therapy) by strategically retreating from the role of transitory attachment figure. This is achieved while maintaining a therapeutic alliance that may be reactivated if necessary.
- consolidate new interpersonal behaviours that the young person has developed during therapy, with a view toward independent functioning.
- assist the young person and parents to be alert for changes that may indicate increase risk of relapse (or a new episode) and develop plans to deal with these possibilities.
- assess the need for and plan the Continuation and Maintenance components of therapy. The therapist is assisted in this by the Response, Remission, and Recovery criteria discussed in Chapter 12.

## Note

1 The therapist strives for a correct balance between this positive focus whilst acknowledging the debilitating effects of the depression. The goal is for the young person to never feel that the therapist is minimising distress associated with his or her symptoms by a premature overemphasis on gains made.

## References

Birmaher, B., Brent, D., et al. (2007). Practice parameter for the assessment and treatment of children and adolescents with depressive disorders. *Journal of the American Academy of Child and Adolescent Psychiatry*, 46(11), 1503–1526.

Mallinckrodt, B., & Jeong, J. (2015). Meta-analysis of client attachment to therapist:

Associations with working alliance and client pre-therapy attachment. *Psychotherapy, 52,* 34–139.

Mufson, L., Moreau, D., Weissman, M., & Klerman, G. (1993). *Interpersonal psychotherapy for depressed adolescents.* New York: Guilford Press.

Mufson, L., Dorta, K., Moreau, D., & Weissman, M. (2004). *Interpersonal psychotherapy for depressed adolescents* (2nd Edition) New York: Guilford Press.

Rey, J. & Birmaher, B. (2009). *Treating child and adolescent depression.* New York: Wolters Kluwer.

# 12 Continuation and Maintenance Therapy

### Contents

| | |
|---|---|
| Continuation Therapy | 331 |
| Maintenance Therapy | 332 |
| Summary | 335 |

## Continuation Therapy

There is a growing body of research that suggests continuation and maintenance therapy significantly reduces relapse in adolescent depression. Kennard et al. (2016) and Kennard et al. (2008) report this in relation to pharmacological intervention. As noted in Chapter 11, the American Academy of Child and Adolescent Psychiatry (AACAP; Birmaher et al., 2007) recommends the treatment of child and adolescent depression should always include an Acute and a Continuation Phase and some young people may also require Maintenance Therapy. "The main goal of the acute phase is to achieve Response and ultimately full symptomatic Remission" (p. 1509). It may be helpful here to reflect on the terminology AACAP use in these parameters:

**Response.** No symptoms or significant reduction in depressive symptoms for at least two weeks

**Remission.** A period of at least two weeks but less than two months with no or few depressive symptoms

**Recovery.** Absence of significant symptoms of depression (that is, no more than one to two symptoms) for more than two months

**Relapse.** A DSM episode of depression during the period of *Remission*

**Recurrence.** The emergence of symptoms of depression during the *Recovery* period (that is, a new episode).

AACAP recommend all depressed young people require additional treatment to consolidate the *Response* to therapy that occurred during the Acute Treatment phase. Although not specifically demonstrated in IPT-A research to date, the recommendations from AACAP parameters would indicate that following *Response* to treatment, treatment should continue from six to twelve months. From an IPT-A perspective, these recommendations suggest that during the conclusion of Acute Treatment (usually after about ten to fourteen sessions), Continuation Therapy should be negotiated with the young person to accommodate the time frame recommended by AACAP.

In IPT-A the Initial and Middle Phases of treatment usually proceed over about eight sessions, which are as close to weekly as possible. The Consolidation Phase is often spaced out as outlined in Chapter 11, so these four to six sessions may stretch over two to three months. When planning Continuation Therapy, the therapist considers if the client has reached *Response*, *Remission*, or *Recovery* criteria. If *Response* or *Remission* criteria have been reached, the therapist negotiates a period of Continuation Therapy at least until *Recovery* criteria have been met. If *Recovery* has been reached, Continuation Therapy will be shorter or may proceed directly to Maintenance. Therefore, the timeframe of Continuation Therapy will depend on the young person's remaining symptomatology after Conclusion of Acute Treatment.

During Continuation Therapy the focus remains on the same Problem Area, usually at monthly intervals, continuing to consolidate the young person's psychosocial improvements and prevent *Relapse*.

The transition from Conclusion of Acute Treatment to Continuation is explicitly discussed with the young person and his or her parents or caregivers, and a new treatment agreement is negotiated. By this time, the therapist will have largely stepped back from the role of transitory attachment figure and continues to assist the young person to meet his or her attachment needs through improved interpersonal relationships.

## Maintenance Therapy

Whilst Continuation Therapy is relevant for young people who have residual symptomatology, Maintenance Therapy is relevant for all IPT-A interventions, even for young people who have achieved complete symptom resolution. The aim of Maintenance sessions is to provide continued support so that the interpersonal gains made during the acute (and continuation) phases of treatment are utilised by the young person in order to minimise the likelihood of *Remission* or *Recurrence*.

Maintenance sessions in IPT-A are scheduled less frequently than sessions in the Acute or Continuation Phases and are also usually less intense. These sessions are scheduled according to the needs of the young person, but typically will occur approximately every eight to twelve weeks. The three specific goals of Maintenance sessions are the following:

1   To maximise the young person's interpersonal functioning
2   To deal with new psychosocial problems that can be dealt with preventatively
3   To provide an ongoing therapeutic relationship that can be adapted should acute symptoms recur

Maximising the young person's interpersonal functioning involves a continuation of the twin tasks of assisting the young person to internalise and generalise the interpersonal strategies learned in the Acute Treatment phase. The original Problem Area remains the focus, and sessions will usually concentrate on reviewing Interpersonal Incidents that have gone well, in order to reinforce these strategies. Outside of therapy, these successes will largely go unnoticed by people who are important to the young person, so the client retelling these stories affords the therapist the opportunity to celebrate these successes and analyse the components of success.

For example, the dialogue in the preceding chapter with **Rachel** would be analysed further so she could understand how her conversation with her mother and father had the effect of reducing the difficulties associated with her Role Transition:

Rachel:     *I just said to Mum, I wish she wouldn't say that stuff about Dad. I think she stopped because she knew it was making things worse for me. Same with Dad.*

Therapist:  *So asking Mum and Dad directly made a difference. That's great, Rachel. Let's have a think about how that happened. Can you remember what you said to Mum?*

Rachel:     *I just said: "Don't say that, Mum! I just wish you and Dad wouldn't keep criticising each other all the time. I have to live with both of you, you know, and I hate it." I said a bit more but that was most of it.*

Therapist:  *So how did you feel when you said that?*

Rachel:     *Well I was pretty annoyed—they were doing it all the time.*

Therapist:  *And how do you think Mum felt?*

Rachel:     *Well, she went quiet, but she's been a bit better since.*

Therapist:  *Okay, so you told Mum how you feel when she was putting Dad down—you said you hate it—and you said you wish she'd stop it. And it was effective. So there were three ingredients there, do you see what they were?*

Rachel:     *Not really.*

Therapist:  *Well number one, you let Mum know how you were feeling (I hate it); number two, you let her know what it was she was doing that got you to feel that way (keep criticising Dad); and number three, you let her know how this could change (Don't say that, Mum). You were clear about those three things. I'm really proud of you, Rachel; that's the sort of thing we've been practicing in our sessions together and it worked well for you. So tell me those three ingredients again and we'll write them down.*

The above dialogue illustrates that the Maintenance Phase is not much different from Conclusion of Acute Treatment and Continuation Therapy. The focus shifts slightly, with the young person reporting interpersonal successes but now with an increased emphasis on analysing the ingredients of these successes. The therapist assists the young person to further understand how these new strategies contribute to a desired interpersonal outcome. In the case of Rachel, the therapist chose to "mark a moment" (see Chapter 4) by getting Rachel to write down the three components that were the key ingredients of her interpersonal success. Alongside this, the therapist continues to link improved interpersonal competencies with improvement in independent functioning and symptom reduction.

Therapist: *You're going really well, Rachel. Each time you use these new strategies, you'll get better at them. And I just want you to keep noticing how much better your anxiety and depression are getting as you're working out how to help people understand what is going on for you.*

In the Maintenance Phase, it is not uncommon for young people to present new psychosocial problems as they arise in everyday life. Most often they do not require acute intervention but instead provide the opportunity to reinforce the interpersonal learning that has already taken place. These new incidents offer the chance for the young person to generalise interpersonal competencies to other situations and other people. For example, the competencies Rachel demonstrated with her parents could equally be appropriately applied if problems arose with her peers, boyfriend, lecturers at university, or other people who are significant for her. The therapist would have a conversation with Rachel about how using these new competencies early in situations can prevent the normal distress of interpersonal problems from developing into abnormal distress or even symptomatology.

During Maintenance, particularly for clients with anxious attachment, the young person may present with interpersonal crises that he or she feels unable to manage. In some cases, these crises may precipitate a return of symptomatology. It may be necessary to return to Acute Treatment, possibly addressing another Problem Area, to effectively manage these situations. IPT-A thus becomes a modular therapy as illustrated in Figure 12.1. If it is necessary to return to the Middle Phase, the therapist will appropriately adjust the nature of the therapeutic relationship to reflect the attachment needs of the young person within the context of *Recurrence*. A new treatment agreement would be collaboratively drawn up to reflect this iteration of therapy.

At the conclusion of Maintenance Therapy, providing the young person and therapist are satisfied with symptom resolution and the degree of independent interpersonal functioning, treatment is complete. However, as noted in relation to Care Maps in Chapter 11, the young person is encouraged to be alert for signs

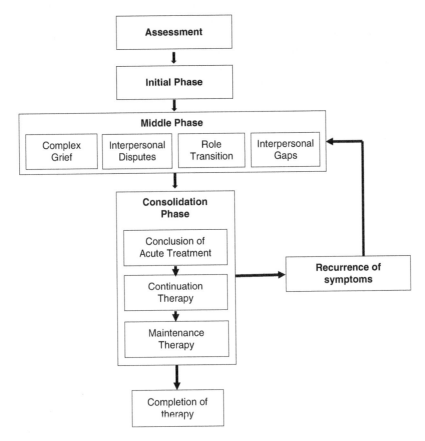

*Figure 12.1* IPT-A as modular therapy.

that symptoms may be returning and, should this occur, to seek further treatment. The young person is encouraged to return for further treatment if a new episode arises.

## Summary

In Continuation and Maintenance Therapy, the therapist continues to step back from the role of transitory attachment figure and, collaboratively with the young person, identifies others from the young person's interpersonal world who may fulfil roles the therapist previously occupied. Whilst accomplishing this objective, therapy proceeds with an ongoing focus on the identified Problem Area. Continuation Therapy will be offered to young people who have reached *Response* or *Remission* criteria, whilst Maintenance will be offered to all young people. By this stage of treatment, the young person will have developed new interpersonal capacities that have been associated with symptom reduction. Continuation and Maintenance Therapy aim to help the young person internalise these new capacities and generalise them so that they are available for future independent functioning, thus reducing the risk of future symptomatology. However, should the young person develop new symptomatology, the modular nature of IPT-A facilitates a return to Acute Treatment. Once symptomatology has resolved, therapy concludes.

## References

Birmaher, B., Brent, D., et al. (2007). Practice parameter for the assessment and treatment of children and adolescents with depressive disorders. *Journal of the American Academy of Child and Adolescent Psychiatry, 46(11)*, 1503–1526.

Kennard, B. D., Emslie, G. J., et al. (2008). Cognitive-behavioural therapy to prevent relapse in paediatric responders to pharmacotherapy for major depressive disorder. *Journal of the American Academy of Child and Adolescent Psychiatry, 47(12)*, 1395–1404.

Kennard, B., Hughes, J. & Foxwell, A. (2016). *CBT for depression in children and adolescents: A guide to relapse prevention.* New York: Guilford.

# Part V
# Closing thoughts

# 13 Closing thoughts

| Contents | |
|---|---|
| Increasing the reach of IPT-A | 339 |
| Practice-based evidence: Clinical implications | 340 |
| Dissemination of IPT-A | 341 |
| Summary | 342 |
| References | 342 |

IPT-A has been demonstrated to be an effective treatment for mental distress and symptomatology in adolescents. In these closing thoughts, we identify three areas for consideration that are relevant to IPT-A but that have not been addressed in the previous chapters: first, extending the reach of IPT-A into public policy; second, reflecting on *practice-based evidence* as an alternative way of thinking about IPT-A that may suggest additional clinical applications; and third, disseminating the practice of IPT-A.

## Increasing the reach of IPT-A

Therapy does not take place in a vacuum. It is a two-way process. The client's world affects therapy and therapy affects the client's world.

The goals of IPT-A are to reduce symptoms of mental distress by enhancing communication skills in significant relationships. In IPT-A, this is accomplished by assisting the young person to develop interpersonal competencies. As these competencies develop, attachment needs are more effectively met, symptoms diminish, and relationships may change. His or her significant others will also benefit from these positive changes. Thus, the impact of therapy stretches beyond the individual to the world outside.

The IPT research and clinical practice cited in this book provide evidence of the role of interpersonal support in mental health and wellbeing for young people. The work of therapy may also be supported by systems-level approaches to address relationship issues. However, these factors have been neglected in health and social policy relative to other key determinants of health and wellbeing such as smoking, alcohol consumption, obesity, and physical inactivity. Mental health professionals with expertise in interpersonal support have an important contribution to make in advocating the principles that inform interpersonal psychotherapy to play a more significant part of the public policy agenda to improve health outcomes for all young people. This is not the responsibility of therapists alone. Mental health outcomes for all might improve if those in positions to influence government and business practice were to factor in the costs of social isolation and adjust policy settings to promote community and work environments that foster supportive interpersonal relationships.

## Practice-based evidence: Clinical implications

We began writing this book in 2013 and for various reasons were delayed in finishing it. This is not the book that would have been published had we completed it earlier. In those intervening years, we learned so much more about IPT-A from clients, clinical work, and the supervision and training we do; from talking to other IPT and IPT-A practitioners; and from reading what others are doing in IPT-A. In completing this book, we are reminded almost daily of the many other instances when IPT-A can be used to help young people negotiate the stresses and strains that may accompany this phase of life. Two examples illustrate this.

1 Complex PTSD
   Three directions emerging independently from current literature may point to the potential usefulness of IPT-A for assisting young people with complex PTSD:

   a   Markowitz and others (Bleiberg and Markowitz, 2005; Markowitz, 2016) have demonstrated the effectiveness of IPT for adults with PTSD.
   b   Current clinical work with adolescents with complex PTSD is suggesting the effectiveness of Imagery Rescripting (ImRs) to manage this condition (Arntz et al., 2013).
   c   ICD 11 (Bottche et al., 2018) identifies three symptom-clusters that comprise complex PTSD: disturbances of affect, disturbances of sense of self, and disturbances in relational functioning.

   Together, these suggest that a combined approach in which ImRs addresses the disturbances of affect and sense of self and IPT-A addresses disturbance in relational functioning via the therapeutic alliance and Problem Area may be productive. Clinical evidence is already supporting the effectiveness of this approach and we await the researchers to see if this is also demonstrated in high-quality studies.

2   Non-suicidal self-injury
    Jacobson and Mufson (2012) reported the use of IPT-A for young people who are self-harming. Building on an interpersonal approach, Nock and Cha (2009) developed a model of conceptualising NSSI that focuses on the functions NSSI are serving for the young person. Their model suggests the functions of NSSI are either *intrapersonal*, for example, reducing toxic emotions (Wolff et al., 2019), and/or *interpersonal*, for example, communicating a need for help or understanding (Muehlenkamp et al., 2013; Victor et al., 2019). In the case of a young person who is self-harming and the NSSI is serving both of these functions, cognitive and schema-focused strategies targeting difficult emotions and core beliefs (*intrapersonal*) can be effectively utilised within a framework in which IPT-A addresses dysfunctional communication patterns (*interpersonal*).

Interpersonal psychotherapy had its origins in clinical practice. Many interventions, such as psychoanalysis, behaviourism, and cognitive therapy, began with the development of a theory and proceeded to clinical practice based on these theoretical underpinnings. IPT, on the other hand, originated when Klerman et al. (1984) stumbled upon a clinical intervention that worked, then spent years developing a theoretical framework around it. That is, theory followed practice. IPT and IPT-A are evolving in a similar manner. The practice-based evidence emerging from clinicians who regularly employ interpersonal psychotherapy consistently suggests the interpersonal framework can easily accommodate psychological skills and strategies derived from other interventions, provided the focus remains on the Problem Area, is attachment based, and occurs within a limited timeframe. This is good news for experienced clinicians as many of their existing clinical skills will be immediately transferable to the interpersonal framework. The two examples above attest to this, as do early studies in IPT-A that demonstrate experienced clinicians can learn IPT-A with relative ease (Mufson et al., 2004; Santor and Kusumakar, 2001). This evolution in IPT-A represents an exciting phase in the development of psychotherapy with young people as it provides greater scope for the clinician to match clinical expertise with the needs of the client. Outcomes from therapists using IPT-A suggest generalist and specific clinical skills are transferrable to an IPT-A framework to individualise treatment for adolescent clients.

All good psychotherapy derives its effectiveness from moving between what works in clinical practice and the research-supported theory that underpins it. Interpersonal Psychotherapy historically began with clinical effectiveness. The challenge now is for researchers to continue to test the efficacy and effectiveness of these ways of working to provide the necessary balance between evidence-based practice and practice-based evidence.

## Dissemination of IPT-A

Training and supervision in IPT-A occurs in a variety of formats. Some countries have been keen to ensure clinician fidelity to the evidence-based model of

IPT-A and have developed formalised accreditation guidelines. In other parts of the world, dissemination has been more informal.

Mufson et al. (2004) have shown IPT-A is relatively easily learned by experienced clinicians. Training in Australia and elsewhere has shown IPT-A is also valued by less experienced clinicians, not least due to the practical, concrete skills that they find are immediately transferable to their clinical work.

Our experience suggests that a two-day introductory training workshop familiarises participants with the theory, framework, and some of the techniques of IPT-A. This, followed by supplementary training, a clinician's guidebook, and supervision, is usually enough for clinicians to begin using IPT-A with clients.

Individual, group, and peer supervision can address clinician as well as agency needs. Guided peer supervision leverages the existing competencies of participants and assumes an ability to apply the IPT framework, at least to some extent, to their own cases and those of their colleagues. When issues are identified that are beyond the expertise of participants, an expert IPT supervisor is consulted. Group peer supervision, when occurring within staff teams, can also play an important teambuilding role. While face-to-face supervision is ideal, phone and video conferencing technology provides a useful alternative.

## Summary

In this book, we have outlined the application of IPT to adolescents and young adults and expanded the range of techniques that can effectively engage young people in the process. We have identified how clinicians can use their existing skills and incorporate them into IPT-A and have stressed the importance of a balance between the evidence arising from studies and evidence from clinical practice. We have also referred to a number of social interventions that can occur outside therapy to complement and support the direct work of the therapist with the young person.

Echoing the horticultural metaphor introduced in Chapter 6, IPT-A provides an accelerated hothouse atmosphere where young people learn to communicate their attachment needs more effectively and enhance their social support networks. Ensuring the growth made in this safe environment survives in the world outside therapy is a crucial task for the therapist, the young people, and their families. Macro level initiatives that assist society to recognise and respond in attuned ways to young people's needs for closeness and support will also assist the work of therapy and have a positive preventative influence.

## References

Arntz, A., Sofi, D., & van Breukelen, G. (2013). Imagery rescripting as treatment for complicated PTSD in refugees: A multiple baseline case series study. *Behaviour Research and Therapy*, 51(6), 274–283.

Bleiberg, K., & Markowitz, J. (2005). Interpersonal psychotherapy for posttraumatic stress disorder. *American Journal of Psychiatry, 162*, 181–183.

Bottche, M., Ehring, T., Kruger-Gottschalk, A., et al. (2018). Testing the ICD proposal for complex PTSD in trauma-exposed adults: Factor structure and symptom profiles. *European Journal of Psychotraumatology, 9*(1); Published online 2018, September 7.

Jacobson, C., & Mufson, L. (2012). Interpersonal psychotherapy for depressed adolescents adapted for self-injury (IPT-ASI): Rationale, overview, and case summary. *American Journal of Psychotherapy, 66*(4), 349–374.

Klerman, G., Weissman, M., Rounsaville, B., & Chevron, M. (1984). *Interpersonal psychotherapy for depression*. New York: Basic Books.

Markowitz, J. (2016). *Interpersonal psychotherapy for posttraumatic stress disorder*. New York: Oxford University Press.

Muehlenkamp, J., Brausch, A., Quigley, K., & Whitlock, J. (2013). Interpersonal features and functions of nonsuicidal self-injury. *Suicide and Life-Threatening Behavior 43*(1), 67–80.

Mufson, L., Dorta, K., Wickramaratne, P., Nomura, Y., Olfson, M., & Weissman, M. (2004). A randomized effectiveness trial of interpersonal psychotherapy for depressed adolescents. *Archives of General Psychiatry, 61*, 577–584.

Nock, M., & Cha, C. (2009). Psychological models of nonsuicidal self-injury. In M. K. Nock (Ed.), *Understanding nonsuicidal self-injury: Origins, assessment, and treatment* (pp. 65–77). Washington, DC: American Psychological Association.

Santor, D., & Kusumakar, V. (2001). Open trial of interpersonal therapy in adolescents with moderate to severe major depression: Effectiveness of novice IPT therapists. *Journal of the American Academy of Child and Adolescent Psychiatry, 40*(2), 236–240.

Victor, S., Hipwell, A., Stepp, S., & Scott, L. (2019). Parent and peer relationships as longitudinal predictors of adolescent non-suicidal self-injury onset. *Child and Adolescent Psychiatry and Mental Health, 13*(1), 2–13.

Wolff, J., Thompson, E., Thomas, S., Nesi, J., Bettis, A., Ransford, B., Scopelliti, K., Frazier, E., & Liu, R. (2019). Emotion dysregulation and non-suicidal self-injury: A systematic review and meta-analysis. *European Psychiatry, 59*, 25–36.

# Index

Aboriginal (Indigenous, First Nations) communities xii, 5; dominant culture effects on 31; eye contact in 284; multiple loss in 171; spirituality in 38
Acceptance and Commitment Therapy 111
activity-based therapy 198–202
acute treatment conclusion 319, 335f; communication of feelings about 321–322; compared to maintenance therapy 334; continuation therapy negotiation in 332; goals of 331–332; improvement markers before 326; penultimate session letters 328–329; primary tasks of 316–329; therapist opportunities 329; transition from to continuation 332
adolescents (young persons): attachment styles 52–55; attachment theory difficulties 51–52; characteristics of 51–52; conflict management for 102–104; cultural differences in understanding and expectations of 208; depression as recurring phenomenon in 322; disputes with parents 207; effects of oppression and abuse on 276; emotional swings in 82; hormonal changes 52; normal disputes with authority figures 208–209; as period of storm and stress 208; questioning of world 52; role transitions 241–276; sex, sexuality and gender identity as role transitions 265–266; social interactions and 279; stepped care for 7f; as transition experience 241–242
affiliation communication dimension (in therapeutic alliance) 76, 77, 322; attachment styles and 77; monitoring of 79f

Ainsworth, M. 52, 53, 54, 54f
American Academy of Child and Adolescent Psychiatry (AACAP) 315, 331; Practice Parameters for Anxiety Disorders 153; Practice Parameters for Depressive Disorders 153; terminology used by 331–332
anger chart 297–298, 300–301, 300f
anticipatory grief 182–183
antidepressants 154
anxious ambivalent style of attachment 52, 53; Clinicians Response Scale (CRS) and 67, 67t–68t
anxious avoidant style of attachment 52–53
Aquinas, Thomas 75
arc of therapy for complex grief 173f
Aristotle 208
assertiveness skills training 290
assessment 9, 10, 119, 335f.
 see also attachment theory, assessment of attachment styles; attachment styles as key factor in 145; holistic 12, 14, 56, 76, 155; of interpersonal gaps 281–285; as ongoing process 162; purposes 45; role transitions 243, 266–267
attachment theory: adolescents and 51–52; anxious ambivalent style 52, 53; anxious avoidant style 52–53; assessment and adaptation of behaviors 4; assessment of attachment styles 55–60; avoidant dismissive style 54, 54f; avoidant fearful style 54, 54f; basis of 50; clinical work based on xii; disorganised style 53; family structure of mental disorder and 28–29; four-dimensional model 53–55, 54f; hypothesis of young person 12; as integral part of IPT-A 49–50; needs of humans in 50; preoccupied style 53, 54f; quality of

narrative as indicator of attachment style 60–61; reaction to ending treatment 322; reasons for care in appraising attachment styles 55–56; secure style 52, 53, 54*f*; style as key factor in assessment and management 145; three-dimensional model 52–53; to understand clients' relationship to world 50; understanding of and influence on therapy 66–67
attention-deficit/hyperactivity disorder (ADHD) 290
Attig, T. 178
avoidant dismissive style of attachment 54, 54*f*; Clinicians Response Scale (CRS) and 67, 67*t*; suspicions of therapist's abilities 77
avoidant fearful style of attachment 54, 67, 54*f*, 67*t*–68*t*; suspicions of therapist's abilities 77

Bartholomew, K. 53, 60
behavioural chain analysis 301
bereavement 171
biological domains of human functioning 17, 18–21; impact of variables on 20–21; role of risk factors 18–20
biopsychosocial assessment model 9; cultural and spiritual domains in 9; exploration of domains in 9; goals of 9
bipolar depression 120
Birmaher, B. 315, 331
blind spots 302, 303, 303*f*
body language 284
Bowlby, J. 29, 50, 51, 52, 53, 63
bullying 276

caregivers *see* significant others (parents, caregivers)
care maps 334, 328*f*
case formulation 40–42; checklist steps 42–45
case studies 6–7
catharsis 197
Cha, C. 341
client suitability 119, 120
clinical techniques: conflict-solving styles 102–104; decrease symptomatology aim 90; effective communication aim of 90; empty chair technique 108–111; exploration and clarification 90; interpersonal mindfulness 111–114; role play 105–108; summary of 114–115
Clinical Tool: Case formulation checklist 42; Clinicians Response Scale (CRS) 64; Ethnocultural identity matrix (ECIM) 31; Feelings Diary 88; Helpful things I can do after loss 196; My tasks following loss 196; Practice sheet for a conversation or complex interaction 298; Practice sheet for a single skill 297; Practice sheet for a specific social skill 299; Questions for a young person's significant others about social competency 310; Resilience grid 24; Role Transition 249; Social skills list 286; Stages of change 41; Suicide risk assessment protocol 26
Clinicians Response Scale (CRS) 63–66, 65*f*; avoidant attachment styles 67, 67*t*–68*t*; preoccupied attachment style 68, 69*t*; secure attachment style 70, 70*t*–71*t*
closeness circles 317, 126*f*, 127*f*, 145, 155, 186, 210, 317
cognitive behavior therapy (CBT) 82
common life stressors 242
communication skills enhancement 4, 284, 292
complex grief 11, 12, 133, 145, 154, 283; arc of therapy in middle phase 173*f*; cultural norms and 188; definition 169–171; different experiences of 190–191, 191*f*; empty chair technique as therapy for 109; essential processes for during middle phase 174–186; experiential and creative activities to help with loss 198–202; indicated processes during middle phase 186–187; mindfulness as therapy for 114; mismatch of experience and expectation in 190–191; potential barriers to discussing loss 181, 187; psychoeducation activities for working on loss 189–198; psychotherapy aims for 169; reduction of symptoms during middle phase 172–173; stepped care approach for 172
confidentiality 150
conflict as suppression and withdrawal 209
conflict curve scale 206, 217, 230, 218*f*, 222*f*
conflict resolution skills 207
conflict-solving styles 206, 229–231; compromise 102, 104, 103*f*; identification of 102, 103*f*; suppression 102, 103, 104, 103*f*; win/lose 102, 104,

103f; win/win 102, 104, 103f; withdrawal 102, 104, 103f
consolidation phase of IPT-A (prev. termination phase) 9, 13–14, 10f, 315–329, 335f; assessment for further treatment as primary task in 329; conclusion of acute treatment 13–14; continuation of maintenance treatment 13, 14; five primary tasks in 316; improvement markers in 326; independent functioning facilitation as primary task in 320–326; not as end of treatment 315–316; recognition of early relapse signs as primary task in 326–329; significant others' involvement towards end of 326–327; therapist steps back as attachment figure as primary task in 316–317; treatment sessions in 332
content affect 86–87
continuation therapy 14, 332, 335f; as aid to reduction in depression 331
continuity of care xii
conversation skills 288–290
coping strategies 22–23
Cornelius, H. 218, 231
criminal justice system 5
Crosby, G. 292
cultural and spiritual dimensions in IPT-A 4
cultural domains of human functioning 17, 30–33; assessment of minority family culture 30–31; expectations and relationships 32–33; family culture 30, impact of Big C culture 30; recognition and experience of depression 32
culture: Big C vs. small c 30; definition 30; impact of Big C culture 30

deliverance individualisation (of IPT-A) 8
depression 5; absence of word in some languages 32; adaptive grief compared to 171; care may to identify 14; continuation therapy to reduce relapse 331; cultural differences in 31–32; diagnosis guidelines 25–26; guidelines for adolescent 7; interpersonal disputes and 207; interpersonal gaps as cause of 280; parental as risk factor 18; as recurring phenomenon in adolescence 322; role transition as problem area for 247; self-esteem as risk factor 21–22; stepped care approach to 7, 8; substance use as risk factor 18, 22, 29; symptoms of compared to traumatic events 22

depressive disorder 109
Derakshan, N. 196
*Diagnostic and Statistical Manual for Mental Disorders: Fifth Edition (DSM-5)* 22, 331
*Diagnostic and Statistical Manual for Mental Disorders: Fourth Edition (DSM-IV)* 39
Dialectical Behaviour Therapy 111
diClemente, C. 41
disorganised style of attachment 53
dispute map 232f, 235f
dispute resolution techniques 228–229
domestic violence 22
dominance communication dimension (in therapeutic alliance) 76, 78, 79, 322; monitoring of 79f
d'Souza, Russell 33

eating disorders 120
education (schools) 29; bullying 276; involvement of during middle phase 167; role of in therapy 153–154
Einstein, Albert 33
electroconvulsive therapy (ECT) 8
Elson, D. M. 120
Emotional Intelligence (EI) skills 292
empty chair technique 183, 186, 257, 292, 317–318; goals of 109
encouragement of affect 82–83, 88–89; personal diagram construction for 82, 83, 84, 85, 84f
Engel, George L. 9, 17
Erikson, E. H. 51
Ethno-Cultural Identity Matrix (ECIM) 33
"An evaluation of youth mental health first aid training in school settings" (Gryglewicz, Childs & Soderstrom) 8
evidence-based intervention (of IPT-A) 3, 40; time-limited therapies and 75
evidence-based practice 4
eye contact 284
Eysenck, M. 196

Faire, S. 218, 231
family structures 28–29
Favazza, A. 27
Feelings Diary 87–88
First Nations *see* Aboriginal (Indigenous, First Nations) communities
Fisher, w. 102, 103f
Flores, P. 49
Fonagy, P. 49
formulation 9, 10, 40–46; interpersonal 147–148; provisional 44–45; purposes 45

Frankl, Viktor 34
Freud, Sigmund 198
Frydenberg, E. 22

Gestalt Therapy 109
Glasser, W. 98
Global Assessment of Functioning (GAF) scale 39; functioning component 39; symptom severity component 39
Goldstein, S. 33
grief and loss problem area 171; stages of 189–190
Grotberg, S. 23
Growing around Grief model 191–192, 191f
Gryglewicz, K. 8
Gunlicks-Stoessel, M. 153

Hall, G. S. 208
Hillin, Anthony 5, 63, 67, xii
holistic model of assessment 120, 19f, 212f, 269f; attachment styles 56; biological domains 17, 18–21; case formulation 45; classification of level of distress 39–40; cultural domains 17, 30–33; moving outside comfort zone 76; psychological domains 17, 21–28; purposes of, 45; reasons for continuation of experiencing distress 40; social domains 17, 28–30; spiritual domains 17, 33–39; stages of change 40–41; summary 18f, 19f, 123f
holistic model of IPT 14, xii; deliverance individualisation 8
homelessness 5
homophobia 276
Horowitz, L. M. 53, 54, 60, 54f

inclusion communication dimension (in therapeutic alliance) 76, 79, 322; monitoring of 79f
Indigenous communities *see* Aboriginal (Indigenous, First Nations) communities
initial phase of IPT-A 9, 14, 335f; aim of first few sessions 119, 10f; collaborative process in 148, 150, 151, 162; interpersonal formulation task 147–148; parental involvement in 151–153; preliminary formulation 10–11; tasks in interpersonal inventory 11; treatment agreement task 148–149
*International Classification of Diseases, 11th edition* (ICD-11) 340

"International Resilience Project: Findings from the research and effectiveness of interventions" (Grotberg) 23
interpersonal competencies 3–4, 327; development of as key goal of IPT-A 49–50; recognition of 324
interpersonal deficits 278
interpersonal disputes 11, 12, 163, 327; approach choice for dealing with 226; conflict assessment stage for dealing with 210–211; cultural differences in nature of 208; as damaging conflicts 209–210; definition 207–208; determination of what and who in 215; dispute issue identification 213–215; expectation mismatch as common cause of 215–216; identification of alternative options for dealing with 224–226; identification of as problem area 210–211; identification of current strategies for dealing with 223–224; impact on mental health by helplessness in 206; integrate strategies into real world for dealing with 227–229; intensity of and strategy for dealing with 217–218; parental involvement in 236–237; parent non-involvement in dealing with 238–239; as recurring theme 216; role play as therapy for 105; role transitions and 246; social skills rehearsal for dealing with 226–227; stages for working on 210–229, 209f; understanding dispute stage for dealing with 211–223
interpersonal formulation 147–148
*The Interpersonal Gap* (Wallen) 292
interpersonal gaps 12, 81, 164, 325; assessment of 281–285; compared to interpersonal deficits 278; confirmation of problem area step for working on 281, 282–283; conversation skills and 288–290; global or specific 279; identification of lack of social skills step for working on 284–287; involvement of significant others in dealing with 308–310; profound effects of 279–280; psychoeducation for 282–283; reasons for development of 280; recognition of distress connection step in working on 287; role play and mindfulness as therapies for 112–113; role play as therapy for 105; as self-maintaining

280–281; social skill development step for working on 287–303; social support networking step for working on 303–308

interpersonal incidents 210; analysis of 95–97; different communication as strategy for 98–100, 100f; five steps to facilitate 100–101; as foundation of clinical techniques in IPT-A 100; grid for 92, 92f; identification of misunderstandings 97, 97f; information collection of specific episode 92–95, 93f; working with 92–93

interpersonal inventory 125–136; attachment style identification task 145–147; attachment styles 56–60; as central to initial phase of IPT-A 155; dispute recognition 210–211; five tasks in 11–12; goals of 125–126; interpersonal map task 126–130; linking life events task 130–134; problem area identification task 134–140; timeline in 87

interpersonal laboratory 79–80

Interpersonal Psychotherapy (IPT): continuity of care 14, xii; family 120; holistic model of 14, xii; patient collaboration 14, xii

Interpersonal Psychotherapy for Adolescents (IPT-A): attachment theory as integral part of 49–50; based on Bowlby's attachment model 63; complexity of therapeutic relationship in 75–76; deliverance individualisation 8; description 3; as evidence-based intervention 3, 14; extension of into public policy 339–340; goals of 339; importance of maintenance xii–xiii; interpersonal disputes as damaging conflict 209–210; as modular therapy 335f; problem area identification in 134–140; psychotherapy to correct distortion as goal of 21–22; stages of intervention in 10f; therapist-client relationship compared to other therapies 62–63; training and supervision in 341–342; young adults, 4–5

interpersonal relationships 71–72; attachment theory and 50, 51; as biologically grounded 50; break down of 49; working model of 51

Jacobson, C. 341
Johari Window 302

Kennard, B. D. 331
Kiesler, D. J. 75, 76, 78
Kipling, Rudyard 289
Kitano, H. 30, 31
Klerman, G. 341

Lawrence, D. 153
Lemma, A. 100
Lerner, R. 60
lesbian, gay, bisexual, transgender, queer or questioning, intersex and asexual (LGBTQIA) 5; role transition and 275
Lewis, R. 22
life stress and stressors 241, 301–302
Likert scale 64

Main, M. 54
maintenance therapy 331, 335f; compared to acute treatment conclusion 334; goals 332–334; new psychosocial problems during 334
major depressive disorder 87
Manson, S. 32
mapping 206, 217; components of 231–233; description 231
markers of improvement 165
Markowitz, J. 340
Marsella, A. 30
Matsumoto, D. 30
maturity 4
McAlpine, Robert 5, 63, 67, xii
media enhanced therapy 291
memories 198
*The mental health of children and adolescents: Report on the second Australian Child and Adolescent Survey of Mental Health and Wellness* (Lawrence, et al.) 153
middle phase of IPT-A 9, 81, 10f, 335f; activity-based therapy for complex grief 198–202; aims of 161–162; arc of therapy for complex grief in 173f; client and therapist roles in 162; collaborative process continuation in 162; concluding 239; consideration of issues before parental involvement 166–167; essential processes for complex grief in 174–186; five-step approach to address role transitions in 246–265; identification and monitoring improvement markers in 165; indicated processes for complex grief in 186–187; interpersonal disputes in 206–238; interpersonal gaps 282, 285, 287–308;

interpersonal support as essential process in 174, 181–186; orientation to 154–155; parental and school involvement during 165–166; plan for maximum gains in 164; positive communication experience about loss as essential process in 174, 175–181; psychoeducation models for complex grief 195–196; reduction of complex grief symptoms in 172–173; social skills in 304–308; understanding complex grief symptoms as essential process in 174–175
mindfulness 296, 301; benefits 111; characteristics 111–112
Mindfulness-Based Cognitive Therapy 111
minority communities xii
mood disorders 242
motivational interviewing techniques 40, 252
*Mourning and melancholia* (Freud) 198
Mufson, L. 4, 9, 150, 171, 320, 341, 342
Mychailyszyn, M. P. 120

National Institute for Health and Care Excellence (NICE) (UK) 7; guidelines for depression diagnosis 25, 7f, 25f
Newton, Isaac 193
Nock, M. 27, 341
non-bereavement loss 171
non-suicidal self-injury (NSSI) 27, 341; *see also* suicide; IPT-A for young people 341
nonverbal communication 284

oral communication 284
Orth, U. 21

Parents and Friends of Lesbians and Gays (PFLAG) 275
parents *see* significant others (parents, caregivers)
patient collaboration 14, xii
Patton, B. 102, 103f
peer groups 21, 28, 29, 243, 275, 325
Perls, Fritz 109
personal diagram: encouragement of affect 82, 83, 84, 85, 84f, 85f; goals of 86; shows link between event and affect 85–86, 85f
physical abuse 22
post-traumatic stress disorder (PTSD) 22, 87; effectiveness of IPT for adults with 340; IPT-A as treatment for complex 340; symptom clusters in complex 340
practice-based evidence 4, 341; clinical implications of 340–341
*Practice Parameters for the Assessment and Treatment of Children and Adolescents with Depressive Disorders* (Birmaher, et al.) 315
preoccupied style of attachment 53, 54f; Clinicians Response Scale (CRS) and 68, 69t; engagement with therapist as friend 77; two-dimensional descriptions of others 61
problem areas 154, 155; collaborative identification of 140–143; complex grief 11, 12, 133, 145, 154, 169–202; grief and loss 171; identification of 134; interpersonal disputes 11, 12, 105, 130, 327; interpersonal gaps 12, 81, 1e3, 105, 325; during middle phase of IPT-A 162–165; role transitions 13, 130, 155, 171, 172, 241–276; strategies and techniques during middle phase 163–164; symptom linking to 143–145; working on interpersonal gaps may help with other 283
process affect 86–87
Prochaska, J. 41
Proctor, E. 34
psychodynamic therapies 63
psychoeducation 8, 17, 119, 166, 214, 296; activities for working on loss 189–198; apps for 290–291; consequences of 121; as essential component of initial phase of IPT-A 125; to help with interpersonal gaps 282–283; in initial phase of IPT-A 11; for insight into distress 21–22; for loss understanding and acceptance 188–189; models for complex grief 195–196; for role transitions 267–268
psychological domains of human functioning 17, 21–28; coping and resilience factors 22–24; role of risk factors 21–23; self-esteem impact on 21–22; traumatic events 22
psychotherapy 8; judgements xi

racism 276
recovery 331, 332
recurrence 332, 334–335
relapse 331, 332
remission 331, 332

repressive coping style 106–197
resilience to stress 23–24; external support characteristics 23, 24; inclusion of to focus on ability 25; internal personal strength characteristics 23, 24; social and interpersonal strength characteristics 23, 24; two-dimensional model 23–25
response (to therapy) 331, 332
Robertson, M. 61, 92, 171
role play 183, 186, 227, 257, 317–318, 325–326; goals of 105; steps for implementing change using 106–108
role transitions 13, 130, 283; assessment of 243, 266–267; characteristics 242, 243; confirmation of as problem area 245–246; definition 242; early indicators of 243; family structures 251f, 255f; identification of as central to symptoms step in approach 246–248; identification of role options as approach step 257–261; involvement of significant others in assessment 265; low self-esteem and impaired social functioning in 243–244; operationalising changes as approach step 261–265; psychoeducation to help 267–268; range of 242; review of aspects of new role as approach step 253–257; review of aspects of old role as approach step 248–252; same-sex attraction as 275, 273f; screening questions to help identify 244–245; sex, sexuality and gender identity as part of 265–266; triggered by loss events 246

*School Mental Health* 8
Schut, H. 193
secure style of attachment 52, 53, 54f, 318–319; Clinicians Response Scale (CRS) and 70, 70t–71t; three-dimensional descriptions of others 61
self-esteem 243, 290
self-harm 341; assessment 28; compared to suicide 27; definition 27; prevalence 27
self-help guidance 8
sexism 276
sexual abuse 22, 37
Sheard, T. 63, 82
significant others (parents, caregivers) 9, 17; disputes with young people 207; involvement in dealing with interpersonal disputes 236–238; involvement in dealing with interpersonal gaps 308–309; involvement in dealing with role transitions 265; involvement in towards end of consolidation phase 326–327; involvement of during middle phase 236; mental health issues experienced by 167, 236; non-involvement in dealing with interpersonal disputes 238–239; normal disputes with young people 208–209; role of in therapy 149, 236
Skillstreaming the Adolescent 290
social domains of human functioning 17, 28–30, 243–244; family structures 28–29
social problem-solving inventory 285
social skills development 261, 276, 294–295; for effective communication 284
Social Skills Improvement System Rating Scales 285
social skills inventory 284, 285
Social Skills Inventory for Adolescents 285
social skills training programs 290
social support networks 303–304
Solomon, J. 54
Sowislo, J. 21
spiritual domains of human functioning 17, 33–39; definition of spirituality 33–34; importance of for understanding of whole person 34–36
stepped care approach (for IPT-A) 7–8; importance of early intervention 8; intervention spectrum 7, 8; in relation to loss 172
stress scales 302
Stroebe, M. 193
Stuart, S. 61, 92, 171
substance use problems 18, 20, 25, 28, 29, 31, 49, 122, 135, 151, 171, 241, 268
suicide 5, 268, 276; *see also* non-suicidal self-injury (NSSI); differentiated from other self-harm types 27; risk assessment of 26–27
Sullivan, H. S. 76
symptomatology 11, 12, 18, 22, 125, 332; decrease of as aim of clinical techniques 90

therapeutic alliance: affiliation aspect of relationship in 76, 77, 78–79; dominance aspect of relationship in 76, 78, 79; inclusion aspect of relationship in 76, 79

therapeutic relationship 74–75; attention to as assistance to therapy 80–81; complexity of in IPT-A 75–76; encouragement of affect 82–83; establishing context for therapy 75; interpersonal issues in 81–82; as interpersonal laboratory 79–80; process affect compared to content affect 86–87; strategic positioning in first meeting 76
therapeutic role 76
therapist-client relationship 62–63; IPT-A compared to other therapies 62–63
therapy: accessibility of 5; continuation and maintenance as core components 5; room as laboratory 13; sequence 9
therapy sessions 321, 332
three-phase model of IPT-A: consolidation phase 9, 13–14; initial phase 9, 14; middle phase 9, 14
Tonkin, L. 191
Transcultural Mental Health Service 237
transference relationship 62–63
transitory attachment figure 10
traumatic events 22
treatment agreement: boundaries and contact component 149, 150–151; expectations of client and therapist component 149, 150; parental role component 149, 151–153; as preparation for middle phase of IPT-A 148; problem area component 149–150; school role component 149, 150; session frequency and duration component 149; session numbers component 149

unipolar depression 120
Ury, R. 102, 103f

Wallen, J. 292
Watkins, L. M. 76, 78
Worden, J. 196
working model of relationships 50, 51, 72; based on real experiences 63

Yalom, I. 74, 75
yin and yang 192–193
young persons see adolescents (young persons)